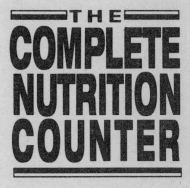

# THE
# COMPLETE
# NUTRITION
# COUNTER

# THE COMPLETE NUTRITION COUNTER

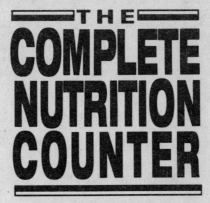

## LYNN SONBERG

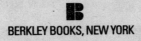

BERKLEY BOOKS, NEW YORK

Research about human nutrition is constantly evolving. While the author has made every effort to include the most accurate and up-to-date information in this book, there can be no guarantee that what we know about this complex subject won't change with time. Please keep in mind that this book is not intended for the purpose of self-diagnosis or self-treatment. The reader should consult his or her physician regarding all health concerns before undertaking any major dietary changes.

THE COMPLETE NUTRITION COUNTER

A Berkley Book / published by arrangement with the author

PRINTING HISTORY
Berkley edition / August 1993

A Lynn Sonberg Book

The Putnam Berkley World Wide Web site address is
http://www.berkley.com

ISBN: 0-425-13859-3

BERKLEY®
Berkley Books are published by The Berkley Publishing Group,
a member of Penguin Putnam Inc.,
200 Madison Avenue, New York, New York 10016.
BERKLEY and the "B" design
are trademarks belonging to Berkley Publishing Corporation.

PRINTED IN THE UNITED STATES OF AMERICA

20   19   18   17   16   15   14   13

# CONTENTS

**Acknowledgments**

The author wishes to thank Shelagh Masline for her invaluable help in researching this book.

# INTRODUCTION

This is truly the only nutrition counter you will ever need. With this handy book as your guide, you can target a variety of foods to supply the nutrients which lead to good health. In addition, you will discover those foods to avoid—products which are high in calories, fat, sodium or cholesterol.

More than four thousand foods are listed here for quick and easy reference. The foods are listed in straight alphabetical order, and both basic and brand-name foods are included. If you are interested in corn, for example, turn to C in the alphabetical listing and you will find information on fresh corn, as well as corn products that are canned and frozen.

Looking for a Mars Bar? An Oreo? Chicken soup? For easiest accessibility, food items such as these are grouped under Candy, Cookies, and Soup. Other broad categories include Bread, Cereal, Cheese, Crackers, Ice Cream, Oils, Pasta, Pudding, and Salad Dressing. In this handy way you can compare and contrast the values of similar products.

Our extensive categories of convenience foods include Frozen Breakfasts, Frozen Dinners and Frozen Entrees. There is also a comprehensive section on fast food. While it's preferable to prepare your own healthy meals, it's clear that many of us simply don't always have the time and energy to do so. In fact, every day one out of five Americans eats at a fast food restaurant. Here you will find the information you need to choose convenience foods most consistent with the most healthful and nutritious meals you would prepare yourself at home.

Included for each food are serving size; calories; protein (in grams); carbohydrates (in grams); fat (in grams); sodium (in milligrams); cholesterol (in milligrams); fiber (in grams); vitamin A; vitamin C; calcium; and iron.

The last four items are given as a percentage of U.S. RDAs, or Recommended Dietary Allowances set by the Food and Nutrition Board of the National Academy of Sciences. These are recommended levels of daily intake of essential nutrients considered appropriate to meet the needs of most healthy

Americans. They are not applicable to children under two or to pregnant or nursing women, whose nutrient needs are above average. Nutrition information on baby food is of course given in the percent of U.S. Recommended Daily Allowances for Infants.

If you're interested in maintaining optimum health and vigor while warding off everyday ailments and serious illness, you should be monitoring the nutrients in this nutrition counter.

## Why You Need This Book

Many Americans today devour too many calories, too much fat, and foods with high levels of cholesterol and sodium. At the same time we are consuming too many of the negatives, we are not eating enough of the positives—such as fruits, vegetables and whole grains—foods rich in complex carbohydrates, and fiber. In addition, studies from the United States Department of Agriculture (USDA) have uncovered calcium and iron deficiencies in the average diets of many women and some men. In short, the average diet of too many Americans puts them at risk for heart disease, high blood pressure, strokes, diabetes, and certain forms of cancer.

You can't always get the information you need to make healthy food choices by looking at product labels. While proposed labelling regulations are much tougher, as this book goes to press it is unclear exactly what form these regulations will take and when they will be phased in. At present some products have no labelling; others have some nutrients, but lack cholesterol and fiber. The Federal Food and Drug Administration and the USDA have made nutrition labelling mandatory on most, but not all, processed foods—and nutrition labelling is voluntary on raw fruits, vegetables, meat, poultry, and seafood.

The good news is that in this book you can simply thumb through the alphabetical listings to discover how nutritious—or not so nutritious—your own diet is. Here you will find the most up-to-date information on products available at this time. If you're like many of us, you will use this book to make the shift to a healthier and more nutritious style of eating.

## What Is a Healthy Diet?

Every five years the U.S. Departments of Health and Human Services and Agriculture issue guidelines for a healthy diet. The 1990 Dietary Guidelines, applicable to Americans over the age of two, recommend that each day we consume:

- 3 to 5 servings of vegetables. Vegetables are rich in vitamin A, vitamin C, and fiber.
- 2 to 4 servings of fruit. Fruits are also rich in fiber and vitamins A and C.
- 6 to 11 servings of pasta, cereal, or bread. These foods are rich in carbohydrates, iron, and fiber.

- 2 to 3 servings of dairy products. Dairy products such as milk and cheese are rich in calcium and protein.
- 2 to 3 servings of meat, poultry, fish, or eggs. These foods are rich in protein and iron.

Serving sizes vary, but one serving of vegetables is roughly one cup of raw leafy greens or half a cup of other vegetables; one serving of fruit could be a medium apple, pear or banana; for grains, a slice of bread or an ounce of cereal; in the dairy department, one cup of milk or 1.5 ounces of cheese; and for meat, poultry and fish, two or three ounces of lean beef or skinless chicken or fish.

## *Dietary Guidelines for Americans*

This book will give you the tools to follow the 1990 Dietary Guidelines for Americans. These are:
- Eat a variety of foods.
- Maintain a healthy weight.
- Choose a diet low in fat, saturated fat, and cholesterol.
- Choose a diet with plenty of vegetables, fruits, and grain products.
- Use sugars only in moderation.
- Use salt and sodium only in moderation.
- If you drink alcoholic beverages, do so in moderation.

Now let's take a closer look at each of the items in this nutrition counter. We'll define each nutrient, and explain its role—positive and negative—in your body. Where relevant, we give the most up-to-date U.S. Dietary Guidelines for the category. And we also provide you with some general tips on how to choose a healthy diet, as well as where to look in this book for food items which are good sources of important nutrients.

Although forty nutrients are needed for the proper functioning of the body, the ten nutrients targeted in this book (plus calories) are of greatest concern to health-conscious Americans. Research has shown that monitoring these nutrients can have the greatest direct effect on maintaining good health and warding off the degenerative diseases that too often accompany our later years.

## *Serving*

Nutritional information on food labels is listed per serving. Be sure to check the serving size provided in our book. Some food containers have more than one serving per package. We have followed serving sizes provided by the USDA and manufacturers. Remember, if you eat a larger serving, you will of course be consuming more of the calories and nutrients listed.

## Calories

A calorie is a measure of energy expressed in terms of heat. It is the amount of heat needed to raise the temperature of one gram of water one degree centigrade. A proper caloric intake will help you maintain a healthy weight. If you currently eat too much, decreasing your caloric intake and/or increasing your activity level may help you lose weight. Following are a few ways you can slim down:

- Use this book to keep track of your daily caloric intake.
- For most people a diet of 1200 calories daily will help you take off those excess pounds; but look at our other categories to make sure that while limiting your calories you are still getting enough nutrients.
- Be more physically active.
- Eat fewer fatty foods.
- Eat more fruits, vegetables, bread, and cereals.
- Skip desserts and second helpings.

## Protein

Protein is an energy-supplying nutrient which should comprise 12% to 20% of your daily caloric intake. Proteins are composed of smaller compounds called amino acids, which are essential to maintain life and support growth.

The U.S. RDA for protein is 45 grams if the protein is complete, that is, from an animal source. Complete proteins are typically found in meat, chicken, fish and dairy products. They contain all of the essential amino acids in significant amounts.

The U.S. RDA for protein is 65 grams if the protein is of an incomplete nature, that is, from a plant source. Grains and vegetables are typical sources of incomplete proteins, or proteins which lack some of the amino acids essential to maintaining life and supporting growth.

Most Americans consume too much protein from animal sources. Health experts today recommend eating smaller portions of meat and poultry—no more than four or five ounces per serving.

## Carbohydrates

Carbohydrates are energy-supplying nutrients which should comprise 55% to 60% of your daily caloric intake. Vegetables, fruits and grains are good sources of complex carbohydrates—and these foods are healthy in other ways as well, such as being generally low in fat and high in dietary fiber.

Complex carbohydrates, such as starches, are common in breads, cereals, pasta, rice, dry beans, and peas, and other vegetables, such as potatoes and corn. Unrefined carbohydrates are best—for example, choose bran cereal instead of corn flakes and brown rice instead of white. And keep in mind that foods rich in carbohydrates can also be an excellent source of much-needed fiber.

Complex carbohydrates should be distinguished from simple carbohydrates, which have a different chemical structure. Simple carbohydrates are sugars, which the 1990 Dietary Guidelines suggest should be used only in moderation. Sugars and the many foods which contain them supply calories but are limited in nutrients, and can also lead to tooth decay.

## Fat

Some fat is necessary in our diet, since our bodies do not produce enough naturally to meet our physiologic needs. But most Americans consume far too much fat. The U.S. Dietary Guidelines recommend that no more than 30% of a person's caloric intake should come from fat, and other major health organizations believe that, for optimal health, fat intake should be no more than 20% of calories. Currently, however, according to the Center for Science in the Public Interest, we get some 37% of our calories from fat.

Diets high in saturated fat raise blood cholesterol, which is linked to heart disease. High fat diets have also been associated with several types of cancer and can cause complications in those with diabetes.

How to cut down on the fat in your diet? You can do this by eating more fruits, vegetables, breads, and cereals. Trim fat from meat, and take skin off poultry. Moderate the use of egg yolks and organ meats, and try to choose skim or lowfat milk, and fat-free or lowfat yogurt and cheese. You may be pleasantly surprised that cutting down on the fat content of your daily caloric intake is also an effective way of eliminating extra pounds.

## Sodium

Table salt contains sodium and chloride, two essential nutrients in our diet. Most Americans, however, consume far more sodium than they need.

The 1990 U.S. Dietary Guidelines recommend that sodium be used only in moderation. They point out that in populations with diets low in salt, high blood pressure is less common. About one in three American adults has high blood pressure; reduced sodium intake will usually cause blood pressure to fall.

Although there is no RDA for sodium, the maximum daily intake suggested by the National Academy of Sciences in 1989 was 2400 milligrams of sodium per day. If you turn to the alphabetical listing for salt in this book, you will discover that one teaspoon of salt contains a whopping 2132 milligrams of sodium.

Try using fresh herbs instead of salt in flavoring your meals. And watch out for canned and processed products—they often contain considerable amounts of sodium. Check the labels and choose those lower in sodium. When cooking pasta or rice, avoid the temptation of tossing in that teaspoon of salt.

## *Cholesterol*

Animal products—such as meat, poultry, fish, shellfish, egg yolks and most dairy products—are the source of dietary cholesterol. High levels of cholesterol in our diets are linked to our increased risk for heart disease.

Cholesterol does not by law have to be listed on the labels of all foods. However, many manufacturers voluntarily supply cholesterol information in terms of milligrams per serving, in order to aid the consumer in planning balanced meals and comparing nutritional values of products. Current dietary guidelines recommend that we consume no more than 300 milligrams of cholesterol each day.

Eating less fat from animal products will help lower cholesterol as well as cutting down on the total fat in your diet. Some foods that contain fat and cholesterol, such as meats, milk, cheese and eggs, also contain high quality protein and valuable vitamins and minerals. But healthier choices are lowfat versions of these foods, such as lean meat and lowfat milk and cheeses.

To keep your cholesterol level under control, eat plenty of vegetables, fruits and grain products; lean meats, fish, and poultry without its fatty skin; choose lowfat dairy products; and use fats and oils sparingly.

## *Fiber*

Dietary fiber is a complex mixture of plant materials which are resistant to human digestion. A high-fiber diet may reduce your risk of developing breast or colon cancer. Fiber promotes normal elimination; helps satisfy the appetite by creating a full feeling; and, in some studies, fiber has been shown to play a role in reducing the level of cholesterol in the blood. Eating foods with fiber can reduce symptoms of chronic constipation, diverticular disease, and hemorrhoids.

A significant source of dietary fiber is a food that contains a substantial amount of fiber in relation to its caloric content, and contributes at least 2 grams of dietary fiber per serving. Many health organizations have stressed the importance of dietary fiber; the National Cancer Institute recommends 20 to 30 grams of fiber per day, with an upper limit of 35 grams.

What are good sources of dietary fiber? As you leaf through this book, you will see that they include whole grain products such as oats, fruits and vegetables, dry beans and peas, and nuts and seeds. Unrefined plant foods are best; a baked potato has more fiber and vitamins as well as considerably less fat than an order of french fries.

## Vitamin A

Vitamin A (retinol) is a fat-soluble vitamin important in the formation and maintenance of healthy skin, hair, and mucous membranes. It is necessary for proper bone growth, tooth development, and reproduction, and helps us to see in dim light. Vitamin A also has antistress benefits.

Exciting new research indicates that nutrients such as vitamin A can strengthen the immune system, which is the body's greatest defense against disease. As well as promoting general resistance to illness, vitamin A has been associated with a lower incidence of heart attack, stroke and hypertension, and decreased cancer rates. Vitamin A actually inhibits tumor growth and protects the body against free radical damage. In addition it supports the production and repair of body cells, and B- and T-cell formation. There is even evidence that vitamin A may reverse precancerous conditions.

The U.S. RDA for vitamin A is 5000 International Units (IU) per day. A good source of vitamin A contains a substantial amount of vitamin A and/or carotenes (which are converted by the body into vitamin A) in relation to its calorie content, and contributes at least 10% of the U.S. RDA.

Fruits and vegetables—especially dark-green vegetables and deep-yellow fruits and vegetables—are excellent sources of vitamin A. Among the many vitamin A–packed items you can choose from in the produce section are apricots, broccoli, cantaloupe, carrots, kale, spinach, squash, and sweet potatoes.

It is important to properly prepare foods which contain vitamin A, since the vitamin can be lost from foods during preparation, cooking or storage. Serving fruits and vegetables raw will help to retain vitamin A. When cooking vegetables, steaming for a brief period in a small amount of water is your best bet. Fruits and vegetables (with the exception of sweet potatoes) should be covered and refrigerated.

Liver and mackerel are also good sources of vitamin A. Like vegetables, they should be steamed, braised, baked or broiled—not fried—in order to retain vitamin A.

Some foods, such as cereal, margarine, lowfat milk, and skim milk, while not natural sources of vitamin A, are often fortified with this nutrient. Since products vary widely, remember to check the label on the package for the percentage of the U.S. RDA.

## Vitamin C

Vitamin C (ascorbic acid) is a water-soluble vitamin important in the formation of collagen, a protein that gives structure to bones, muscles, cartilage and blood vessels. It aids in the maintenance of capillaries, bones and teeth, and is vital to iron absorption.

Vitamin C is also famous for its role as an immune-boosting nutrient, probably best known for fighting the common cold. Like vitamin A, vitamin C has antistress benefits and encourages general resistance to illness. In addition, this valuable nutrient in our diet works as an anticarcinogen and antioxidant, and promotes antibody production.

The U.S. RDA for vitamin C is 60 milligrams per day. A good source of vitamin C contains a substantial amount of vitamin C in relation to its calorie content, and contributes at least 10% of the U.S. RDA.

What are good sources of vitamin C? Fruits and vegetables—especially citrus fruits and tomatoes—contributed 67% of the vitamin C in women's diets in a recent USDA study. Eating a variety of foods that contain vitamin C is the best way to get an adequate amount. These include apples, bananas, berries, grapefruit, melons, oranges, peaches, pears, plums, asparagus, broccoli, brussel sprouts, cauliflower, onions, potatoes, spinach, squash, and sweet potatoes.

As in the case of vitamin A, it is important to properly prepare foods which contain vitamin C, since the nutrient can be lost from foods during preparation, cooking or storage. Serving fruits and vegetables raw will help to retain vitamin C. When cooking vegetables, steaming for a brief period in a small amount of water is your best bet. Potatoes should be cooked in their skins. Cut raw fruits and vegetables should be stored in an airtight container and refrigerated. Do not soak or store in water, because vitamin C will be dissolved in water.

Liver, clams, mussels, and oysters are also good sources of vitamin C. Some foods, such as cereal and juice, are often fortified with vitamin C. Since products vary, remember to check the label on the package for the percentage of the U.S. RDA.

## Calcium

Calcium is an important mineral, used in building and maintaining bones and teeth. Muscle contraction, blood clotting, and cell membrane maintenance are functions of calcium. Calcium is also an immune booster, promoting general resistance to illness. Health experts recommend high intakes of calcium to prevent the onset of osteoporosis, a brittle bone condition that affects mainly older women.

Recent USDA surveys have shown that women and younger men do not get enough calcium in their diet. Women and men from 19 to 24 years of age require 1200 milligrams of calcium per day, while the RDA for people from 25 to 50 is 800 milligrams. Pregnant and nursing women have greater calcium needs, and should check with their doctor to ensure that they are meeting them.

Consult the entries in this book to make sure that you are meeting your own daily calcium requirement. Milk and milk products provided almost half the calcium requirement for women in one USDA survey. Green vegetables, such as broccoli and spinach, are also good sources of calcium, as are canned salmon and sardines when the bones are crushed and eaten.

Proper preparation of calcium-rich vegetables is important, since this nutrient is lost in cooking. Your best bet is to steam vegetables for a short time in a minimal amount of water.

Some foods, such as bread, cereal and orange juice, are not normally good sources of calcium but are often fortified with this mineral. Most instant-prepared cereals are fortified with calcium. Since products vary in the amount of calcium included, check the label on the package for the percentage of the U.S. RDA.

## *Iron*

Iron is an important mineral which carries oxygen through our bodies. It is a part of hemoglobin in the blood and of myoglobin in the muscles. Like the other nutrients we include here, iron enhances general resistance to illness. In addition, it has antistress benefits and promotes antibacterial activity.

There is concern that women do not get enough iron in their diet. In a recent USDA survey, more than 75% of American women between the ages of 19 and 50 had iron intakes below 80% of the RDA. The U.S. RDA for adults is 18 milligrams per day.

Pregnant or nursing women should consult their doctors about their iron intake, as doctors usually prescribe iron supplements to meet their even greater requirements. Likewise doctors often recommend feeding a fortified milk formula or breakfast cereal or giving an iron supplement to infants and toddlers, since it is also especially difficult to meet their iron needs.

The ability of the body to absorb and use iron varies with different foods. For example, the iron in meat, poultry, and fish is absorbed more easily than iron from other food sources. If you eat these animal products in a meal, the availability of iron from other foods is increased. The presence of vitamin C (ascorbic acid) also increases iron absorption with a meal. Our bodies naturally increase or decrease iron absorption according to need. An inadequate intake of iron can lead to iron deficiency anemia, in which the size and number of red blood cells are reduced.

Eating a variety of foods that contain iron is the best way to make sure you are getting an adequate amount. People who eat a healthy balanced diet rarely need iron supplements. But intakes of iron tend to be low in relation to recommendations, and only a limited amount of foods are good sources; therefore it's especially important to ensure that you are getting an adequate intake.

Meat, poultry, fish, beans, peas, kale, spinach and tofu are good sources of iron. Iron is lost in cooking some foods, so care must be taken in their preparation. Your best bet is to cook iron-rich foods for the shortest possible time in a minimal amount of water.

Pasta, white rice, bread and cereal are often enriched or fortified with iron, since iron is one of the nutrients lost in processing. Enriched products or products made from enriched flour are labeled accordingly. Fortified ready-to-eat cereals usually contain at least 25% of the U.S. RDA for iron. Consult the entries in this book to make sure that you are meeting your daily iron requirement.

## KEY TO
## ABBREVIATIONS AND SYMBOLS
## USED WITHIN

g = grams
< = less than
* = less than 2% of U.S. RDA
med = medium
mg = milligrams
0 = none
na = not available
oz = ounce
pkt = packet
% = percentage of the U.S. RDA
pc = piece
sl = slice
Tr = trace, less than 0.5

THE A TO Z NUTRITION COUNTER
FOR BRAND-NAME AND BASIC FOODS,
INCLUDING CALORIES, PROTEIN, CARBOHYDRATES,
FAT, SODIUM, CHOLESTEROL,
FIBER, VITAMIN A, VITAMIN C,
CALCIUM, AND IRON

| FOOD NAME<br>(All foods are prepared, unless otherwise noted.) | Serving Size | Calories |
|---|---|---|
| ACORN SQUASH  Baked | ½ cup | 60 |
| ALMONDS | | |
| Shelled, sliced | 1 cup | 560 |
| Shelled, whole | 1 cup | 850 |
| ANCHOVIES  Canned in olive oil | 5 med | 42 |
| APPLE | | |
| Raw with skin | 1 med | 80 |
| Raw with skin | 1 large | 125 |
| Dried | 1 cup | 353 |
| APPLE BUTTER | 1 tbsp | 33 |
| APPLE JUICE | | |
| Canned or bottled | 1 cup | 120 |
| Mott's | 6 fl oz | 88 |
| Mott's Natural Style | 6 fl oz | 76 |
| APPLE-GRAPE JUICE | | |
| Frozen and reconstituted | 6 fl oz | 90 |
| APPLESAUCE | | |
| Canned (Del Monte) | ½ cup | 90 |
| Canned (Del Monte Lite) | ½ cup | 50 |
| Canned (Mott's) | ½ cup | 230 |
| Canned (Mott's Natural Style) | ½ cup | 100 |
| APRICOTS | | |
| Raw with skin | 3 med | 52 |
| Dried (Del Monte) | 2 oz | 140 |
| Canned, halves (Del Monte) | ½ cup | 100 |

| Protein (g) | Carbohydrates (g) | Fat (g) | Sodium (mg) | Cholesterol (mg) | Fiber (g) | Vitamin A (%) | Vitamin C (%) | Calcium (%) | Iron (%) |
|---|---|---|---|---|---|---|---|---|---|
| 1 | 15 | Tr | 4 | 0 | 2 | 85 | 23 | 3 | 4 |
| | | | | | | | | | |
| 19 | 19 | 49 | 4 | 0 | 4.4 | * | * | 20 | 25 |
| 25 | 28 | 77 | 6 | 0 | na | * | * | 35 | 35 |
| 6 | 0 | 2 | 734 | na | 0 | * | * | 4 | 4 |
| | | | | | | | | | |
| 0 | 15 | <1 | 1 | 0 | 3 | 2 | 10 | * | 2 |
| 0 | 31 | 1 | 2 | 0 | 5 | 4 | 13 | 2 | 3 |
| 1 | 92 | 2 | 7 | Tr | na | na | 17 | 4 | 11 |
| 0 | 8 | 0 | 1 | na | 0 | * | * | * | 1 |
| | | | | | | | | | |
| 0 | 30 | 0 | 5 | 29 | 0 | * | 3 | 2 | 8 |
| 0 | 22 | 0 | 13 | 0 | 0 | * | 6 | * | 2 |
| 0 | 19 | 0 | 28 | 0 | 0 | * | 6 | * | 2 |
| | | | | | | | | | |
| * | 23 | 0 | 5 | 0 | 0 | * | * | * | * |
| | | | | | | | | | |
| 0 | 24 | 0 | 3 | 0 | na | * | 2 | * | 2 |
| 0 | 13 | 0 | 5 | 0 | na | * | 15 | * | * |
| * | 55 | 0 | 3 | 0 | na | * | 10 | * | 2 |
| * | 22 | 0 | 3 | 0 | na | * | 10 | * | 2 |
| | | | | | | | | | |
| <2 | 12 | Tr | 1 | 0 | 1.4 | 60 | 20 | 2 | 2 |
| 2 | 35 | 0 | 9 | 0 | na | 90 | * | 2 | 15 |
| 0 | 26 | 0 | 9 | 0 | na | 10 | 6 | * | 2 |

| FOOD NAME | Serving Size | Calories |
|---|---|---|
| Canned, whole (Del Monte) | ½ cup | 100 |
| APRICOT NECTAR (Del Monte) | 6 fl oz | 100 |
| ARTICHOKE | 1 med | 30 |
| ARTICHOKE HEARTS | | |
| Frozen (Birds Eye Deluxe) | 3 oz | 30 |
| ASPARAGUS | | |
| Fresh, boiled | 4 spears | 13 |
| Canned, spears and tips (Del Monte) | ½ cup | 20 |
| Canned, cut (Green Giant) | ½ cup | 20 |
| Frozen, spears (Birds Eye) | 3.3 oz | 25 |
| Frozen, spears (cut) in | | |
| butter sauce (Green Giant) | ½ cup | 70 |
| AVOCADO | | |
| California | 1 med | 306 |
| California, pureed | ½ cup | 204 |
| Florida | 1 med | 339 |
| Florida, pureed | ½ cup | 129 |
| BABY FOOD | | |
| *Baked Products* | | |
| Arrowroot cookie | 1 | 25 |
| Pretzel | 1 | 24 |
| Zwieback | 1 | 30 |
| *Cereal* | | |
| Barley, dry | 1 tbsp | 15 |
| High protein, dry | 1 tbsp | 15 |

| Protein (g) | Carbohydrates (g) | Fat (g) | Sodium (mg) | Cholesterol (mg) | Fiber (g) | Vitamin A (%) | Vitamin C (%) | Calcium (%) | Iron (%) |
|---|---|---|---|---|---|---|---|---|---|
| 0 | 27 | 0 | 9 | 0 | na | 10 | 4 | * | 2 |
| 1 | 26 | 0 | 9 | 0 | na | 40 | 50 | * | 4 |
| 3 | 12 | 0 | 36 | 0 | 1.5 | 4 | 17 | 6 | 7 |
| | | | | | | | | | |
| 2 | 7 | 0 | 140 | 0 | 3 | 2 | 8 | * | 4 |
| | | | | | | | | | |
| 2 | 2 | Tr | 1 | 0 | 0.6 | 10 | 25 | 2 | 2 |
| 2 | 3 | 0 | 355 | 0 | na | 10 | 25 | * | 2 |
| 2 | 3 | 0 | 420 | 0 | 1.2 | 6 | 25 | 0 | 4 |
| 3 | 4 | 0 | 0 | 0 | na | 15 | 50 | 2 | 4 |
| | | | | | | | | | |
| 4 | 6 | 4 | 725 | na | na | 15 | 45 | 2 | 6 |
| | | | | | | | | | |
| <4 | 12 | 30 | 21 | 0 | 4.7 | 12 | 50 | 4 | 8 |
| 2 | 8 | 20 | 14 | 0 | 3.1 | 6 | 25 | 2 | 4 |
| 5 | 27 | 27 | 14 | 0 | 6.4 | 16 | 70 | 4 | 8 |
| 2 | 10 | 10 | 6 | 0 | 2.4 | 4 | 18 | 1 | 2 |
| | | | | | | | | | |
| Tr | 4 | 1 | 21 | Tr | 0 | * | * | * | * |
| <1 | 5 | 0 | 16 | na | 0.1 | * | * | * | 3 |
| <1 | 5 | 1 | 16 | 1 | 0 | * | * | * | 1 |
| | | | | | | | | | |
| Tr | 3 | Tr | 1 | na | 0.1 | * | * | 4 | 11 |
| <2 | <2 | Tr | <1 | na | 0.1 | * | * | 4 | 11 |

| FOOD NAME | Serving Size | Calories |
|---|---|---|
| Mixed, dry | 1 tbsp | 15 |
| Oatmeal, dry | 1 tbsp | 12 |
| Rice, dry | 1 tbsp | 15 |
| *Dinners, junior* | | |
| Beef & Egg Noodles with Vegetables | 1 jar | 140 |
| Chicken & Noodles | 1 jar | 120 |
| Macaroni & Cheese | 1 jar | 140 |
| Macaroni, Tomato & Beef | 1 jar | 125 |
| Spaghetti, Tomato Sauce & Meat | 1 jar | 130 |
| Split Peas & Ham | 1 jar | 152 |
| Turkey & Rice with Vegetables | 1 jar | 120 |
| Vegetables & Bacon | 1 jar | 170 |
| Vegetables & Beef | 1 jar | 140 |
| Vegetables & Chicken | 1 jar | 110 |
| Vegetables & Ham | 1 jar | 120 |
| Vegetables & Lamb | 1 jar | 130 |
| *Dinners, strained* | | |
| Beef and Egg Noodles | 1 jar | 60 |
| Cereal and Egg Yolk | 1 jar | 70 |
| Chicken and Noodles | 1 jar | 80 |
| Chicken Soup | 1 jar | 70 |
| Macaroni & Cheese | 1 jar | 90 |
| Macaroni, Tomato & Beef | 1 jar | 75 |
| Turkey Rice with Vegetables | 1 jar | 60 |
| Vegetables & Bacon | 1 jar | 88 |

| Protein (g) | Carbohydrates (g) | Fat (g) | Sodium (mg) | Cholesterol (mg) | Fiber (g) | Vitamin A (%) | Vitamin C (%) | Calcium (%) | Iron (%) |
|---|---|---|---|---|---|---|---|---|---|
| Tr | <3 | Tr | 4 | na | 0.1 | * | * | 4 | 11 |
| Tr | 2 | Tr | 1 | na | 0.1 | * | * | 5 | 11 |
| Tr | 4 | Tr | 1 | na | 0 | * | * | 4 | 11 |
| | | | | | | | | | |
| 7 | 20 | 4 | 36 | na | 1 | 80 | 10 | 2 | 6 |
| 4 | 19 | 3 | 28 | na | 0.4 | 70 | 8 | 6 | 4 |
| 6 | 19 | 4 | 168 | na | 0.4 | 6 | 6 | 20 | 4 |
| 5 | 22 | 2 | 34 | na | 1.1 | 100 | 10 | 4 | 6 |
| 5 | 22 | 3 | 42 | na | 1.1 | 45 | * | 6 | 8 |
| 7 | 24 | 3 | 36 | na | 1.7 | 100 | 8 | 6 | 6 |
| 4 | 20 | 3 | 60 | na | 0.9 | 120 | 6 | 8 | 6 |
| 4 | 20 | 8 | 121 | na | 1.5 | 170 | 10 | 4 | 4 |
| 5 | 21 | 4 | 25 | na | 1.1 | 90 | 6 | 2 | 4 |
| 5 | 17 | 3 | 21 | na | 0.6 | 100 | 10 | 6 | 4 |
| 4 | 15 | 4 | 37 | na | 0.9 | 65 | 8 | 2 | 6 |
| 4 | 18 | 5 | 25 | na | 0.9 | 130 | 8 | 2 | 4 |
| | | | | | | | | | |
| 3 | 10 | 2 | 37 | na | na | 20 | * | * | 2 |
| 3 | 10 | 2 | 17 | na | na | 6 | 2 | 6 | 2 |
| 3 | 12 | 2 | 20 | na | na | 45 | 6 | 6 | 2 |
| 3 | 9 | 2 | 20 | na | na | 40 | * | 6 | 2 |
| 3 | 11 | 3 | 102 | na | na | 2 | 4 | 10 | 2 |
| 3 | 12 | 2 | 18 | na | na | 50 | 6 | 2 | 2 |
| 2 | 10 | 1 | na | na | na | 30 | * | 6 | 2 |
| 2 | 11 | 3 | 55 | 4 | na | 120 | * | 2 | 2 |

| FOOD NAME | Serving Size | Calories |
|---|---|---|
| Vegetables & Beef | 1 jar | 70 |
| Vegetables & Chicken | 1 jar | 70 |
| Vegetables & Ham | 1 jar | 60 |
| Vegetables & Lamb | 1 jar | 67 |
| Vegetables & Liver | 1 jar | 60 |
| Vegetables & Turkey | 1 jar | 60 |
| *Beech-Nut Baby's First Fruit* | | |
| Applesauce | 2.5 oz | 50 |
| Bananas | 2.5 oz | 70 |
| Peaches | 2.5 oz | 45 |
| Pears | 2.5 oz | 50 |
| *Beech-Nut Baby's First Vegetable* | | |
| Butternut Squash | 2.5 oz | 30 |
| Carrots | 2.5 oz | 25 |
| Peas | 2.5 oz | 40 |
| Sweet Potatoes | 2.5 oz | 50 |
| *Beech-Nut Stage 1 Cereal* | | |
| Barley (Dry) | ½ oz | 60 |
| Barley, Mixed with Formula | 2.4 fl oz | 120 |
| Oatmeal (Dry) | ½ oz | 70 |
| Oatmeal, Mixed with Formula | 2.4 fl oz | 120 |
| Rice (Dry) | ½ oz | 60 |
| Rice, Mixed with Formula | 2.4 fl oz | 120 |
| *Beech-Nut Stage 1 Juice* | | |
| Apple | 4 fl oz | 60 |

| Protein (g) | Carbohydrates (g) | Fat (g) | Sodium (mg) | Cholesterol (mg) | Fiber (g) | Vitamin A (%) | Vitamin C (%) | Calcium (%) | Iron (%) |
|---|---|---|---|---|---|---|---|---|---|
| <3 | 8 | 2 | 27 | na | na | 160 | 2 | 2 | 2 |
| 3 | 9 | 2 | 14 | na | na | 50 | 2 | 4 | 2 |
| 2 | 9 | 1 | 15 | na | na | 45 | * | 6 | 4 |
| <3 | 9 | <3 | 26 | na | na | 140 | * | 4 | 4 |
| 3 | 10 | 1 | 19 | na | na | 120 | 10 | * | 20 |
| 2 | 10 | 2 | 20 | na | na | 50 | 4 | 2 | 2 |
| | | | | | | | | | |
| 0 | 11 | 0 | 0 | na | na | * | 35 | * | * |
| 0 | 16 | 0 | 0 | na | na | 2 | 45 | * | * |
| 0 | 10 | 0 | 0 | na | na | 20 | 45 | * | * |
| 0 | 12 | 0 | 0 | na | na | * | 45 | * | * |
| | | | | | | | | | |
| 0 | 7 | 0 | 0 | na | na | 150 | * | * | * |
| 0 | 6 | 0 | 80 | na | na | 650 | * | 2 | * |
| 2 | 7 | 0 | 0 | na | na | 100 | * | * | * |
| 0 | 11 | 0 | 10 | na | na | 230 | * | * | * |
| | | | | | | | | | |
| 1 | 12 | 0 | 10 | na | na | * | * | 20 | 45 |
| 2 | 18 | 4 | 25 | na | na | 6 | 4 | 25 | 50 |
| 1 | 11 | 2 | 15 | na | na | * | * | 20 | 45 |
| 2 | 16 | 5 | 25 | na | na | 6 | 4 | 25 | 50 |
| 1 | 13 | 0 | 0 | na | na | * | * | 20 | 45 |
| 2 | 18 | 4 | 20 | na | na | 6 | 4 | 25 | 50 |
| | | | | | | | | | |
| 0 | 14 | 0 | 10 | na | na | * | 120 | * | 2 |

| FOOD NAME | Serving Size | Calories |
|---|---|---|
| Grape | 4 fl oz | 90 |
| Pear | 4 fl oz | 70 |
| *Beech-Nut Stage 1 Fruit* | | |
| Applesauce | 4.5 oz | 70 |
| Bananas | 4.5 oz | 120 |
| Peaches | 4.5 oz | 70 |
| Pears | 4.5 oz | 80 |
| *Beech-Nut Stage 1 Vegetables* | | |
| Butternut Squash | 4.5 oz | 60 |
| Carrots | 4.5 oz | 45 |
| Green Beans | 4.25 oz | 40 |
| Peas | 4.5 oz | 70 |
| Sweet Potatoes | 4.5 oz | 90 |
| *Beech-Nut Stage 1 Meat* | | |
| Beef and Broth | 2.5 oz | 80 |
| Chicken and Broth | 2.5 oz | 70 |
| Lamb and Broth | 2.5 oz | 60 |
| Turkey and Broth | 2.5 oz | 90 |
| Veal and Broth | 2.5 oz | 70 |
| *Beech-Nut Stage 2 Cereal* | | |
| Mixed (Dry) | ½ oz | 60 |
| Mixed with Formula | 2.4 fl oz | 120 |
| Oatmeal and Bananas (Dry) | ½ oz | 70 |
| Oatmeal and Bananas, Mixed with Formula | 2.4 fl oz | 120 |

| Protein (g) | Carbohydrates (g) | Fat (g) | Sodium (mg) | Cholesterol (mg) | Fiber (g) | Vitamin A (%) | Vitamin C (%) | Calcium (%) | Iron (%) |
|---|---|---|---|---|---|---|---|---|---|
| 0 | 22 | 0 | 10 | na | na | * | 120 | 2 | * |
| 0 | 17 | 0 | 0 | na | na | * | 120 | * | * |
| | | | | | | | | | |
| 0 | 17 | 0 | 0 | na | na | * | 45 | * | * |
| 0 | 27 | 0 | 0 | na | na | 4 | 45 | * | 2 |
| 0 | 16 | 0 | 0 | na | na | 35 | 45 | * | * |
| 0 | 20 | 0 | 0 | na | na | * | 45 | 2 | * |
| | | | | | | | | | |
| 1 | 12 | 0 | 0 | na | na | 250 | 2 | 2 | 2 |
| 0 | 10 | 0 | 65 | na | na | 700 | * | 4 | * |
| 1 | 8 | 0 | 0 | na | na | 30 | * | 8 | 6 |
| 3 | 13 | 0 | 0 | na | na | 35 | 6 | 2 | 8 |
| 1 | 20 | 0 | 55 | na | na | 450 | 4 | 2 | 2 |
| | | | | | | | | | |
| 9 | 0 | 5 | 40 | na | na | * | * | * | 6 |
| 9 | 0 | 4 | 55 | na | na | * | * | 2 | 8 |
| 9 | 0 | 3 | 50 | na | na | * | * | * | 6 |
| 8 | 0 | 6 | 40 | na | na | * | * | 6 | 4 |
| 10 | 0 | 3 | 50 | na | na | * | * | * | 4 |
| | | | | | | | | | |
| 1 | 12 | 0 | 10 | na | na | * | * | 20 | 45 |
| 2 | 17 | 4 | 25 | na | na | 6 | 4 | 25 | 50 |
| 1 | 12 | 0 | 0 | na | na | * | * | 15 | 35 |
| | | | | | | | | | |
| 2 | 18 | 4 | 20 | na | na | 6 | 4 | 20 | 40 |

| FOOD NAME | Serving Size | Calories |
|---|---|---|
| Rice and Apples (Dry) | ½ oz | 70 |
| Rice and Apples, Mixed with Formula | 2.4 fl oz | 120 |
| Rice and Bananas (Dry) | ½ oz | 70 |
| Rice and Bananas, Mixed with Formula | 2.4 fl oz | 120 |
| *Beech-Nut Stage 2 Jar Cereal* | | |
| Mixed with Apples and Bananas | 4.5 oz | 90 |
| Oatmeal with Apples and Bananas | 4.5 oz | 90 |
| Rice with Apples and Bananas | 4.5 oz | 90 |
| *Beech-Nut Stage 2 Juice* | | |
| Apple Cherry | 4 fl oz | 70 |
| Apple Cranberry | 4 fl oz | 60 |
| Apple Grape | 4 fl oz | 70 |
| Juice Plus (Iron-Fortified Grape) | 4 fl oz | 90 |
| Mango Nectar with Grape and Pear | 4 fl oz | 80 |
| Mixed Fruit | 4 fl oz | 70 |
| Papaya Nectar with Grape and Pear | 4 fl oz | 70 |
| Peach Nectar with Pear and Grape | 4 fl oz | 70 |
| Tropical Blend | 4 fl oz | 90 |
| Tropical Blend Nectar | 4 fl oz | 90 |
| *Beech-Nut Stage 2 Fruit* | | |
| Apples & Apricots | 4.5 oz | 80 |
| Apples & Bananas | 4.5 oz | 80 |
| Apples & Cherries | 4.5 oz | 70 |
| Apples & Pears | 4.5 oz | 80 |
| Apples, Pears & Bananas | 4.5 oz | 90 |

| Protein (g) | Carbohydrates (g) | Fat (g) | Sodium (mg) | Cholesterol (mg) | Fiber (g) | Vitamin A (%) | Vitamin C (%) | Calcium (%) | Iron (%) |
|---|---|---|---|---|---|---|---|---|---|
| 0 | 14 | 0 | 0 | na | na | * | * | 15 | 35 |
| 1 | 19 | 4 | 20 | na | na | 6 | 4 | 20 | 40 |
| 0 | 13 | 0 | 0 | na | na | * | * | 15 | 35 |
| 1 | 19 | 4 | 20 | na | na | 4 | 4 | 20 | 40 |
| | | | | | | | | | |
| 2 | 19 | 1 | 0 | na | na | * | 45 | 2 | 45 |
| 2 | 17 | 1 | 5 | na | na | * | 45 | 2 | 45 |
| 1 | 20 | 0 | 10 | na | na | * | 45 | 2 | 45 |
| | | | | | | | | | |
| 0 | 16 | 0 | 10 | na | na | * | 120 | * | 2 |
| 0 | 15 | 0 | 10 | na | na | * | 120 | * | 2 |
| 0 | 17 | 0 | 15 | na | na | * | 120 | * | 2 |
| 0 | 22 | 0 | 10 | na | na | * | 100 | * | 15 |
| 0 | 19 | 0 | 5 | na | na | * | 120 | * | * |
| 0 | 16 | 0 | 10 | na | na | 10 | 120 | * | 2 |
| 0 | 17 | 0 | 10 | na | na | 2 | 120 | * | * |
| 0 | 17 | 0 | 10 | na | na | 15 | 120 | * | 2 |
| 0 | 21 | 0 | 10 | na | na | 4 | 120 | 2 | * |
| 0 | 21 | 0 | 10 | na | na | 4 | 120 | 2 | * |
| | | | | | | | | | |
| 0 | 19 | 0 | 0 | na | na | 40 | 45 | * | 2 |
| 0 | 18 | 0 | 0 | na | na | 2 | 45 | * | * |
| 0 | 18 | 0 | 5 | na | na | 4 | 45 | * | 2 |
| 0 | 20 | 0 | 0 | na | na | * | 45 | * | * |
| 0 | 21 | 0 | 0 | na | na | 2 | 45 | * | * |

| FOOD NAME | Serving Size | Calories |
|---|---|---|
| Apricots with Pears & Apples | 4.5 oz | 90 |
| Bananas with Pears & Apples | 4.5 oz | 100 |
| Fruit Dessert | 4.5 oz | 80 |
| Pears & Pineapple | 4.5 oz | 90 |
| Plums with Apples & Rice | 4.5 oz | 70 |
| Prunes with Rice | 4.5 oz | 110 |
| *Beech-Nut Stage 2 Vegetables* | | |
| Carrots & Peas | 4.5 oz | 50 |
| Creamed Corn | 4.5 oz | 100 |
| Garden Vegetables | 4.5 oz | 60 |
| Mixed Vegetables | 4.5 oz | 60 |
| *Beech-Nut Stage 2 Dinners* | | |
| Beef & Egg Noodle | 4.5 oz | 90 |
| Chicken & Rice | 4.5 oz | 80 |
| Chicken Noodle | 4.5 oz | 90 |
| Chicken Soup | 4.5 oz | 90 |
| Macaroni & Beef | 4.5 oz | 100 |
| Turkey Rice | 4.5 oz | 70 |
| Vegetable Beef | 4.5 oz | 80 |
| Vegetable Chicken | 4.5 oz | 90 |
| Vegetable Ham | 4.5 oz | 90 |
| Vegetable Lamb | 4.5 oz | 100 |
| *Beech-Nut Stage 2 Dinners Supreme* | | |
| Beef | 4.5 oz | 130 |
| Turkey | 4.5 oz | 110 |

| Protein (g) | Carbohydrates (g) | Fat (g) | Sodium (mg) | Cholesterol (mg) | Fiber (g) | Vitamin A (%) | Vitamin C (%) | Calcium (%) | Iron (%) |
|---|---|---|---|---|---|---|---|---|---|
| 0 | 21 | 0 | 0 | na | na | 80 | 45 | 2 | 2 |
| 0 | 24 | 0 | 0 | na | na | 4 | 45 | * | 2 |
| 0 | 20 | 0 | 0 | na | na | 6 | 45 | * | * |
| 0 | 21 | 0 | 0 | na | na | * | 45 | 2 | 2 |
| 0 | 16 | 0 | 10 | na | na | 15 | 45 | * | 2 |
| 0 | 27 | 0 | 15 | na | na | 6 | * | 2 | 2 |
| | | | | | | | | | |
| 2 | 10 | 0 | 100 | na | na | 500 | * | 4 | 2 |
| 2 | 20 | 1 | 25 | na | na | 6 | * | 2 | * |
| 2 | 11 | 0 | 20 | na | na | 140 | 2 | 4 | 6 |
| 1 | 12 | 0 | 30 | na | na | 320 | 2 | 2 | 2 |
| | | | | | | | | | |
| 2 | 11 | 4 | 35 | na | na | 300 | * | 2 | 2 |
| 2 | 11 | 3 | 40 | na | na | 230 | * | 4 | 2 |
| 2 | 13 | 3 | 35 | na | na | 210 | * | 4 | 2 |
| 3 | 16 | 1 | 25 | na | na | 170 | * | * | 2 |
| 2 | 13 | 4 | 50 | na | na | 290 | * | 4 | 4 |
| 2 | 12 | 2 | 30 | na | na | 100 | * | 4 | 2 |
| 2 | 10 | 4 | 35 | na | na | 240 | * | 2 | 2 |
| 3 | 12 | 3 | 50 | na | na | 160 | * | 10 | 2 |
| 3 | 12 | 3 | 35 | na | na | 250 | * | 2 | 2 |
| 2 | 13 | 4 | 35 | na | na | 200 | * | 2 | 2 |
| | | | | | | | | | |
| 3 | 13 | 7 | 35 | na | na | 140 | * | 2 | 2 |
| 4 | 11 | 6 | 35 | na | na | 120 | * | 6 | 4 |

| FOOD NAME | Serving Size | Calories |
|---|---|---|
| *Beech-Nut Stage 2 Dessert* | | |
| Apple, Peach & Strawberry | 4.5 oz | 100 |
| Apple & Strawberry | 4.5 oz | 90 |
| Apple Yogurt | 4.5 oz | 120 |
| Banana Pineapple | 4.5 oz | 110 |
| Banana Pudding | 4.5 oz | 100 |
| Banana Yogurt | 4.5 oz | 120 |
| Cottage Cheese with Pineapple | 4.5 oz | 130 |
| Dutch Apple | 4.5 oz | 100 |
| Mixed Fruit Yogurt | 4.5 oz | 130 |
| Peach Yogurt | 4.5 oz | 120 |
| Pear Yogurt | 4.5 oz | 130 |
| Vanilla Custard Pudding | 4.5 oz | 140 |
| *Beech-Nut Stage 2 Tropical Fruit Dessert* | | |
| Guava | 4.5 oz | 100 |
| Island Fruit | 4.5 oz | 90 |
| Mango | 4.5 oz | 110 |
| Papaya | 4.5 oz | 100 |
| *Beech-Nut Stage 3 Juice* | | |
| Orange | 4 fl oz | 70 |
| *Beech-Nut Stage 3 Fruit* | | |
| Applesauce | 6 oz | 90 |
| Apples & Bananas | 6 oz | 100 |
| Apples & Cherries | 6 oz | 100 |
| Apricots with Pears & Apples | 6 oz | 120 |

| Protein (g) | Carbohydrates (g) | Fat (g) | Sodium (mg) | Cholesterol (mg) | Fiber (g) | Vitamin A (%) | Vitamin C (%) | Calcium (%) | Iron (%) |
|---|---|---|---|---|---|---|---|---|---|
| 0 | 24 | 0 | 0 | na | na | 10 | 45 | * | * |
| 0 | 22 | 0 | 0 | na | na | 2 | 45 | * | 2 |
| 1 | 25 | 2 | 25 | na | na | * | 45 | 8 | * |
| 0 | 27 | 0 | 15 | na | na | 2 | 45 | * | * |
| 0 | 25 | 0 | 10 | na | na | 2 | 45 | * | 2 |
| 1 | 26 | 2 | 30 | na | na | * | 45 | 8 | * |
| 2 | 26 | 1 | 15 | na | na | 2 | 45 | 2 | * |
| 0 | 24 | 0 | 15 | na | na | * | 45 | 2 | * |
| 1 | 28 | 1 | 20 | na | na | 2 | 45 | 6 | * |
| 1 | 25 | 2 | 30 | na | na | 15 | 45 | 8 | * |
| 1 | 29 | 2 | 35 | na | na | * | 45 | 8 | * |
| 2 | 24 | 4 | 60 | na | na | 2 | * | 10 | * |
| 0 | 24 | 0 | 10 | na | na | 4 | 45 | * | 2 |
| 0 | 22 | 0 | 10 | na | na | 15 | 45 | * | * |
| 0 | 27 | 0 | 15 | na | na | 30 | 45 | * | * |
| 0 | 24 | 0 | 15 | na | na | 20 | 45 | * | * |
| 0 | 15 | 0 | 0 | na | na | 8 | 120 | 2 | * |
| 0 | 22 | 0 | 0 | na | na | * | 45 | * | * |
| 0 | 25 | 0 | 0 | na | na | * | 45 | * | * |
| 0 | 24 | 0 | 0 | na | na | 2 | 45 | * | 2 |
| 1 | 27 | 0 | 0 | na | na | 90 | 45 | 2 | 2 |

| FOOD NAME | Serving Size | Calories | |
|---|---|---|---|
| Bananas with Pears & Apples | 6 oz | 130 | |
| Fruit Dessert | 6 oz | 120 | |
| Peaches | 6 oz | 90 | |
| Pears | 6 oz | 100 | |
| *Beech-Nut Stage 3 Vegetables* | | | |
| Carrots | 6 oz | 60 | |
| Green Beans | 5.75 oz | 45 | |
| Sweet Potatoes | 6 oz | 110 | |
| *Beech-Nut Stage 3 Dinners* | | | |
| Beef & Egg Noodle | 6 oz | 120 | |
| Chicken Noodle | 6 oz | 100 | |
| Macaroni & Beef | 6 oz | 130 | |
| Spaghetti & Beef | 6 oz | 130 | |
| Turkey Rice | 6 oz | 100 | |
| Vegetable Beef | 6 oz | 120 | |
| Vegetable Chicken | 6 oz | 110 | |
| *Beech-Nut Stage 3 Dessert* | | | |
| Cottage Cheese Pineapple | 6 oz | 170 | |
| Mixed Fruit Yogurt | 6 oz | 160 | |
| Vanilla Custard Pudding | 6 oz | 180 | |
| BACON | | | |
| Cooked | 1 slice | 35 | |
| Cooked (Oscar Mayer) | 1 slice | 35 | |
| Canadian | 1 slice | 35 | |
| Canadian (Oscar Mayer) | 1 slice | 35 | |

| Protein (g) | Carbohydrates (g) | Fat (g) | Sodium (mg) | Cholesterol (mg) | Fiber (g) | Vitamin A (%) | Vitamin C (%) | Calcium (%) | Iron (%) |
|---|---|---|---|---|---|---|---|---|---|
| 0 | 31 | 0 | 0 | na | na | 6 | 45 | * | 2 |
| 0 | 28 | 0 | 5 | na | na | 8 | 45 | * | * |
| 1 | 22 | 0 | 0 | na | na | 40 | 45 | * | * |
| 0 | 24 | 0 | 0 | na | na | * | 45 | * | * |
| | | | | | | | | | |
| 1 | 13 | 0 | 170 | na | na | 900 | * | 4 | 2 |
| 2 | 10 | 0 | 0 | na | na | 30 | * | 8 | 8 |
| 1 | 26 | 0 | 80 | na | na | 600 | 2 | 4 | 2 |
| | | | | | | | | | |
| 4 | 14 | 5 | 50 | na | na | 280 | * | 4 | 4 |
| 4 | 14 | 3 | 55 | na | na | 240 | * | 6 | 4 |
| 4 | 16 | 6 | 70 | na | na | 330 | * | 6 | 4 |
| 4 | 16 | 6 | 65 | na | na | 320 | * | 4 | 4 |
| 3 | 14 | 3 | 80 | na | na | 250 | * | 6 | 2 |
| 3 | 16 | 5 | 60 | na | na | 350 | * | 2 | 4 |
| 4 | 14 | 4 | 75 | na | na | 320 | * | 6 | 4 |
| | | | | | | | | | |
| 3 | 36 | 2 | 20 | na | na | * | 45 | 4 | * |
| 1 | 36 | 2 | 30 | na | na | 4 | 45 | 8 | * |
| 3 | 30 | 5 | 80 | na | na | 2 | * | 15 | 2 |
| | | | | | | | | | |
| 2 | Tr | 3 | 120 | 5 | 0 | * | * | * | * |
| 2 | Tr | 3 | 140 | 5 | 0 | na | 3 | * | * |
| 6 | Tr | 1 | 350 | 12 | 0 | * | 12 | * | * |
| 6 | Tr | 1 | 389 | 12 | 0 | na | 12 | * | * |

| FOOD NAME | Serving Size | Calories | |
|---|---|---|---|
| **BACON SUBSTITUTE** | | | |
| Oscar Mayer Lean 'N Tasty Beef | 1 slice | 46 | |
| Vegetarian, Morningstar Breakfast Strips | 1 slice | 38 | |
| **BAGEL** | | | |
| Plain | 1 | 150 | |
| Egg | 1 | 165 | |
| **BANANA  Raw** | 1 med | 100 | |
| **BARBECUE SAUCE** | | | |
| *French's* | | | |
| Cattlemen's Regular | 1 tbsp | 25 | |
| Cattlemen's Smoky | 1 tbsp | 25 | |
| *Heinz* | 1 tbsp | 20 | |
| Hickory Smoke | 1 tbsp | 20 | |
| Hot | 1 tbsp | 20 | |
| Mushroom | 1 tbsp | 20 | |
| Onion | 1 tbsp | 20 | |
| *Hunt's* | | | |
| All Natural Hickory | 1 tbsp | 25 | |
| All Natural Hot & Zesty | 1 tbsp | 25 | |
| All Natural Onion | 1 tbsp | 20 | |
| All Natural Original | 1 tbsp | 20 | |
| *Kraft* | 2 tbsp | 45 | |
| Garlic | 2 tbsp | 40 | |
| Hickory Smoke | 2 tbsp | 45 | |
| Hickory Smoke Onion Bits | 2 tbsp | 50 | |

| Protein (g) | Carbohydrates (g) | Fat (g) | Sodium (mg) | Cholesterol (mg) | Fiber (g) | Vitamin A (%) | Vitamin C (%) | Calcium (%) | Iron (%) |
|---|---|---|---|---|---|---|---|---|---|
| 3 | Tr | 4 | 190 | 13 | 0 | na | 5 | * | * |
| 1 | Tr | 4 | 99 | 0 | 0 | * | * | * | 1 |
| | | | | | | | | | |
| 6 | 30 | 1 | 320 | 0 | na | * | * | * | 6 |
| 6 | 28 | 2 | 360 | 5 | na | 1 | * | 1 | 7 |
| 1 | 27 | <1 | 1 | 0 | 1.8 | 4 | 20 | * | 4 |
| | | | | | | | | | |
| 0 | 5 | 0 | 255 | na | na | * | * | * | * |
| 0 | 5 | 0 | 295 | na | na | * | * | * | * |
| 0 | 5 | 0 | 230 | 0 | na | na | na | na | na |
| 0 | 5 | 0 | 220 | 0 | na | na | na | na | na |
| 0 | 5 | 0 | 220 | 0 | na | na | na | na | na |
| 0 | 5 | 0 | 220 | 0 | na | na | na | na | na |
| 0 | 5 | 0 | 200 | 0 | na | na | na | na | na |
| | | | | | | | | | |
| 0 | 6 | 0 | 195 | na | na | 4 | 6 | * | * |
| 0 | 6 | 0 | 195 | na | na | 4 | 4 | * | * |
| 0 | 5 | 0 | 195 | na | na | 4 | 4 | * | * |
| 0 | 5 | 0 | 195 | na | na | 4 | 4 | * | * |
| 0 | 10 | 1 | 460 | 0 | na | 4 | * | * | * |
| 0 | 9 | 0 | 420 | 0 | na | 4 | * | * | * |
| 0 | 10 | 1 | 440 | 0 | na | 4 | * | * | * |
| 0 | 11 | 1 | 340 | 0 | na | 4 | * | * | * |

| FOOD NAME | Serving Size | Calories | |
|---|---|---|---|
| Hot | 2 tbsp | 45 | |
| Hot Hickory Smoke | 2 tbsp | 45 | |
| Italian Seasonings | 2 tbsp | 50 | |
| Kansas City Style | 2 tbsp | 50 | |
| Mesquite Smoke | 2 tbsp | 45 | |
| Onion Bits | 2 tbsp | 50 | |
| Thick 'n Spicy Chunky | 2 tbsp | 60 | |
| Thick 'n Spicy Hickory Smoke | 2 tbsp | 50 | |
| Thick 'n Spicy with Honey | 2 tbsp | 60 | |
| Thick 'n Spicy Mesquite Smoke | 2 tbsp | 50 | |
| Thick 'n Spicy Original | 2 tbsp | 50 | |
| BARLEY Cooked | 1 cup | 193 | |
| BASS Striped, fried | 3 oz | 170 | |
| BEANS, BAKED | | | |
| Barbecue Beans (Campbell's) | 7⅞ oz | 210 | |
| Beans 'n' Franks (Heinz) | 7¾ oz | 330 | |
| Home Style (Campbell's) | 8 oz | 220 | |
| Hot Chili (Campbell's) | 7¾ oz | 180 | |
| Old Fashioned in Molasses & Brown Sugar (Campbell's) | 8 oz | 230 | |
| Pork & Beans in Tomato Sauce (Campbell's) | 8 oz | 200 | |
| Red Kidney (B & M) | 8 oz | 330 | |
| Small Pea (B & M) | 8 oz | 330 | |
| Vegetarian (Campbell's) | 7¾ oz | 170 | |

| Protein (g) | Carbohydrates (g) | Fat (g) | Sodium (mg) | Cholesterol (mg) | Fiber (g) | Vitamin A (%) | Vitamin C (%) | Calcium (%) | Iron (%) |
|---|---|---|---|---|---|---|---|---|---|
| 0 | 9 | 1 | 520 | 0 | na | 4 | * | * | * |
| 0 | 9 | 1 | 360 | 0 | na | 4 | * | * | * |
| 0 | 10 | 1 | 280 | 0 | na | 4 | * | * | * |
| 0 | 11 | 1 | 270 | 0 | na | 2 | * | 2 | 4 |
| 0 | 10 | 1 | 410 | 0 | na | 6 | * | * | * |
| 0 | 11 | 1 | 340 | 0 | na | 2 | * | * | * |
| 0 | 13 | 1 | 420 | 0 | na | 4 | * | * | 2 |
| 0 | 12 | 1 | 430 | 0 | na | 6 | * | * | 2 |
| 0 | 13 | 1 | 340 | 0 | na | 4 | * | 2 | 2 |
| 0 | 13 | 1 | 270 | 0 | na | 2 | * | 2 | 2 |
| 0 | 12 | 1 | 430 | 0 | na | 4 | * | * | 2 |
| 4 | 44 | <1 | 5 | 0 | 0.4 | * | 5 | * | 5 |
| 15 | 6 | 8 | 66 | 60 | 0 | * | * | 2 | 4 |
|  |  |  |  |  |  |  |  |  |  |
| 10 | 43 | 4 | 900 | na | na | 10 | 8 | 8 | 15 |
| na | 34 | 15 | 905 | na | na | na | na | na | na |
| 11 | 48 | 4 | 820 | na | na | 6 | 8 | 10 | 20 |
| 10 | 38 | 4 | 870 | na | na | 15 | 10 | 10 | 20 |
|  |  |  |  |  |  |  |  |  |  |
| 11 | 49 | 3 | 730 | na | na | 2 | 10 | 10 | 20 |
|  |  |  |  |  |  |  |  |  |  |
| 10 | 43 | 3 | 770 | na | na | 10 | 4 | 10 | 15 |
| na | 50 | 7 | 776 | na | na | * | * | 4 | 35 |
| na | 49 | 8 | 848 | na | na | * | * | 10 | 40 |
| 11 | 40 | 1 | 780 | na | na | 15 | * | 10 | 20 |

| FOOD NAME | Serving Size | Calories | |
|---|---|---|---|
| Vegetarian (Heinz) | 8 oz | 230 | |
| Yellow-Eyed (B & M) | 8 oz | 330 | |
| BEEF | | | |
| *Bottom round* | | | |
| Braised, simmered or pot roasted | | | |
| Lean and fat | 3 oz | 220 | |
| Lean only | 2.8 oz | 175 | |
| *Chuck blade* | | | |
| Braised, simmered, or pot roasted | | | |
| Lean and fat | 3 oz | 325 | |
| Lean only | 2.2 oz | 170 | |
| *Ground,* broiled patty | | | |
| Lean | 3 oz | 230 | |
| Regular | 3 oz | 245 | |
| *Heart,* lean, braised | 3 oz | 150 | |
| *Liver,* fried slice | 3 oz | 185 | |
| *Rib,* roasted | | | |
| Lean and fat | 3 oz | 315 | |
| Lean only | 2.2 oz | 150 | |
| *Round, eye of,* roasted | | | |
| Lean and fat | 3 oz | 205 | |
| Lean only | 2.6 oz | 135 | |
| *Sirloin steak,* broiled | | | |
| Lean and fat | 3 oz | 240 | |
| Lean only | 2.5 oz | 150 | |

| Protein (g) | Carbohydrates (g) | Fat (g) | Sodium (mg) | Cholesterol (mg) | Fiber (g) | Vitamin A (%) | Vitamin C (%) | Calcium (%) | Iron (%) |
|---|---|---|---|---|---|---|---|---|---|
| na | 43 | 2 | 980 | na | na | na | na | na | na |
| na | 50 | 4 | 968 | na | na | * | * | 10 | 20 |
| 25 | 0 | 13 | 43 | 81 | 0 | * | * | * | 16 |
| 25 | 0 | 8 | 40 | 75 | 0 | * | * | * | 15 |
| 22 | 0 | 26 | 53 | 87 | 0 | * | * | 2 | 14 |
| 19 | 0 | 9 | 44 | 66 | 0 | * | * | 2 | 13 |
| 21 | 0 | 16 | 65 | 74 | 0 | * | * | * | 10 |
| 20 | 0 | 18 | 70 | 76 | 0 | * | * | * | 12 |
| 24 | 0 | 5 | 54 | 164 | 0 | * | * | * | 36 |
| 23 | 7 | 7 | 90 | 410 | 0 | 900 | 38 | <1 | 38 |
| 19 | 0 | 26 | 54 | 72 | 0 | * | * | * | 11 |
| 17 | 0 | 9 | 45 | 49 | 0 | * | * | * | 9 |
| 23 | 0 | 12 | 50 | 62 | 0 | * | * | * | 8 |
| 22 | 0 | 5 | 46 | 52 | 0 | * | * | * | 8 |
| 23 | 0 | 15 | 53 | 77 | 0 | * | * | * | 14 |
| 22 | 0 | 6 | 48 | 64 | 0 | * | * | * | 13 |

| FOOD NAME | Serving Size | Calories |
|---|---|---|
| *Canned,* corned beef | 3 oz | 185 |
| *Dried,* chipped beef | 2.5 oz | 145 |
| BEER | 12 fl oz | 150 |
| Lite | 12 fl oz | 100 |
| BEETS | | |
| Sliced, cooked | 1 cup | 55 |
| Sliced, canned (Del Monte) | ½ cup | 35 |
| Sliced, canned (Del Monte No Salt Added) | ½ cup | 35 |
| BISCUITS | | |
| Ballard Ovenready | 1 | 50 |
| 1869 Brand Butter Tastin' | 1 | 100 |
| Hungry Jack Butter Tastin' Flaky | 1 | 90 |
| Pillsbury Good 'N Buttery Fluffy | 1 | 90 |
| 1869 Brand, baking powder | 1 | 100 |
| Ballard Ovenready, buttermilk | 1 | 50 |
| 1869 Brand, buttermilk | 1 | 100 |
| Hungry Jack Extra Rich, buttermilk | 1 | 50 |
| Pillsbury, buttermilk | 1 | 50 |
| Pillsbury Heat 'n Eat, buttermilk | 2 pieces | 170 |
| BLACKBERRIES | ½ cup | 37 |
| BLUEBERRIES | ½ cup | 41 |
| BLUEBERRY TURNOVER  (Pepperidge Farm) | 1 | 310 |
| BLUEFISH | | |
| Baked or broiled with butter | 3 oz | 140 |
| Fried | 3 oz | 140 |

| Protein (g) | Carbohydrates (g) | Fat (g) | Sodium (mg) | Cholesterol (mg) | Fiber (g) | Vitamin A (%) | Vitamin C (%) | Calcium (%) | Iron (%) |
|---|---|---|---|---|---|---|---|---|---|
| 22 | 0 | 10 | 802 | 80 | 0 | * | * | * | 21 |
| 24 | 0 | 4 | 3053 | 46 | 0 | * | * | * | 13 |
| 1 | 14 | 0 | 25 | 0 | 0 | * | * | 2 | * |
| 0 | 6 | 0 | na | 0 | 0 | * | * | * | * |
|  |  |  |  |  |  |  |  |  |  |
| 2 | 12 | 0 | 73 | 0 | 4 | 6 | 27 | 6 | 4 |
| 1 | 8 | 0 | 290 | 0 | na | * | 4 | * | 2 |
| 1 | 8 | 0 | 100 | 0 | na | * | 4 | * | 2 |
|  |  |  |  |  |  |  |  |  |  |
| 1 | 10 | 1 | 180 | 0 | na | * | * | * | 3 |
| 2 | 12 | 5 | 300 | 0 | na | * | * | 1 | 3 |
| 2 | 12 | 4 | 300 | 0 | na | * | * | * | 3 |
| 1 | 11 | 5 | 270 | 0 | na | * | * | * | 3 |
| 12 | 12 | 5 | 300 | 0 | na | * | * | 1 | 3 |
| 1 | 10 | 1 | 180 | na | na | * | * | * | 3 |
| 2 | 12 | 5 | 300 | 0 | na | * | * | 1 | 3 |
| 1 | 9 | 1 | 170 | 0 | na | * | * | * | 2 |
| 1 | 10 | 1 | 180 | 0 | na | * | * | * | 3 |
| 4 | 27 | 5 | 530 | 0 | na | * | * | 1 | 3 |
| <1 | 9 | Tr | Tr | 0 | 3.3 | 3 | 25 | 3 | 4 |
| <1 | 10 | Tr | 5 | 0 | 1.7 | <2 | 17 | 1 | 4 |
| 3 | 19 | 19 | 230 | na | na | * | 10 | * | 4 |
|  |  |  |  |  |  |  |  |  |  |
| 21 | 0 | 4 | 88 | 150 | 0 | * | * | 2 | 4 |
| 20 | 4 | 9 | 124 | 50 | 0 | 2 | * | 2 | 4 |

| FOOD NAME | Serving Size | Calories |
|---|---|---|
| BOK CHOY  Cooked | 1 cup | 25 |
| BOLOGNA | 1 slice | 80 |
|    Eckrich German Brand | 1 slice | 80 |
|    Oscar Mayer | 1 slice | 90 |
|    Eckrich, Beef | 1 slice | 90 |
|    Oscar Mayer, Beef | 1 slice | 90 |
|    Oscar Mayer, Beef Lebanon | 1 slice | 45 |
|    Oscar Mayer, Beef Light | 1 slice | 65 |
|    Eckrich, Garlic | 1 slice | 90 |
|    Oscar Mayer, Garlic | 1 slice | 130 |
|    Oscar Mayer, Garlic Beef | 1 slice | 90 |
|    Oscar Mayer, Light | 1 slice | 65 |
|    Eckrich, Bologna with Cheese | 1 slice | 90 |
|    Oscar Mayer, Bologna with Cheese | 1 slice | 75 |
|    Oscar Mayer, Wisconsin Made Ring | 1 slice | 90 |
| BONITO  Raw | 3 oz | 111 |
| BOUILLON | | |
|    Beef | 1 cube | 6 |
|    Chicken | 1 cube | 8 |
|    Onion | 1 cube | 8 |
| BRAZIL NUTS | ⅓ cup | 305 |
| BREAD | | |
|    Apple Cinnamon (Pepperidge Farm) | 2 slices | 140 |
|    Apple Walnut (Arnold) | 2 slices | 128 |
|    Bran'nola | 2 slices | 180 |

| Protein (g) | Carbohydrates (g) | Fat (g) | Sodium (mg) | Cholesterol (mg) | Fiber (g) | Vitamin A (%) | Vitamin C (%) | Calcium (%) | Iron (%) |
|---|---|---|---|---|---|---|---|---|---|
| 2 | 4 | 0 | na | 0 | na | 105 | 43 | 25 | 6 |
| 4 | <1 | 7 | 250 | 15 | 0 | * | 6 | * | 2 |
| 4 | 1 | 7 | 300 | na | 0 | * | 10 | * | 2 |
| 3 | <1 | 8 | 310 | 20 | 0 | * | 6 | * | * |
| 3 | 1 | 8 | 230 | na | 0 | * | 10 | * | 2 |
| 3 | <1 | 8 | 305 | 20 | 0 | * | 6 | * | * |
| 5 | <1 | 3 | 300 | 15 | 0 | * | na | * | na |
| 3 | <1 | 5 | 305 | 15 | 0 | * | na | * | na |
| 3 | 1 | 9 | 230 | na | 0 | * | 10 | * | 2 |
| 5 | 1 | 12 | 475 | 25 | 0 | * | na | * | na |
| 3 | <1 | 8 | 300 | 20 | 0 | * | na | * | na |
| 3 | <1 | 6 | 300 | 15 | 0 | * | na | * | na |
| 3 | 1 | 9 | 250 | na | 0 | * | 10 | * | 2 |
| 3 | 1 | 7 | 230 | 15 | 0 | * | 6 | * | * |
| 3 | <1 | 8 | 240 | 20 | 0 | * | na | * | na |
| 22 | Tr | <2 | 36 | 0 | 0 | na | na | na | na |
| <1 | 1 | <1 | 930 | 0 | Tr | * | * | * | * |
| <1 | 1 | <1 | 900 | 0 | Tr | * | * | * | * |
| <1 | 1 | <1 | 670 | 0 | Tr | * | * | * | * |
| 7 | 5 | 31 | 0 | 0 | 5 | * | na | 8 | 10 |
| 4 | 26 | 3 | 210 | 0 | na | * | * | 6 | 2 |
| 4 | 25 | <3 | 206 | 2 | 2.6 | * | * | na | na |
| 7 | 31 | 3 | 355 | 0 | 5.6 | * | * | 2 | 10 |

| FOOD NAME | Serving Size | Calories |
|---|---|---|
| Brown & Serve Italian Enriched (Pepperidge Farm) | 1 oz | 80 |
| Cinnamon (Pepperidge Farm) | 2 slices | 180 |
| Cinnamon Oatmeal (Oatmeal Goodness) | 2 slices | 180 |
| Cinnamon Raisin (Arnold) | 2 slices | 134 |
| Cinnamon Raisin (Pepperidge Farm) | 2 slices | 180 |
| Cracked Wheat (Wonder) | 2 slices | 140 |
| Date Walnut (Pepperidge Farm) | 2 slices | 150 |
| French (DiCarlo Parisian) | 2 slices | 140 |
| French Enriched, Twin (Pepperidge Farm) | 1 oz | 80 |
| French Extra Sour (Colombo) | 2 oz | 153 |
| French Fully Baked (Pepperidge Farm) | 2 oz | 150 |
| Garlic (Colombo) | 2 oz | 185 |
| Grain, Nutty (Arnold) | 2 slices | 170 |
| Granola, Oat and Honey (Pepperidge Farm) | 2 slices | 120 |
| Hollywood Dark | 2 slices | 140 |
| Hollywood White | 2 slices | 140 |
| Italian | 2 slices | 170 |
| Italian (Brownberry Light) | 2 slices | 88 |
| Italian (Wonder) | 2 slices | 140 |
| Multi-Grain (Pepperidge Farm Very Thin) | 2 slices | 80 |
| Oat (Arnold) | 2 slices | 180 |
| Oat, Crunchy (Pepperidge Farm) | 2 slices | 190 |
| Oatmeal (Pepperidge Farm) | 2 slices | 140 |

| Protein (g) | Carbohydrates (g) | Fat (g) | Sodium (mg) | Cholesterol (mg) | Fiber (g) | Vitamin A (%) | Vitamin C (%) | Calcium (%) | Iron (%) |
|---|---|---|---|---|---|---|---|---|---|
| 2 | 14 | 1 | 150 | 0 | 0 | * | * | 2 | 4 |
| 4 | 30 | 6 | 220 | 0 | 4 | * | * | * | 8 |
| 8 | 30 | 4 | 280 | 0 | 2 | * | * | na | na |
| 4 | 26 | 3 | 172 | 4 | <2 | * | * | 4 | 8 |
| 4 | 32 | 4 | 200 | 0 | 2 | * | * | 4 | 8 |
| 6 | 26 | 2 | 360 | 0 | 1.6 | * | * | 8 | 2 |
| 4 | 23 | 5 | 215 | 0 | 4 | * | * | na | na |
| 6 | 28 | 2 | 360 | 0 | 1.4 | * | * | 3 | 9 |
| 3 | 15 | 1 | 160 | 0 | 0 | * | * | 2 | 4 |
| 8 | 27 | <2 | 180 | 0 | 0.7 | * | * | na | na |
| 5 | 28 | 2 | 320 | 0 | 0.5 | * | * | 4 | 8 |
| 6 | 17 | 10 | 331 | 0 | na | * | * | na | na |
| 8 | 35 | 3 | 288 | Tr | 6 | * | * | * | 8 |
| 4 | 24 | 4 | 210 | 0 | 4 | * | * | na | na |
| 6 | 38 | 2 | 375 | 0 | 1.6 | * | * | 10 | 15 |
| 6 | 26 | 2 | 335 | 0 | 1.4 | * | * | 8 | 10 |
| 6 | 34 | 0 | 59 | Tr | 2 | * | * | 1 | 8 |
| 5 | 20 | <1 | 178 | Tr | 4 | * | * | na | na |
| 4 | 26 | 2 | 320 | 0 | 1.4 | * | * | na | na |
| 2 | 14 | 1 | 150 | 0 | 2 | 8 | * | * | 4 |
| 16 | 68 | 4 | 342 | 0 | 5.6 | * | * | 4 | 8 |
| 8 | 34 | 4 | 290 | 0 | 3 | * | * | na | na |
| 4 | 24 | 2 | 320 | 0 | 2 | * | * | 4 | 8 |

| FOOD NAME | Serving Size | Calories | |
|---|---|---|---|
| Oatmeal (Pepperidge Farm Very Thin Sliced) | 2 slices | 80 | |
| Oatmeal Light (Arnold) | 2 slices | 88 | |
| Pita (Sahara Oat Bran) | ½ pc | 66 | |
| Pita (Sahara White) | ½ pc | 79 | |
| Pita (Sahara Whole Wheat) | ½ pc | 150 | |
| Potato (Eddy's) | 2 slices | 140 | |
| Profile Dark | 2 slices | 150 | |
| Profile Light | 2 slices | 150 | |
| Pumpernickel (Arnold) | 2 slices | 140 | |
| Pumpernickel (Pepperidge Farm) | 2 slices | 160 | |
| Pumpernickel (Pepperidge Farm Party) | 4 slices | 70 | |
| Raisin | 2 slices | 130 | |
| Raisin Tea (Arnold) | 2 slices | 140 | |
| Round Top (Roman Meal) | 2 slices | 140 | |
| Rye (Beefsteak) | 2 slices | 140 | |
| Rye, Jewish Seeded (Arnold) | 2 slices | 150 | |
| Rye, Jewish Seeded (Levy's) | 2 slices | 152 | |
| Rye (Pepperidge Farm) | 2 slices | 170 | |
| Rye (Pepperidge Farm Party) | 4 slices | 70 | |
| Rye (Pepperidge Farm Very Thin) | 2 slices | 90 | |
| Seven Grain (Home Pride) | 2 slices | 140 | |
| Wheat (Arnold Brick Oven) | 2 slices | 114 | |
| Wheat (Beefsteak) | 2 slices | 140 | |
| Wheat (Brownberry Natural) | 2 slices | 160 | |

| Protein (g) | Carbohydrates (g) | Fat (g) | Sodium (mg) | Cholesterol (mg) | Fiber (g) | Vitamin A (%) | Vitamin C (%) | Calcium (%) | Iron (%) |
|---|---|---|---|---|---|---|---|---|---|
| 2 | 16 | 2 | 160 | 0 | 0 | * | * | * | 4 |
| 5 | 20 | 1 | 196 | Tr | 3.8 | * | * | na | na |
| 2 | 15 | <1 | 163 | 0 | 1.8 | * | * | na | na |
| 3 | 16 | <1 | 147 | 0 | na | * | * | na | na |
| 6 | 28 | 2 | 320 | 0 | 1.4 | * | * | na | na |
| na | 28 | 2 | 340 | 0 | na | * | * | 2 | 4 |
| 6 | 25 | 3 | 310 | 0 | na | * | * | 4 | 10 |
| 5 | 26 | 2 | 340 | 0 | na | * | * | 4 | 10 |
| 5 | 30 | 2 | 396 | 0 | 2.6 | * | * | 4 | 10 |
| 6 | 30 | 2 | 230 | 0 | 4 | * | * | 4 | 10 |
| 2 | 12 | 1 | 160 | 0 | 1 | * | * | 2 | 4 |
| 4 | 26 | 2 | 91 | 0 | 2.4 | * | * | 4 | 7 |
| 3 | 26 | 3 | 225 | 0 | na | * | * | * | 2 |
| 6 | 27 | 2 | 320 | 0 | 1.2 | * | * | 6 | 10 |
| 6 | 26 | 2 | 360 | 0 | 1.4 | * | * | 4 | 10 |
| 5 | 28 | 2 | 425 | 0 | 2 | * | * | 4 | 4 |
| 6 | 32 | 2 | 362 | 0 | 2.8 | * | * | na | na |
| 6 | 30 | 2 | 420 | 0 | 4 | * | * | 4 | 10 |
| 2 | 12 | 1 | 250 | 0 | 1 | * | * | 2 | 4 |
| 2 | 17 | 2 | 285 | 0 | 1 | * | * | na | na |
| na | 25 | 2 | 270 | 0 | 1.6 | * | * | 4 | 10 |
| 2 | 11 | <2 | 208 | 0 | 3.4 | * | * | 2 | 8 |
| 6 | 22 | 2 | 320 | 0 | 2.8 | * | * | na | na |
| 6 | 34 | <3 | 366 | 0 | 4.6 | * | * | na | na |

| FOOD NAME | Serving Size | Calories |
|---|---|---|
| Wheat (Fresh & Natural) | 2 slices | 140 |
| Wheat (Home Pride Butter Top) | 2 slices | 140 |
| Wheat (Pepperidge Farm Family) | 2 slices | 140 |
| Wheat (Pepperidge Farm Very Thin) | 2 slices | 70 |
| Wheat (Roman Meal) | 2 slices | 140 |
| Wheat (Wonder Family) | 2 slices | 150 |
| Wheat, Cracked (Eddy's) | 2 slices | 140 |
| Wheat, Cracked (Pepperidge Farm) | 2 slices | 140 |
| Wheat, Cracked (Wonder) | 2 slices | 140 |
| Wheat, Hearty (Arnold) | 2 slices | 176 |
| Wheat, Honey Wheatberry (Home Pride) | 2 slices | 140 |
| Wheat, Honey Wheatberry (Pepperidge Farm) | 2 slices | 140 |
| Wheat, Honey Wheatberry (Roman Light) | 2 slices | 78 |
| Wheat, Light (Butter-Nut) | 2 slices | 100 |
| Wheat, Light (Millbrook) | 2 slices | 100 |
| Wheat, Sprouted (Pepperidge Farm) | 2 slices | 140 |
| Wheat, Whole (Arnold Stoneground 100%) | 2 slices | 96 |
| Wheat, Whole (Home Pride 100%) | 2 slices | 140 |
| Wheat, Whole (Pepperidge Farm Thin Sliced) | 2 slices | 130 |
| Wheat, Whole (Wonder 100%) | 2 slices | 140 |
| White (Arnold Brick Oven) | 2 slices | 130 |
| White (Home Pride Butter Top) | 2 slices | 150 |
| White (Pepperidge Farm Sandwich) | 2 slices | 130 |

| Protein (g) | Carbohydrates (g) | Fat (g) | Sodium (mg) | Cholesterol (mg) | Fiber (g) | Vitamin A (%) | Vitamin C (%) | Calcium (%) | Iron (%) |
|---|---|---|---|---|---|---|---|---|---|
| 6 | 26 | 2 | 270 | 0 | 3.6 | * | * | 2 | 8 |
| 6 | 26 | 3 | 310 | 0 | 1.6 | * | * | 6 | 8 |
| 4 | 26 | 2 | 270 | 0 | 4 | * | * | 4 | 10 |
| 4 | 14 | 0 | 150 | 0 | 0 | * | * | 4 | 4 |
| 4 | 25 | 2 | 280 | 0 | na | * | * | 6 | 10 |
| 6 | 27 | 2 | 300 | 0 | 1.6 | * | * | 8 | 10 |
| 6 | 26 | 2 | 360 | 0 | na | * | * | * | 2 |
| 4 | 26 | 2 | 280 | 0 | 2 | * | * | * | 8 |
| 6 | 26 | 2 | 360 | 0 | 1.6 | * | * | na | na |
| 8 | 34 | 4 | 394 | Tr | 5.4 | * | * | na | na |
| 5 | 26 | 2 | 310 | 0 | na | * | * | 4 | 8 |
| | | | | | | | | | |
| 4 | 28 | 2 | 280 | 0 | 2 | * | * | na | na |
| 5 | 20 | <1 | 216 | 0 | 5.8 | * | * | na | na |
| 5 | 22 | 0 | 350 | 0 | na | * | * | 2 | 4 |
| 5 | 22 | 0 | 350 | 0 | na | * | * | 2 | 4 |
| 6 | 22 | 4 | 200 | 0 | 4 | * | * | 2 | 10 |
| 5 | 20 | <2 | 196 | Tr | 3.2 | * | * | na | na |
| na | 24 | 2 | 280 | 0 | na | * | * | 4 | 10 |
| | | | | | | | | | |
| 2 | 24 | 2 | 220 | 0 | 4 | * | * | 4 | 10 |
| 6 | 24 | 2 | 240 | 0 | 3.6 | * | * | 2 | 8 |
| 4 | 22 | 2 | 205 | Tr | 0.8 | * | * | 4 | 6 |
| 5 | 26 | 3 | 305 | 0 | 1.4 | * | * | 6 | 8 |
| 4 | 24 | 2 | 260 | 0 | 0 | * | * | 4 | 8 |

| FOOD NAME | Serving Size | Calories |
|---|---|---|
| White (Pepperidge Farm Toasting) | 2 slices | 180 |
| White (Pepperidge Farm Thin Sliced Enriched) | 2 slices | 160 |
| White (Sweetheart) | 2 slices | 140 |
| White (Wonder) | 2 slices | 140 |
| White with Buttermilk (Wonder) | 2 slices | 140 |
| **BREAD CRUMBS** | | |
| (Devonsheer) | 1 oz | 108 |
| (Pepperidge Farm Premium) | 1 oz | 110 |
| Italian Style (Devonsheer) | 1 oz | 104 |
| Seasoned (Pepperidge Farm) | 1 oz | 110 |
| **BREADFRUIT** | ½ cup | 114 |
| **BROCCOLI** | | |
| Fresh, cooked | 1 cup | 40 |
| *Frozen* | | |
| Birds Eye Baby Spears | 3.3 oz | 30 |
| Birds Eye Chopped | 3.3 oz | 25 |
| Birds Eye Cuts | 3.3 oz | 25 |
| Birds Eye Florets | 3.3 oz | 25 |
| Birds Eye Spears | 3.3 oz | 25 |
| Green Giant Cuts | ½ cup | 16 |
| Green Giant Harvest Fresh Spears | ½ cup | 20 |
| *Frozen, in cheese sauce* | | |
| Birds Eye | 5 oz | 130 |

| Protein (g) | Carbohydrates (g) | Fat (g) | Sodium (mg) | Cholesterol (mg) | Fiber (g) | Vitamin A (%) | Vitamin C (%) | Calcium (%) | Iron (%) |
|---|---|---|---|---|---|---|---|---|---|
| 6 | 34 | 2 | 400 | 0 | 2 | * | * | 4 | 12 |
| | | | | | | | | | |
| 4 | 28 | 4 | 260 | 0 | 0 | * | * | 4 | 8 |
| 6 | 28 | 2 | 300 | 0 | na | * | * | 2 | 4 |
| 6 | 26 | 2 | 280 | 0 | 1.4 | * | * | 6 | 8 |
| 4 | 26 | 2 | 320 | 0 | 1.4 | * | * | 6 | 8 |
| | | | | | | | | | |
| 4 | 22 | 1 | 272 | 0 | 0.9 | * | * | 2 | 6 |
| na | 22 | 1 | 260 | 0 | na | * | * | 2 | 6 |
| 4 | 21 | 1 | 408 | 0 | 0.9 | * | * | na | na |
| na | 22 | 1 | 260 | 0 | na | * | * | 2 | 6 |
| 1 | 30 | Tr | 2 | 0 | 1.6 | na | na | na | na |
| | | | | | | | | | |
| 5 | 7 | 0 | 16 | 0 | 4 | 78 | 230 | 14 | 7 |
| | | | | | | | | | |
| 3 | 5 | 0 | 15 | 0 | 3 | 25 | 120 | 4 | 4 |
| 3 | 5 | 0 | 15 | 0 | 3 | 45 | 90 | 4 | 2 |
| 3 | 5 | 0 | 25 | 0 | 3 | 40 | 90 | 6 | 4 |
| 3 | 5 | 0 | 20 | 0 | 3 | 25 | 90 | 4 | 4 |
| 3 | 5 | 0 | 20 | 0 | 3 | 25 | 90 | 4 | 4 |
| 2 | 3 | 0 | 15 | 0 | 2 | 8 | 60 | 2 | * |
| | | | | | | | | | |
| 2 | 4 | 0 | 190 | 0 | 2.4 | 25 | 80 | 2 | 2 |
| | | | | | | | | | |
| 6 | 12 | 7 | 560 | 10 | 2 | 70 | 70 | 15 | 4 |

| FOOD NAME | Serving Size | Calories |
|---|---|---|
| Green Giant | ½ cup | 70 |
| *Frozen combinations* | | |
| Broccoli, Baby Carrots and | | |
| Water Chestnuts (Birds Eye) | 4 oz | 45 |
| Broccoli, Cauliflower and | | |
| Carrots (Birds Eye) | 4 oz | 35 |
| Broccoli, Cauliflower and | | |
| Red Peppers (Birds Eye) | 4 oz | 30 |
| Broccoli, Corn and | | |
| Red Peppers (Birds Eye) | 4 oz | 60 |
| Broccoli, Green Beans, Pearl Onions | | |
| and Red Peppers (Birds Eye) | 4 oz | 35 |
| Broccoli, Red Peppers, Bamboo Shoots | | |
| and Straw Mushrooms (Birds Eye) | 4 oz | 30 |
| Broccoli and Carrots | | |
| (Green Giant Fanfare) | ½ cup | 25 |
| Broccoli and Cauliflower | | |
| (Green Giant Medley) | ½ cup | 60 |
| Broccoli and Cauliflower | | |
| (Green Giant Supreme) | ½ cup | 20 |
| BRUSSELS SPROUTS | | |
| Fresh, cooked | 1 cup | 55 |
| *Frozen* | | |
| Birds Eye | 3.3 oz | 35 |
| Green Giant | ½ cup | 30 |

| Protein (g) | Carbohydrates (g) | Fat (g) | Sodium (mg) | Cholesterol (mg) | Fiber (g) | Vitamin A (%) | Vitamin C (%) | Calcium (%) | Iron (%) |
|---|---|---|---|---|---|---|---|---|---|
| 4 | 8 | 3 | 425 | 2 | 2.2 | 30 | 70 | 6 | 2 |
| 2 | 10 | 0 | 35 | 0 | 3 | 150 | 60 | 4 | 4 |
| 2 | 7 | 0 | 40 | 0 | 3 | 180 | 70 | 4 | 4 |
| 3 | 5 | 0 | 25 | 0 | 3 | 35 | 100 | 4 | 4 |
| 3 | 14 | 1 | 15 | 0 | 3 | 35 | 60 | 2 | 4 |
| 2 | 7 | 0 | 15 | 0 | 3 | 30 | 60 | 6 | 6 |
| 3 | 5 | 0 | 20 | 0 | 3 | 45 | 90 | 4 | 6 |
| 3 | 5 | 0 | 20 | 0 | 2 | 50 | 70 | 2 | 4 |
| 3 | 10 | 1 | 470 | 0 | 3 | 40 | 80 | 2 | 2 |
| 3 | 4 | 0 | 30 | 0 | 2.1 | 40 | 60 | 2 | 2 |
| 7 | 10 | 1 | 16 | 0 | 7 | 16 | 230 | 5 | 9 |
| 3 | 7 | 0 | 15 | 0 | 3 | 15 | 110 | 2 | 4 |
| 2 | 5 | 0 | 15 | 0 | 1.6 | 6 | 25 | * | 2 |

| FOOD NAME | Serving Size | Calories |
|---|---|---|
| Green Giant, in butter sauce | ½ cup | 60 |
| Green Giant, in cheese sauce | ½ cup | 80 |
| Birds Eye, baby, in cheese sauce | 4.5 oz | 130 |
| *Frozen combinations* | | |
| Brussels Sprouts, Cauliflower and Carrots (Birds Eye) | 4 oz | 40 |
| BULGUR Cooked | 1 cup | 152 |
| BUTTER | 1 tbsp | 100 |
| Whipped | 1 tbsp | 65 |
| BUTTERMILK | 1 cup | 100 |
| CABBAGE | | |
| Raw, shredded | 1 cup | 16 |
| Cooked | 1 cup | 32 |
| Chinese, raw, shredded | 1 cup | 10 |
| Red, raw, shredded | 1 cup | 20 |
| Savoy, raw, shredded | 1 cup | 20 |
| CAKE | | |
| Angel Food (Dolly Madison) | ⅙ | 120 |
| Boston Creme (Pepperidge Farm) | 2⅞ oz | 290 |
| Carrot (Pepperidge Farm) | 1½ oz | 150 |
| Chocolate Fudge (Pepperidge Farm) | 1⅝ oz | 180 |
| Chocolate Fudge Stripe (Pepperidge Farm) | 1⅝ oz | 170 |
| Cholesterol Free Pound Cake (Pepperidge Farm) | 1 oz | 110 |

| Protein (g) | Carbohydrates (g) | Fat (g) | Sodium (mg) | Cholesterol (mg) | Fiber (g) | Vitamin A (%) | Vitamin C (%) | Calcium (%) | Iron (%) |
|---|---|---|---|---|---|---|---|---|---|
| 3 | 8 | 1 | 280 | 5 | 4.1 | 15 | 90 | 2 | 2 |
| 3 | 13 | 2 | 475 | na | na | 10 | 90 | 6 | 2 |
| 6 | 12 | 7 | 500 | 5 | 2 | 50 | 90 | 10 | 4 |
| | | | | | | | | | |
| 3 | 8 | 0 | 30 | 0 | 4 | 110 | 90 | 2 | 4 |
| 6 | 34 | Tr | 9 | 0 | 0.6 | * | 5 | 3 | 11 |
| 0 | 0 | 12 | 116 | 31 | 0 | 9 | * | * | * |
| 0 | 0 | 12 | 74 | 20 | 0 | 6 | * | * | * |
| 8 | 12 | 2 | 257 | 15 | 0 | 2 | 3 | 29 | 1 |
| | | | | | | | | | |
| 1 | 4 | Tr | 12 | 0 | 0.8 | 2 | 60 | 4 | 2 |
| 1 | 7 | Tr | 28 | 0 | 1 | 4 | 80 | 6 | 2 |
| 1 | <2 | Tr | 46 | 0 | 0.8 | 2 | 30 | 4 | 2 |
| 1 | 4 | Tr | 8 | 0 | 1.4 | * | 70 | 2 | 4 |
| 1 | 4 | Tr | 20 | 0 | 0.6 | 2 | 60 | 4 | 4 |
| | | | | | | | | | |
| 2 | 17 | 5 | 150 | na | na | * | * | 4 | 2 |
| 3 | 39 | 14 | 190 | 50 | na | * | * | 4 | 4 |
| 1 | 19 | 9 | 160 | 15 | na | 15 | 2 | * | 2 |
| 1 | 23 | 10 | 140 | 20 | 0 | * | * | * | 4 |
| | | | | | | | | | |
| 2 | 20 | 9 | 140 | 20 | na | * | * | * | 4 |
| | | | | | | | | | |
| 1 | 13 | 6 | 85 | 0 | na | * | * | * | * |

| FOOD NAME | Serving Size | Calories |
|---|---|---|
| Coconut (Pepperidge Farm) | 1⅝ oz | 180 |
| Devil's Food (Pepperidge Farm) | 1⅝ oz | 180 |
| German Chocolate (Pepperidge Farm) | 1⅝ oz | 180 |
| Golden (Pepperidge Farm) | 1⅝ oz | 180 |
| Lemon Coconut (Pepperidge Farm) | 3 oz | 280 |
| Lemon Cream (Pepperidge Farm) | 1⅝ oz | 170 |
| Pineapple Cream (Pepperidge Farm) | 2 oz | 190 |
| Pound (Dolly Madison) | ⅙ | 220 |
| Strawberry Cream (Pepperidge Farm) | 2 oz | 190 |
| Strawberry Stripe (Pepperidge Farm) | 1½ oz | 160 |
| Vanilla (Pepperidge Farm) | 1⅝ oz | 190 |
| Vanilla Fudge Swirl | | |
| (Pepperidge Farm) | 2¼ oz | 250 |
| *From Mix* | | |
| Angel Food (Betty Crocker) | 1/12 | 130 |
| Angel Food (Betty Crocker Chocolate) | 1/12 | 140 |
| Angel Food (Betty Crocker One-Step) | 1/12 | 140 |
| Angel Food (Betty Crocker Strawberry) | 1/12 | 150 |
| Angel Food (Pillsbury Lovin' Loaf) | ⅛ | 90 |
| Banana (Pillsbury) | 1/12 | 250 |
| Banana Walnut (Snackin' Cake) | 1/9 | 190 |
| Black Forest Cherry (Pillsbury Bundt) | 1/16 | 279 |
| Blueberry Streusel (Pillsbury) | 1/16 | 260 |
| Boston Creme (Pillsbury Bundt) | 1/16 | 260 |
| Butter Recipe (Pillsbury) | 1/12 | 260 |

| Protein (g) | Carbohydrates (g) | Fat (g) | Sodium (mg) | Cholesterol (mg) | Fiber (g) | Vitamin A (%) | Vitamin C (%) | Calcium (%) | Iron (%) |
|---|---|---|---|---|---|---|---|---|---|
| 1 | 24 | 8 | 120 | 20 | na | * | * | 2 | 2 |
| 1 | 24 | 9 | 135 | 20 | 0 | * | * | * | 2 |
| 1 | 22 | 10 | 170 | 20 | na | * | * | 2 | 2 |
| 1 | 24 | 9 | 110 | 20 | na | * | * | 2 | 2 |
| 3 | 38 | 13 | 220 | 30 | na | * | 4 | 2 | 4 |
| 2 | 221 | 9 | 120 | 20 | na | * | * | * | * |
| 2 | 28 | 7 | 130 | 7 | na | * | * | 2 | 4 |
| 4 | 33 | 8 | 290 | 50 | 0 | * | * | 4 | 6 |
| 1 | 30 | 7 | 120 | 20 | na | * | * | 2 | 4 |
| 1 | 21 | 8 | 120 | 20 | na | * | * | * | 2 |
| 1 | 25 | 8 | 120 | 20 | 0 | * | * | * | * |
| | | | | | | | | | |
| 2 | 33 | 11 | 160 | 35 | na | * | * | * | * |
| | | | | | | | | | |
| 3 | 30 | 0 | 140 | na | na | * | * | 4 | * |
| 3 | 32 | 0 | 275 | na | na | * | * | * | * |
| 3 | 32 | 0 | 250 | na | na | * | * | 4 | * |
| 3 | 34 | 0 | 270 | na | na | * | * | 4 | * |
| 2 | 20 | 0 | 210 | 0 | na | * | * | 2 | * |
| 3 | 35 | 11 | 280 | 55 | na | * | * | 4 | 4 |
| 2 | 31 | 6 | 260 | na | na | * | * | 4 | 2 |
| 3 | 41 | 12 | 320 | 40 | na | * | * | 2 | 8 |
| 3 | 39 | 11 | 200 | 40 | na | * | * | 2 | 4 |
| 3 | 42 | 10 | 290 | 40 | na | * | * | 4 | 4 |
| 3 | 35 | 12 | 370 | 75 | na | 6 | * | 8 | 4 |

## Cake *Mix*

| FOOD NAME | Serving Size | Calories |
|---|---|---|
| Butter Recipe Chocolate (Pillsbury) | 1/12 | 250 |
| Carrot (Pillsbury) | 1/12 | 260 |
| Carrot Nut (Snackin' Cake) | 1/9 | 180 |
| Cheesecake (Jell-O) | 1/8 | 280 |
| Cheesecake (Jell-O Lemon) | 1/8 | 270 |
| Cheesecake (Jell-O NY Style) | 1/8 | 280 |
| Chocolate, Sour Cream (Duncan Hines) | 1/12 | 200 |
| Chocolate Caramel (Pillsbury Bundt) | 1/16 | 290 |
| Chocolate Chip (Pillsbury) | 1/12 | 240 |
| Chocolate Eclair (Pillsbury Bundt) | 1/16 | 260 |
| Chocolate Macaroon (Pillsbury Bundt) | 1/16 | 280 |
| Chocolate Mousse (Pillsbury) | 1/16 | 260 |
| Cinnamon (Stir 'n Streusel) | 1/6 | 240 |
| Cinnamon Streusel (Pillsbury) | 1/16 | 260 |
| Coffee (Pillsbury Cinnamon Swirl with Icing) | 1 | 230 |
| Coffee (Pillsbury Pecan Crumb with Icing) | 1 | 230 |
| Dark Chocolate (Pillsbury) | 1/12 | 250 |
| Devil's Food (Pillsbury) | 1/12 | 270 |
| Devil's Food (Pillsbury Lovin' Light) | 1/12 | 170 |
| Double Chocolate Chip (Moist & Easy) | 1/9 | 180 |
| Fudge (Duncan Hines) | 1/12 | 270 |
| Fudge Swirl (Pillsbury) | 1/12 | 270 |
| Funfetti (Pillsbury) | 1/12 | 230 |

| Protein (g) | Carbohydrates (g) | Fat (g) | Sodium (mg) | Cholesterol (mg) | Fiber (g) | Vitamin A (%) | Vitamin C (%) | Calcium (%) | Iron (%) |
|---|---|---|---|---|---|---|---|---|---|
| 4 | 32 | 13 | 420 | 75 | na | 6 | * | 10 | 8 |
| 3 | 34 | 12 | 300 | 55 | na | 50 | * | 4 | 4 |
| 2 | 30 | 6 | 240 | na | na | 4 | * | 8 | 4 |
| 5 | 36 | 13 | 350 | 30 | na | 8 | * | 15 | * |
| 5 | 36 | 13 | 400 | 13 | na | 8 | * | 15 | 2 |
| 6 | 38 | 12 | 420 | 30 | na | 6 | * | 15 | 2 |
| 3 | 34 | 6 | 330 | na | na | * | * | 10 | 6 |
| 3 | 43 | 13 | 370 | 45 | na | * | * | 2 | 8 |
| 3 | 34 | 10 | 280 | 35 | na | * | * | 8 | 4 |
| 3 | 42 | 10 | 290 | 40 | na | * | * | 4 | 4 |
| 3 | 37 | 14 | 340 | 40 | na | * | * | * | 6 |
| 3 | 37 | 12 | 310 | 40 | na | * | * | 2 | 6 |
| 3 | 42 | 7 | 230 | na | na | * | * | * | 4 |
| 3 | 38 | 11 | 200 | 40 | na | * | * | 2 | 4 |
| 3 | 29 | 11 | 240 | 0 | na | * | * | * | 6 |
| 3 | 29 | 12 | 240 | 0 | na | * | * | * | 6 |
| 3 | 32 | 12 | 340 | 55 | na | * | * | 10 | 6 |
| 4 | 32 | 14 | 350 | 55 | na | * | * | 10 | 8 |
| 4 | 32 | 3 | 380 | 35 | na | * | * | 10 | 8 |
| 3 | 32 | 5 | 340 | na | na | * | * | 6 | 6 |
| 4 | 34 | 13 | 350 | na | na | 6 | * | 2 | 6 |
| 3 | 36 | 12 | 300 | 55 | na | * | * | 8 | 4 |
| 3 | 35 | 9 | 290 | 0 | na | * | * | 2 | 2 |

# Cake Mix

| FOOD NAME | Serving Size | Calories |
|---|---|---|
| German Chocolate (Pillsbury) | 1/12 | 250 |
| German Chocolate (Snackin' Cake) | 1/9 | 180 |
| Gingerbread (Pillsbury) | 1/9 | 180 |
| Golden (Duncan Hines) | 1/12 | 270 |
| Golden Chocolate Chip (Snackin' Cake) | 1/9 | 190 |
| Lemon (Pillsbury) | 1/12 | 240 |
| Lemon (Stir 'n Frost) | 1/6 | 230 |
| Lemon Chiffon (Betty Crocker) | 1/6 | 190 |
| Lemon Supreme (Pillsbury) | 1/16 | 260 |
| Pineapple Creme (Pillsbury) | 1/16 | 280 |
| Pound (Dromedary) | 1/12 | 210 |
| Pudding Cake, Chocolate (Betty Crocker) | 1/6 | 230 |
| Pudding Cake, Lemon (Betty Crocker) | 1/6 | 230 |
| Spice (Stir 'n Frost) | 1/6 | 270 |
| Strawberry (Pillsbury) | 1/12 | 250 |
| Strawberry Supreme (Duncan Hines) | 1/12 | 200 |
| Sunshine Vanilla (Pillsbury) | 1/12 | 260 |
| Supermoist, Butter Brickle (Betty Crocker) | 1/12 | 260 |
| Supermoist, Butter Pecan (Betty Crocker) | 1/12 | 250 |
| Supermoist, Carrot (Betty Crocker) | 1/12 | 250 |
| Supermoist, Chocolate Fudge (Betty Crocker) | 1/12 | 250 |
| Supermoist, Marble (Betty Crocker) | 1/12 | 270 |
| Supermoist, Orange (Betty Crocker) | 1/12 | 260 |
| Tunnel of Fudge (Pillsbury) | 1/16 | 310 |
| Tunnel of Lemon (Pillsbury) | 1/16 | 270 |

| Protein (g) | Carbohydrates (g) | Fat (g) | Sodium (mg) | Cholesterol (mg) | Fiber (g) | Vitamin A (%) | Vitamin C (%) | Calcium (%) | Iron (%) |
|---|---|---|---|---|---|---|---|---|---|
| 3 | 34 | 11 | 280 | 55 | na | * | * | 2 | 4 |
| 2 | 30 | 6 | 255 | na | na | * | * | 6 | 4 |
| 2 | 32 | 5 | 300 | 0 | na | * | * | * | 2 |
| 3 | 36 | 13 | 270 | na | na | 4 | * | 4 | 4 |
| 2 | 34 | 5 | 255 | na | na | * | * | 6 | 4 |
| 3 | 34 | 10 | 280 | 55 | na | * | * | 6 | 4 |
| 2 | 39 | 7 | 210 | na | na | * | * | 2 | 2 |
| 4 | 35 | 4 | 190 | na | na | * | * | 2 | 4 |
| 3 | 37 | 11 | 300 | 40 | na | * | * | 4 | 4 |
| 2 | 42 | 11 | 280 | 40 | na | * | * | 4 | 4 |
| 3 | 29 | 9 | na | na | na | 2 | * | 2 | 2 |
| 2 | 45 | 5 | 255 | na | na | 2 | * | 4 | 6 |
| 1 | 45 | 5 | 270 | na | na | 2 | * | 4 | 2 |
| 2 | 47 | 8 | 305 | na | na | * | * | 2 | 4 |
| 3 | 35 | 11 | 310 | 55 | na | * | * | 6 | 4 |
| 3 | 35 | 5 | 240 | na | na | * | * | 6 | 4 |
| 3 | 34 | 12 | 300 | 55 | na | * | * | 8 | 4 |
| 3 | 37 | 11 | 255 | na | na | * | * | 6 | 4 |
| 3 | 35 | 11 | 250 | na | na | * | * | 4 | 4 |
| 3 | 35 | 11 | 255 | na | na | * | * | 4 | 4 |
| 3 | 35 | 11 | 450 | na | na | * | * | 6 | 6 |
| 3 | 40 | 11 | 280 | na | na | * | * | 6 | 6 |
| 3 | 36 | 11 | 280 | na | na | * | * | 6 | 4 |
| 3 | 42 | 16 | 340 | 40 | na | * | * | * | 8 |
| 2 | 44 | 9 | 280 | 40 | na | * | * | 4 | 4 |

| FOOD NAME | Serving Size | Calories |
|---|---|---|
| Upside Down Cake (Betty Crocker) | ⅑ | 270 |
| Vienna Dream Bar (Betty Crocker) | 1/24 | 90 |
| White (Pillsbury) | 1/12 | 220 |
| White (Pillsbury Lovin' Lite) | 1/12 | 180 |
| White (Stir 'n Frost) | ⅙ | 220 |
| Yellow (Pillsbury) | 1/12 | 260 |
| Yellow (Pillsbury Lovin' Light) | 1/12 | 180 |
| Yellow (Stir 'n Frost) | ⅙ | 220 |
| CAKE, SNACK | | |
| Big Wheels (Hostess) | 1 | 170 |
| Chip Flips (Hostess) | 1 | 330 |
| Choco-Diles (Hostess) | 1 | 240 |
| Coffee Cake (Hostess) | 1 | 220 |
| Crumb Cake (Hostess) | 1 | 130 |
| Cupcake, Chocolate (Hostess) | 1 | 170 |
| Cupcake, Orange (Hostess) | 1 | 150 |
| Dessert Cup (Hostess) | 1 | 60 |
| Devil Dog (Drake's) | 1 | 170 |
| Ding Dong (Hostess) | 1 | 170 |
| Fruit Loaf (Hostess) | 1 | 400 |
| Ho Ho (Hostess) | 1 | 120 |
| Kandy Kake, Chocolate (Tastykake) | 1 | 95 |
| Kandy Kake, Peanut Butter (Tastykake) | 1 | 105 |
| Lil' Angel (Hostess) | 1 | 90 |
| Peanut Putters, filled (Hostess) | 1 | 360 |

| Protein (g) | Carbohydrates (g) | Fat (g) | Sodium (mg) | Cholesterol (mg) | Fiber (g) | Vitamin A (%) | Vitamin C (%) | Calcium (%) | Iron (%) |
|---|---|---|---|---|---|---|---|---|---|
| 2 | 43 | 10 | 215 | na | na | 4 | * | 4 | 2 |
| 1 | 10 | 5 | 65 | na | na | * | * | * | * |
| 3 | 34 | 9 | 290 | 0 | na | * | * | 2 | 2 |
| 3 | 35 | 3 | 310 | 35 | na | * | * | 8 | 4 |
| 2 | 38 | 7 | 235 | na | na | * | * | 4 | 2 |
| 3 | 34 | 12 | 300 | 55 | na | * | * | 8 | 4 |
| 3 | 35 | 3 | 300 | 35 | na | * | * | 8 | 4 |
| 2 | 38 | 7 | 210 | na | na | * | * | 2 | 2 |
| | | | | | | | | | |
| 2 | 21 | 9 | 130 | na | na | * | * | 2 | 2 |
| 3 | 47 | 16 | 165 | na | na | * | * | 2 | 6 |
| 2 | 35 | 11 | 280 | na | na | * | * | 2 | 4 |
| 4 | 32 | 9 | 220 | na | na | * | * | 2 | 6 |
| 2 | 22 | 4 | 95 | na | na | * | * | 2 | 4 |
| 2 | 29 | 5 | 290 | na | na | * | * | * | 4 |
| 2 | 28 | 5 | 175 | na | na | * | * | 2 | 2 |
| 2 | 14 | 0 | 120 | na | na | * | * | 2 | 2 |
| 2 | 22 | 8 | 165 | na | na | * | * | * | 4 |
| 2 | 21 | 9 | 130 | na | na | * | * | 2 | 2 |
| 4 | 77 | 9 | 520 | na | na | * | * | 4 | 10 |
| 2 | 17 | 6 | 90 | na | na | * | * | 2 | 2 |
| 1 | 12 | 4 | 64 | na | na | * | * | na | na |
| 2 | 11 | 6 | 48 | na | na | * | * | na | na |
| 2 | 14 | 2 | 95 | na | na | * | * | 2 | 2 |
| 5 | 46 | 15 | 240 | na | na | * | * | 4 | 8 |

| FOOD NAME | Serving Size | Calories |
|---|---|---|
| Peanut Putters, unfilled (Hostess) | 1 | 410 |
| Ring Ding (Drake's) | 1 | 160 |
| Sno Ball (Hostess) | 1 | 150 |
| Suzy Q (Hostess) | 1 | 240 |
| Tiger Tail (Hostess) | 1 | 210 |
| Twinkies (Hostess) | 1 | 160 |
| Yankee Doodle (Drake's) | 1 | 110 |
| CANDY | | |
| Almond Joy | 1 bar | 242 |
| Baby Ruth | 1 bar | 260 |
| Butterfinger | 1 bar | 220 |
| Caramello | 1 bar | 173 |
| Caramels | 1 oz | 115 |
| Chocolate Bar (Cadbury) | 1 bar | 300 |
| Chocolate Bar (Hershey) | 1 bar | 220 |
| Chocolate Bar, Almond (Cadbury) | 1 bar | 310 |
| Chocolate Bar, Almond (Hershey) | 1 bar | 230 |
| Chocolate Bar, Brazil Nut (Cadbury) | 1 bar | 310 |
| Chocolate Bar, Fruit and Nut (Cadbury) | 1 bar | 300 |
| Chocolate Bar, Hazelnut (Cadbury) | 1 bar | 310 |
| Chocolate Coated Bridge Mix (Deran) | 1 oz | 130 |
| Chocolate Fudge (Deran) | 1 oz | 115 |
| Chocolate Malted Milk Balls (Deran) | 1 oz | 140 |
| Golden Almond Bar (Hershey) | 1 bar | 160 |
| Gum Drops | 1 oz | 100 |

| Protein (g) | Carbohydrates (g) | Fat (g) | Sodium (mg) | Cholesterol (mg) | Fiber (g) | Vitamin A (%) | Vitamin C (%) | Calcium (%) | Iron (%) |
|---|---|---|---|---|---|---|---|---|---|
| 6 | 43 | 21 | 240 | na | na | * | * | 4 | 6 |
| 2 | 20 | 9 | 120 | na | na | * | * | * | 4 |
| 2 | 28 | 4 | 170 | na | na | * | * | 2 | 2 |
| 2 | 37 | 10 | 300 | na | na | * | * | 2 | 4 |
| 2 | 38 | 6 | 240 | na | na | * | * | 2 | 4 |
| 2 | 26 | 5 | 150 | na | na | * | * | 2 | 2 |
| 2 | 15 | 5 | 130 | na | na | * | * | * | 2 |
|  |  |  |  |  |  |  |  |  |  |
| 3 | 30 | 13 | 90 | na | na | * | * | 2 | 2 |
| 6 | 31 | 11 | 100 | na | na | * | * | 2 | 2 |
| 6 | 31 | 11 | 100 | na | na | * | * | 2 | 2 |
| 2 | 20 | 10 | 70 | na | na | * | * | 7 | 4 |
| 1 | 22 | 3 | 74 | na | na | * | * | 4 | 2 |
| 3 | 34 | 16 | 90 | 0 | 0 | 2 | * | 14 | 8 |
| 2 | 23 | 13 | 35 | na | na | * | * | 8 | 4 |
| 3 | 31 | 18 | 80 | na | na | 2 | * | 14 | 4 |
| 2 | 22 | 14 | 35 | na | na | * | * | 8 | 2 |
| 3 | 32 | 18 | 80 | na | na | * | * | 14 | 4 |
| 3 | 33 | 16 | 80 | na | na | 2 | * | 12 | 6 |
| 3 | 32 | 17 | 90 | na | na | * | * | 14 | 4 |
| <1 | 20 | 5 | 25 | na | na | * | * | * | 2 |
| 1 | 21 | 3 | 54 | na | 0 | * | * | 2 | 2 |
| <1 | 20 | 6 | 70 | na | na | * | * | 2 | 2 |
| 1 | 12 | 11 | 20 | na | na | * | * | 6 | 4 |
| 0 | 25 | 0 | 10 | na | 0 | * | * | * | 1 |

| FOOD NAME | Serving Size | Calories | |
|---|---|---|---|
| Hard | 1 oz | 110 | |
| Kisses (Hershey) | 6 | 150 | |
| Kit Kat (Hershey) | 1 bar | 160 | |
| Krackel (Hershey) | 1 bar | 160 | |
| M&M's, plain | 1 pkg | 240 | |
| M&M's, peanut | 1 pkg | 240 | |
| Mars Bar | 1 bar | 230 | |
| Marshmallows | 2 large | 40 | |
| Milky Way | 1 bar | 260 | |
| Mints, plain | 1 oz | 105 | |
| Mounds | 1 bar | 235 | |
| Mr. Goodbar | 1 bar | 200 | |
| Nestle Crunch | 1 bar | 150 | |
| Peanut Brittle | 1 oz | 140 | |
| Peanut Clusters | 1 oz | 150 | |
| Peppermint Patty | 1 | 161 | |
| Power House | 1 bar | 262 | |
| Reese's Peanut Butter Chips | ¼ cup | 230 | |
| Reese's Peanut Butter Cups | 2 | 240 | |
| Reese's Pieces | 35 pc | 140 | |
| Rolo | 5 pc | 140 | |
| Rum Wafers | 1 oz | 150 | |
| Snickers | 1 bar | 270 | |
| Special Dark Chocolate Bar (Hershey) | 1 bar | 160 | |
| Starburst | 1 pkg | 240 | |

| Protein (g) | Carbohydrates (g) | Fat (g) | Sodium (mg) | Cholesterol (mg) | Fiber (g) | Vitamin A (%) | Vitamin C (%) | Calcium (%) | Iron (%) |
|---|---|---|---|---|---|---|---|---|---|
| 0 | 28 | 0 | 9 | na | 0 | * | * | 1 | 3 |
| 2 | 16 | 9 | 25 | na | 0 | * | * | 6 | 2 |
| 2 | 19 | 8 | 30 | na | na | * | * | 6 | 2 |
| 2 | 17 | 10 | 30 | na | na | * | * | 6 | 2 |
| 3 | 33 | 10 | 41 | na | na | * | * | 8 | 4 |
| 5 | 28 | 12 | 29 | na | na | * | * | 4 | 2 |
| 4 | 29 | 10 | 71 | na | na | * | * | 6 | 2 |
| 0 | 10 | 0 | 10 | na | 0 | * | * | * | * |
| 3 | 43 | 9 | 119 | na | 0 | * | * | 6 | 2 |
| 0 | 25 | 1 | 56 | na | 0 | * | * | * | 2 |
| 2 | 32 | 11 | 90 | na | na | * | * | * | 4 |
| 5 | 18 | 12 | 20 | na | na | * | * | 6 | 4 |
| 2 | 18 | 8 | 45 | na | na | * | * | 4 | * |
| 3 | 20 | 5 | 145 | na | na | * | * | * | * |
| 3 | 13 | 9 | 15 | na | na | * | * | 2 | 2 |
| 1 | 33 | 3 | 13 | na | 0 | * | * | * | 3 |
| 5 | 38 | 10 | 210 | na | na | * | * | 4 | 4 |
| 7 | 19 | 13 | 90 | na | na | * | * | 6 | 4 |
| 4 | 23 | 14 | 145 | na | na | * | * | 4 | 2 |
| 2 | 17 | 6 | 45 | na | na | * | * | 4 | 2 |
| 1 | 16 | 9 | 65 | na | 0 | * | * | 8 | 2 |
| 0 | 20 | 7 | 15 | na | na | * | * | * | 2 |
| 6 | 33 | 13 | 139 | na | na | * | * | 6 | 2 |
| 1 | 19 | 9 | 1 | na | 0 | * | * | * | 2 |
| 0 | 49 | 5 | 26 | na | 0 | * | * | * | * |

| FOOD NAME | Serving Size | Calories | |
|---|---|---|---|
| Summit | 1 pkg | 110 | |
| Toffee | 1 pc | 30 | |
| Whatchamacallit | 1 bar | 170 | |
| CANTALOUPE | ½ | 94 | |
| CARROTS | | | |
| Raw | 1 | 30 | |
| Fresh, cooked | 1 cup | 50 | |
| Grated raw | 1 cup | 45 | |
| Canned | 1 cup | 45 | |
| *Frozen* | | | |
| (Birds Eye Parisienne) | 2.6 oz | 30 | |
| (Birds Eye Sliced) | 3.2 oz | 35 | |
| (Birds Eye Whole Baby) | 3.3 oz | 40 | |
| *Frozen combinations* | | | |
| Broccoli, Baby Carrots and Water Chestnuts (Birds Eye) | 4 oz | 45 | |
| Broccoli, Cauliflower and Carrots (Birds Eye) | 4 oz | 35 | |
| Brussels Sprouts, Cauliflower and Carrots (Birds Eye) | 4 oz | 40 | |
| Cauliflower, Whole Baby Carrots and Snow Pea Pods (Birds Eye) | 4 oz | 40 | |
| Cauliflower, Zucchini, Carrots and Red Peppers (Birds Eye) | 4 oz | 30 | |
| Sugar Snap Peas, Baby Carrots and Water Chestnuts (Birds Eye) | 3.2 oz | 50 | |

| Protein (g) | Carbohydrates (g) | Fat (g) | Sodium (mg) | Cholesterol (mg) | Fiber (g) | Vitamin A (%) | Vitamin C (%) | Calcium (%) | Iron (%) |
|---|---|---|---|---|---|---|---|---|---|
| 2 | 12 | 7 | 30 | na | na | * | * | 2 | * |
| 0 | 5 | 1 | 20 | na | na | * | * | * | * |
| 3 | 18 | 10 | 70 | na | na | * | * | 4 | * |
| 2 | 22 | <1 | 23 | 0 | 2.1 | 180 | 150 | 4 | 6 |
| | | | | | | | | | |
| 1 | 7 | 0 | 34 | 0 | 3 | 159 | 10 | 3 | 3 |
| 1 | 11 | 0 | 51 | 0 | 5 | 330 | 15 | 5 | 5 |
| 1 | 11 | 0 | 52 | 0 | 4 | 240 | 15 | 4 | 4 |
| 1 | 10 | 0 | 500 | 0 | 5 | 386 | 5 | 5 | 6 |
| | | | | | | | | | |
| 1 | 7 | 0 | 35 | 0 | 2 | 240 | 8 | 2 | 2 |
| 1 | 8 | 0 | 40 | 0 | 1 | 300 | 8 | 2 | 4 |
| 1 | 9 | 0 | 45 | 0 | 2 | 300 | 10 | 2 | 4 |
| | | | | | | | | | |
| 2 | 10 | 0 | 35 | 0 | 3 | 150 | 60 | 4 | 4 |
| 2 | 7 | 0 | 40 | 0 | 3 | 180 | 70 | 4 | 4 |
| | | | | | | | | | |
| 3 | 8 | 0 | 30 | 0 | 4 | 110 | 90 | 2 | 4 |
| | | | | | | | | | |
| 2 | 8 | 0 | 35 | 0 | 3 | 150 | 60 | 4 | 4 |
| | | | | | | | | | |
| 2 | 6 | 0 | 25 | 0 | 2 | 100 | 60 | 2 | 4 |
| | | | | | | | | | |
| 2 | 11 | 0 | 20 | 0 | 4 | 100 | 25 | 6 | 4 |

| FOOD NAME | Serving Size | Calories | |
|---|---|---|---|
| Zucchini, Carrots, Pearl Onions and Mushrooms (Birds Eye) | 4 oz | 30 | |
| Broccoli, Cauliflower and Carrots in Butter Sauce (Birds Eye) | 3.3 oz | 45 | |
| Broccoli, Cauliflower and Carrots in Cheese Sauce (Birds Eye) | 5 oz | 110 | |
| Broccoli, Cauliflower & Carrots (Green Giant One Serving) | 1 pkg | 30 | |
| Broccoli, Cauliflower & Carrots in Cheese Flavored Sauce (Green Giant One Serving) | 1 pkg | 80 | |
| Broccoli, Carrots & Rotini in Cheese Flavored Sauce (Green Giant One Serving) | 1 pkg | 100 | |
| CASABA MELON | 1 wedge | 40 | |
| CASHEWS | ⅓ cup | 260 | |
| CAULIFLOWER | | | |
| Raw | 1 cup | 25 | |
| Fresh, cooked | 1 cup | 30 | |
| *Frozen* | | | |
| (Birds Eye) | 3.3 oz | 25 | |
| (Green Giant) | ½ cup | 12 | |
| *Frozen combinations* | | | |
| Broccoli, Cauliflower and Carrots (Birds Eye) | 4 oz | 35 | |
| Broccoli, Cauliflower and Red Peppers (Birds Eye) | 4 oz | 30 | |

| Protein (g) | Carbohydrates (g) | Fat (g) | Sodium (mg) | Cholesterol (mg) | Fiber (g) | Vitamin A (%) | Vitamin C (%) | Calcium (%) | Iron (%) |
|---|---|---|---|---|---|---|---|---|---|
| 1 | 7 | 0 | 15 | 0 | 1 | 130 | 8 | 2 | 4 |
| 2 | 6 | 2 | 290 | 5 | 2 | 90 | 50 | 2 | 2 |
| 6 | 11 | 5 | 410 | 5 | 2 | 120 | 60 | 10 | 4 |
| 3 | 7 | 0 | 40 | 0 | 3 | 70 | 50 | 4 | 4 |
| 3 | 13 | 2 | 650 | 5 | 2 | 70 | 30 | 8 | 2 |
| 5 | 17 | 2 | 440 | 5 | 3 | 170 | 10 | 6 | 6 |
| 2 | 9 | Tr | 17 | 0 | 0.8 | * | 30 | 2 | 4 |
| 8 | 14 | 21 | 7 | 0 | 2.5 | * | * | 2 | 10 |
| 3 | 5 | Tr | 11 | 0 | 2.4 | 2 | 110 | 2 | 4 |
| 3 | 5 | Tr | 11 | 0 | 2.8 | 2 | 120 | 2 | 4 |
| 2 | 5 | 0 | 20 | 0 | 2 | * | 80 | 2 | 2 |
| 1 | 3 | 0 | 25 | 0 | 2 | * | 40 | * | * |
| 2 | 7 | 0 | 40 | 0 | 3 | 180 | 70 | 4 | 4 |
| 3 | 5 | 0 | 25 | 0 | 3 | 35 | 100 | 4 | 4 |

| FOOD NAME | Serving Size | Calories | |
|-----------|:---:|:---:|---|
| Cauliflower, Baby Whole Carrots and Snow Pea Pods (Birds Eye) | 4 oz | 40 | |
| Cauliflower, Zucchini, Carrots and Red Peppers (Birds Eye) | 4 oz | 30 | |
| Broccoli, Cauliflower and Carrots in Butter Sauce (Birds Eye) | 3.3 oz | 45 | |
| Broccoli, Cauliflower and Carrots in Cheese Sauce (Birds Eye) | 5 oz | 110 | |
| In Cheese Flavored Sauce (Green Giant One Serving) | 1 pkg | 80 | |
| Broccoli, Cauliflower & Carrots (Green Giant One Serving) | 1 pkg | 30 | |
| Broccoli, Cauliflower and Carrots in Cheese Flavored Sauce (Green Giant) | 1 pkg | 80 | |
| CAVIAR | 2 tbsp | 75 | |
| CELERY | 1 stalk | 5 | |
| Chopped | 1 cup | 20 | |
| CEREAL | | | |
| All-Bran (Kellogg's) | ⅓ cup | 70 | |
| All-Bran with Extra Fiber (Kellogg's) | ½ cup | 50 | |
| 100% Bran (Nabisco) | ⅓ cup | 47 | |
| Alpha-bits | 1 cup | 110 | |
| Apple Cinnamon Squares | ½ cup | 90 | |
| Apple Jacks | 1 cup | 110 | |
| Apple Raisin Crisp | ⅔ cup | 130 | |

| Protein (g) | Carbohydrates (g) | Fat (g) | Sodium (mg) | Cholesterol (mg) | Fiber (g) | Vitamin A (%) | Vitamin C (%) | Calcium (%) | Iron (%) |
|---|---|---|---|---|---|---|---|---|---|
| 2 | 8 | 0 | 35 | 0 | 3 | 150 | 60 | 4 | 4 |
| 2 | 6 | 0 | 25 | 0 | 2 | 100 | 60 | 2 | 4 |
| 2 | 6 | 2 | 290 | 5 | 2 | 90 | 50 | 2 | 2 |
| 6 | 11 | 5 | 410 | 5 | 2 | 120 | 60 | 10 | 4 |
| 3 | 14 | 2 | 640 | 5 | 2 | 30 | 50 | 8 | 2 |
| 3 | 7 | 0 | 40 | 0 | 3 | 70 | 50 | 4 | 4 |
| 3 | 13 | 2 | 650 | 5 | 2 | 70 | 30 | 8 | 2 |
| 8 | 1 | 4 | 625 | 190 | 0 | * | * | 8 | 18 |
| 0 | 2 | 0 | 50 | 0 | 1 | 2 | 7 | 2 | 1 |
| 1 | 5 | 0 | 150 | 0 | 4 | 6 | 18 | 5 | 2 |
| 4 | 21 | 1 | 260 | 0 | 9 | 15 | 25 | 2 | 25 |
| 4 | 22 | 0 | 140 | 0 | 14 | 15 | 25 | 2 | 25 |
| 2 | 14 | 1 | 140 | 0 | 6 | * | 30 | 1 | 10 |
| 2 | 24 | 1 | 195 | 0 | na | 25 | na | * | 10 |
| 2 | 23 | 0 | 5 | 0 | 2 | * | * | * | 45 |
| 2 | 26 | 0 | 125 | 0 | 1 | 15 | 25 | * | 25 |
| 2 | 32 | 0 | 230 | 0 | 3 | 15 | * | * | 10 |

| FOOD NAME | Serving Size | Calories |
|---|---|---|
| Blueberry Squares | ½ cup | 90 |
| Body Buddies, brown sugar & honey | 1 cup | 110 |
| Body Buddies, fruit flavor | 1 cup | 110 |
| Boo Berry | 1 cup | 110 |
| Bran Buds | ⅓ cup | 70 |
| Bran Chex | ⅔ cup | 90 |
| Bran Flakes | ⅔ cup | 90 |
| Buc Wheats | ⅔ cup | 97 |
| Cap'n Crunch | 1 cup | 146 |
| Cap'n Crunch with Peanut Butter | 1 cup | 173 |
| Cheerios | 1 cup | 88 |
| Cheerios Honey Nut | 1 cup | 146 |
| Chocolate Donutz | 1 cup | 120 |
| Cinnamon Mini Buns | ¾ cup | 110 |
| Cocoa Pebbles | 1 cup | 126 |
| Cocoa Puffs | 1 cup | 110 |
| Cocoa Krispies | ¾ cup | 110 |
| Common Sense Oat Bran | ¾ cup | 100 |
| Common Sense Oat Bran with Raisins | ¾ cup | 130 |
| Corn Bran (Quaker) | ⅔ cup | 110 |
| Corn Chex | 1 cup | 110 |
| Corn Flakes (Kellogg's) | 1 cup | 100 |
| Corn Pops (Kellogg's) | 1 cup | 110 |
| Corn Total | ⅔ cup | 73 |
| Count Chocula | 1 cup | 110 |

| Protein (g) | Carbohydrates (g) | Fat (g) | Sodium (mg) | Cholesterol (mg) | Fiber (g) | Vitamin A (%) | Vitamin C (%) | Calcium (%) | Iron (%) |
|---|---|---|---|---|---|---|---|---|---|
| 2 | 23 | 0 | 5 | 0 | 3 | * | * | * | 45 |
| 2 | 24 | 1 | 290 | 0 | na | 25 | 25 | 10 | 45 |
| 2 | 24 | 1 | 285 | 0 | na | 25 | 25 | 10 | 45 |
| 1 | 24 | 1 | 210 | 0 | na | 25 | 25 | 2 | 25 |
| 3 | 23 | 1 | 200 | 0 | 11 | 15 | 25 | * | 25 |
| 3 | 23 | 0 | 300 | 0 | 6 | * | 25 | * | 25 |
| 3 | 22 | 0 | 220 | 0 | 5 | 15 | * | * | 100 |
| 2 | 21 | 1 | 208 | 0 | na | 40 | 40 | 5 | 40 |
| 1 | 32 | 3 | 223 | 0 | na | * | * | * | 33 |
| 3 | 28 | 5 | 333 | na | na | * | * | * | 33 |
| 3 | 16 | 2 | 264 | 0 | na | 20 | 20 | 3 | 20 |
| 4 | 31 | 1 | 340 | na | na | 33 | 33 | 3 | 33 |
| 2 | 23 | 2 | 185 | na | na | 25 | 25 | * | 25 |
| 2 | 25 | 1 | 220 | 0 | 1 | 15 | 25 | * | 25 |
| 1 | 29 | 2 | 189 | na | na | 29 | na | * | 11 |
| 1 | 25 | 1 | 205 | na | na | * | 25 | * | 25 |
| 1 | 25 | 0 | 190 | 0 | 0 | 15 | 25 | * | 10 |
| 4 | 22 | 1 | 250 | 0 | 3 | 15 | * | * | 45 |
| 4 | 29 | 1 | 250 | 0 | 3 | 15 | * | 2 | 45 |
| 2 | 23 | 1 | 295 | 0 | na | * | * | 2 | 25 |
| 2 | 25 | 0 | 310 | 0 | 4 | * | 25 | * | 10 |
| 2 | 24 | 0 | 290 | 0 | 1 | 15 | 25 | * | 10 |
| 1 | 26 | 0 | 90 | 0 | 1 | 15 | 25 | * | 10 |
| 1 | 16 | 1 | 206 | 0 | na | 67 | 67 | 3 | 67 |
| 2 | 24 | 1 | 205 | na | na | 25 | 25 | 2 | 25 |

| FOOD NAME | Serving Size | Calories |
|---|---|---|
| Cracklin' Bran | ⅔ cup | 147 |
| Cracklin' Oat Bran | ½ cup | 110 |
| Crispix | 1 cup | 110 |
| Double Dip Crunch | ⅔ cup | 120 |
| Fiberwise | ⅔ cup | 90 |
| Froot Loops | 1 cup | 110 |
| Frosted Flakes (Kellogg's) | ¾ cup | 110 |
| Frosted Krispies | ¾ cup | 110 |
| Frosted Mini-Wheats | 4 | 100 |
| Frosted Mini-Wheats, Bite Size | ½ cup | 100 |
| Fruit & Fibre, Apple Cinnamon | ⅔ cup | 120 |
| Fruit & Fibre, Date Raisin | ⅔ cup | 120 |
| Fruit Brute | 1 cup | 110 |
| Fruitful Bran | ⅔ cup | 120 |
| Fruity Marshmallow Krispies | 1¼ cup | 140 |
| Golden Grahams | ⅔ cup | 97 |
| Granola (Post) | ⅓ cup | 173 |
| Grape-Nuts | ⅓ cup | 133 |
| Grape-Nuts Flakes | ⅔ cup | 76 |
| Honey Bran | ⅔ cup | 76 |
| Just Right with Fiber Nuggets | ⅔ cup | 100 |
| Just Right with Raisins, Dates & Nuts | ¾ cup | 140 |
| Kenmei Rice Bran | ¾ cup | 110 |
| Kix | 1 cup | 110 |
| Life | ⅔ cup | 110 |

| Protein (g) | Carbohydrates (g) | Fat (g) | Sodium (mg) | Cholesterol (mg) | Fiber (g) | Vitamin A (%) | Vitamin C (%) | Calcium (%) | Iron (%) |
|---|---|---|---|---|---|---|---|---|---|
| 3 | 27 | 5 | 227 | 0 | 5 | 33 | 33 | 2 | 13 |
| 3 | 21 | 3 | 140 | 0 | 4 | 15 | 25 | * | 10 |
| 2 | 25 | 0 | 220 | 0 | 1 | 15 | 25 | * | 10 |
| 2 | 23 | 2 | 160 | 0 | 0 | 15 | 25 | * | 10 |
| 3 | 23 | 1 | 140 | 0 | 5 | 15 | 25 | 2 | 25 |
| 2 | 25 | 1 | 125 | 0 | 1 | 15 | 100 | * | 25 |
| 1 | 26 | 0 | 200 | 0 | 1 | 15 | 25 | * | 10 |
| 1 | 26 | 0 | 220 | 0 | 0 | 15 | 25 | * | 10 |
| 3 | 24 | 0 | 0 | 0 | 3 | * | * | * | 10 |
| 3 | 24 | 0 | 0 | 0 | 3 | * | * | * | 10 |
| 4 | 29 | 1 | 260 | 0 | 4 | 33 | na | * | 33 |
| 4 | 28 | 1 | 227 | 0 | 4 | 33 | na | * | 33 |
| 2 | 24 | 1 | 215 | na | na | 25 | 25 | 4 | 25 |
| 3 | 31 | 0 | 240 | 0 | 5 | 15 | * | * | 25 |
| 2 | 32 | 0 | 210 | 0 | 0 | 15 | 25 | * | 10 |
| 2 | 21 | 1 | 306 | 0 | na | 22 | 22 | * | 22 |
| 3 | 27 | 5 | 73 | <1 | 4 | 33 | na | * | 33 |
| 4 | 31 | 1 | 260 | 0 | 5 | 33 | na | * | 5 |
| 2 | 18 | 1 | 149 | 0 | 3 | 19 | na | * | 19 |
| 2 | 18 | 1 | 152 | 0 | na | 19 | 19 | * | 19 |
| 2 | 24 | 1 | 200 | 0 | 2 | 100 | * | * | 100 |
| 3 | 30 | 1 | 190 | 0 | 2 | 100 | * | * | 100 |
| 2 | 24 | 1 | 230 | 0 | 1 | 15 | * | 6 | 2 |
| 2 | 24 | 1 | 315 | na | na | 25 | 25 | 4 | 25 |
| 5 | 20 | 1 | 175 | na | na | * | * | 6 | 25 |

| FOOD NAME | Serving Size | Calories |
|---|---|---|
| Lucky Charms | 1 cup | 110 |
| Most | ⅔ cup | 133 |
| Mueslix Crispy Blend | ⅔ cup | 160 |
| Mueslix Golden Crunch | ½ cup | 120 |
| Nut & Honey Crunch | ⅔ cup | 110 |
| Nut & Honey Crunch O's | ⅔ cup | 110 |
| Nutri-Grain Almond Raisin | ⅔ cup | 140 |
| Nutri-Grain Raisin Bran | 1 cup | 130 |
| Nutri-Grain Wheat | ⅔ cup | 90 |
| Oatbake Honey Bran | ⅓ cup | 110 |
| Oatbake Raisin Nut | ⅓ cup | 110 |
| Product 19 | 1 cup | 100 |
| Puffed Rice | 1 cup | 60 |
| Puffed Wheat | 1 cup | 55 |
| Quisp | 1 cup | 94 |
| Raisin Bran (Kellogg's) | ¾ cup | 120 |
| Raisin Squares | ½ cup | 90 |
| Rice Chex | 1 cup | 98 |
| Rice Krispies | 1 cup | 110 |
| Shredded Wheat, Spoon Size | ⅔ cup | 120 |
| Smacks | ¾ cup | 110 |
| Special K | 1 cup | 110 |
| Strawberry Squares | ½ cup | 90 |
| Sugar Corn Pops | 1 cup | 110 |
| Super Sugar Crisp | 1 cup | 126 |

| Protein (g) | Carbohydrates (g) | Fat (g) | Sodium (mg) | Cholesterol (mg) | Fiber (g) | Vitamin A (%) | Vitamin C (%) | Calcium (%) | Iron (%) |
|---|---|---|---|---|---|---|---|---|---|
| 2 | 24 | 1 | 185 | na | na | 25 | 25 | 2 | 25 |
| 5 | 29 | 0 | 193 | 0 | 5 | 133 | 133 | 2 | 133 |
| 3 | 33 | 2 | 150 | 0 | 3 | 15 | * | 4 | 25 |
| 3 | 25 | 2 | 170 | 0 | 3 | 15 | * | 2 | 25 |
| 2 | 24 | 1 | 200 | 0 | 0 | 15 | 25 | * | 10 |
| 2 | 22 | 2 | 190 | 0 | 1 | 15 | 25 | 2 | 10 |
| 3 | 31 | 2 | 220 | 0 | 3 | * | * | * | 4 |
| 4 | 31 | 1 | 200 | 0 | 5 | * | * | 20 | 10 |
| 3 | 23 | 0 | 170 | 0 | 3 | * | 25 | * | 4 |
| 2 | 21 | 3 | 190 | 0 | 3 | 15 | 25 | * | 25 |
| 2 | 21 | 3 | 190 | 0 | 3 | 15 | 25 | * | 25 |
| 3 | 24 | 0 | 320 | 0 | 1 | 15 | 100 | * | 100 |
| 1 | 13 | 0 | 1 | 0 | na | * | * | * | 2 |
| 2 | 0 | 12 | 1 | 0 | 3 | * | * | * | 3 |
| 1 | 19 | 2 | 197 | na | na | * | * | * | 13 |
| 3 | 31 | 1 | 210 | 0 | 5 | 25 | * | * | 45 |
| 2 | 23 | 0 | 0 | 0 | 2 | * | * | * | 45 |
| 1 | 22 | 0 | 249 | 0 | 1 | * | 22 | * | 9 |
| 2 | 25 | 0 | 290 | 0 | 0 | 15 | 25 | * | 10 |
| 3 | 27 | 1 | 4 | 0 | 4 | * | * | 2 | 7 |
| 2 | 25 | 1 | 70 | 0 | 1 | 15 | 25 | * | 10 |
| 6 | 20 | 0 | 230 | 0 | 1 | 15 | 25 | * | 25 |
| 2 | 23 | 0 | 5 | 0 | 3 | * | * | * | 45 |
| 1 | 26 | 0 | 105 | na | 0 | 25 | 25 | * | 10 |
| 2 | 30 | 1 | 40 | na | na | 29 | na | * | 11 |

| FOOD NAME | Serving Size | Calories | |
|---|---|---|---|
| Team | ⅔ cup | 73 | |
| Total | ⅔ cup | 73 | |
| Trix | 1 cup | 110 | |
| Wheat Chex | ⅔ cup | 110 | |
| Wheat Germ | ¼ cup | 100 | |
| Wheaties | ⅔ cup | 73 | |
| Whole Grain Shredded Wheat | ½ cup | 90 | |
| *Hot* | | | |
| Cream of Wheat | ⅔ cup | 76 | |
| Farina (Pillsbury) | ⅔ cup | 80 | |
| Grits (Quaker Instant Plain) | 1 pkg | 80 | |
| Grits (Quaker Quick) | 3 tbsp | 100 | |
| Oatmeal (Harvest Brand Instant) | 1 pkg | 110 | |
| Oatmeal (Harvest Brand Instant with Apples and Cinnamon) | 1 pkg | 140 | |
| Oatmeal (Harvest Brand Instant with Cinnamon and Spice) | 1 pkg | 180 | |
| Oatmeal (Harvest Brand Instant with Maple and Brown Sugar) | 1 pkg | 170 | |
| Oatmeal (Harvest Brand Instant with Peaches and Cream) | 1 pkg | 140 | |
| Oats (Quaker Instant Apple Cinnamon) | 1 pkg | 140 | |
| Oats (Quaker Instant Cinnamon Spice) | 1 pkg | 164 | |
| Oats (Quaker Instant Raisin Bran) | 1 pkg | 150 | |
| Oats (Quaker Instant Raisin Spice) | 1 pkg | 160 | |

| Protein (g) | Carbohydrates (g) | Fat (g) | Sodium (mg) | Cholesterol (mg) | Fiber (g) | Vitamin A (%) | Vitamin C (%) | Calcium (%) | Iron (%) |
|---|---|---|---|---|---|---|---|---|---|
| 1 | 16 | 1 | 123 | na | na | 17 | 17 | * | 5 |
| 2 | 15 | 1 | 250 | 0 | 2 | 67 | 67 | 3 | 67 |
| 1 | 25 | 1 | 170 | na | na | 25 | 25 | * | 25 |
| 3 | 23 | 0 | 200 | na | na | * | 25 | * | 25 |
| 9 | 12 | 3 | 0 | 0 | 3 | * | * | * | 10 |
| 2 | 15 | 1 | 246 | 0 | 2 | 17 | 17 | 3 | 17 |
| 3 | 23 | 0 | 0 | 0 | 4 | * | * | * | 10 |
| 2 | 17 | 0 | 10 | 0 | 1 | * | * | * | 34 |
| 2 | 17 | <1 | 265 | 0 | 3 | * | * | * | 4 |
| 2 | 18 | 0 | 520 | 0 | 1 | * | * | * | 4 |
| 2 | 22 | 0 | 9 | 0 | 1 | * | * | * | 4 |
| 3 | 18 | 2 | 220 | 0 | 3 | * | * | * | 6 |
| 3 | 26 | 2 | 230 | 0 | 2.5 | * | * | * | 6 |
| 3 | 35 | 2 | 300 | 0 | 2.5 | * | * | * | 6 |
| 3 | 32 | 2 | 290 | 0 | 2.5 | * | * | * | 8 |
| 2 | 27 | 2 | 200 | 0 | 2.5 | * | * | * | 4 |
| 4 | 26 | 2 | 260 | 0 | 3 | 20 | * | 10 | 25 |
| 5 | 35 | 2 | 322 | 0 | 3.1 | 20 | * | 10 | 25 |
| 4 | 29 | 2 | 340 | 0 | 2.8 | 20 | * | 10 | 25 |
| 4 | 31 | 2 | 310 | 0 | 2.8 | 20 | * | 10 | 25 |

| FOOD NAME | Serving Size | Calories | |
|---|---|---|---|
| Oats (Quaker Instant Regular) | 1 pkg | 110 | |
| Oats (Quaker Quick) | ⅔ cup | 110 | |
| Wheat | 1 cup | 110 | |
| CHEESE | | | |
| American, processed (Borden) | 1 oz | 110 | |
| American, processed (Kraft Deluxe Loaf) | 1 oz | 110 | |
| American, processed (Kraft Deluxe Slices) | 1 oz | 110 | |
| American, processed (Kraft Free Singles Nonfat) | 1 oz | 45 | |
| American, processed (Kraft Light Singles) | 1 oz | 70 | |
| American, processed (Kraft Light Singles, White) | 1 oz | 70 | |
| American, processed (Land O' Lakes) | 1 oz | 110 | |
| American, processed (Land O' Lakes Sharp) | 1 oz | 100 | |
| American, processed (Land O' Lakes with Swiss) | 1 oz | 100 | |
| American, processed (Light 'n Lively Singles) | 1 oz | 70 | |
| American, processed (Light 'n Lively Singles, White) | 1 oz | 70 | |

| Protein (g) | Carbohydrates (g) | Fat (g) | Sodium (mg) | Cholesterol (mg) | Fiber (g) | Vitamin A (%) | Vitamin C (%) | Calcium (%) | Iron (%) |
|---|---|---|---|---|---|---|---|---|---|
| 4 | 18 | 2 | 400 | 0 | 2.8 | 20 | * | 10 | 25 |
| 5 | 18 | 2 | 9 | 0 | 2.8 | * | * | * | 4 |
| 4 | 23 | 1 | 2 | 0 | na | * | * | 2 | 7 |
| 6 | 1 | 9 | 460 | 25 | 0 | 4 | * | 20 | * |
| 6 | 1 | 9 | 430 | 25 | 0 | 6 | * | 15 | * |
| 6 | 1 | 9 | 450 | 25 | 0 | 6 | * | 15 | * |
| 7 | 4 | 0 | 420 | 5 | 0 | 10 | * | 20 | * |
| 6 | 2 | 4 | 420 | 15 | 0 | 6 | * | 20 | * |
| 6 | 2 | 4 | 410 | 15 | 0 | 6 | * | 20 | * |
| 6 | 1 | 9 | 450 | 30 | 0 | 6 | * | 15 | * |
| 6 | 1 | 9 | 360 | 30 | 0 | 6 | * | 15 | * |
| 7 | 1 | 8 | 400 | 25 | 0 | 6 | * | 20 | * |
| 6 | 2 | 4 | 420 | 15 | 0 | 6 | * | 20 | * |
| 6 | 2 | 4 | 410 | 15 | 0 | 6 | * | 20 | * |

| FOOD NAME | Serving Size | Calories | |
|---|---|---|---|
| American, processed | | | |
| (Old English Sharp Loaf) | 1 oz | 110 | |
| American, processed | | | |
| (Old English Sharp Slices) | 1 oz | 110 | |
| Blue (Kraft) | 1 oz | 100 | |
| Brick (Kraft) | 1 oz | 110 | |
| Brick (Land O' Lakes) | 1 oz | 110 | |
| Camembert | 1 wedge | 115 | |
| Cheddar (Kraft) | 1 oz | 110 | |
| Cheddar (Land O' Lakes) | 1 oz | 110 | |
| Cheddar (Land O' Lakes | | | |
| Chedarella) | 1 oz | 100 | |
| Cheddar, Natural Reduced Fat | | | |
| (Cracker Barrel Light Sharp White) | 1 oz | 80 | |
| Cheddar, Natural Reduced Fat | | | |
| (Kraft Light Naturals Mild) | 1 oz | 80 | |
| Cheddar, Natural Reduced Fat | | | |
| (Kraft Light Naturals Sharp) | 1 oz | 80 | |
| Cheddar, Processed | | | |
| (Kraft Light Singles Sharp) | 1 oz | 70 | |
| Cheddar, Processed | | | |
| (Light 'n Lively Singles Sharp) | 1 oz | 70 | |
| Cheez 'n Bacon Singles (Kraft) | 1 oz | 90 | |
| Colby (Kraft) | 1 oz | 110 | |
| Colby (Land O' Lakes) | 1 oz | 110 | |

| Protein (g) | Carbohydrates (g) | Fat (g) | Sodium (mg) | Cholesterol (mg) | Fiber (g) | Vitamin A (%) | Vitamin C (%) | Calcium (%) | Iron (%) |
|---|---|---|---|---|---|---|---|---|---|
| 6 | 1 | 9 | 400 | 30 | 0 | 8 | * | 20 | * |
| 6 | 1 | 9 | 440 | 30 | 0 | 6 | * | 15 | * |
| 6 | 1 | 9 | 330 | 30 | 0 | 6 | * | 15 | * |
| 7 | 0 | 9 | 180 | 30 | 0 | 6 | * | 20 | * |
| 7 | 1 | 8 | 160 | 25 | 0 | 6 | * | 20 | * |
| 8 | 0 | 9 | 324 | 20 | 0 | 7 | * | 15 | 1 |
| 7 | 1 | 9 | 180 | 30 | 0 | 6 | * | 20 | * |
| 7 | <1 | 9 | 180 | 30 | 0 | 6 | * | 20 | * |
| 7 | <1 | 8 | 180 | 25 | 0 | 6 | * | 20 | * |
| 9 | 1 | 5 | 220 | 20 | 0 | 6 | * | 25 | * |
| 9 | 0 | 5 | 220 | 20 | 0 | 6 | * | 25 | * |
| 9 | 1 | 5 | 220 | 20 | 0 | 6 | * | 25 | * |
| 6 | 2 | 4 | 380 | 15 | 0 | 6 | * | 20 | * |
| 6 | 2 | 4 | 380 | 15 | 0 | 6 | * | 20 | * |
| 6 | 2 | 7 | 400 | 25 | 0 | 6 | * | 15 | * |
| 7 | 1 | 9 | 180 | 30 | 0 | 6 | * | 20 | * |
| 7 | 1 | 9 | 170 | 25 | 0 | 6 | * | 20 | * |

| FOOD NAME | Serving Size | Calories |
|---|---|---|
| Colby, Natural Reduced Fat (Kraft Light Naturals) | 1 oz | 80 |
| Colby, Natural Reduced Fat (Kraft Light Naturals, Shredded with Monterey Jack) | 1 oz | 80 |
| Cottage, large curd, 4% milkfat | 1 cup | 235 |
| Cottage, small curd, 4% milkfat | 1 cup | 220 |
| Cottage, dry curd | 1 cup | 125 |
| Cottage, lowfat 2% | 1 cup | 205 |
| Cream Cheese (Philadelphia Brand) | 1 oz | 100 |
| Cream Cheese with Chives (Philadelphia Brand) | 1 oz | 90 |
| Cream Cheese with Pimento (Philadelphia Brand) | 1 oz | 90 |
| Cream Cheese Light Neufchatel (Philadelphia Brand) | 1 oz | 80 |
| Cream Cheese (Philadelphia Brand Light Pasteurized Process) | 1 oz | 60 |
| Cream Cheese (Philadelphia Brand Soft) | 1 oz | 100 |
| Cream Cheese with Chives and Onion (Philadelphia Brand Soft) | 1 oz | 100 |
| Cream Cheese with Herb and Garlic (Philadelphia Brand Soft) | 1 oz | 100 |
| Cream Cheese with Olives and Pimento (Philadelphia Brand Soft) | 1 oz | 90 |

| Protein (g) | Carbohydrates (g) | Fat (g) | Sodium (mg) | Cholesterol (mg) | Fiber (g) | Vitamin A (%) | Vitamin C (%) | Calcium (%) | Iron (%) |
|---|---|---|---|---|---|---|---|---|---|
| 9 | 0 | 5 | 220 | 20 | 0 | 6 | * | 25 | * |
| | | | | | | | | | |
| 8 | 1 | 5 | 220 | 20 | 0 | 6 | * | 25 | * |
| 28 | 6 | 10 | 910 | 30 | 0 | 7 | * | 14 | 2 |
| 26 | 6 | 9 | 850 | 30 | 0 | 7 | * | 13 | 2 |
| 25 | 0 | 3 | 17 | 20 | 0 | 1 | * | 5 | 2 |
| 31 | 8 | 4 | 915 | 30 | 0 | 3 | * | 16 | 2 |
| 2 | 1 | 10 | 90 | 30 | 0 | 6 | * | 2 | * |
| 2 | 1 | 9 | 125 | 30 | 0 | 8 | * | 2 | * |
| 2 | 1 | 9 | 150 | 30 | 0 | 8 | * | 2 | * |
| 3 | 1 | 7 | 115 | 25 | 0 | 6 | * | 2 | * |
| 3 | 2 | 5 | 160 | 10 | 0 | 6 | * | 4 | * |
| 1 | 2 | 10 | 100 | 30 | 0 | 6 | * | 4 | * |
| 2 | 2 | 9 | 100 | 30 | 0 | 8 | * | 2 | * |
| 1 | 2 | 9 | 160 | 25 | 0 | 6 | * | 4 | * |
| 2 | 2 | 8 | 160 | 25 | 0 | 8 | * | 2 | * |

| FOOD NAME | Serving Size | Calories |
|---|---|---|
| Cream Cheese with Pineapple (Philadelphia Brand Soft) | 1 oz | 90 |
| Cream Cheese with Smoked Salmon (Philadelphia Brand Soft) | 1 oz | 90 |
| Cream Cheese with Strawberries (Philadelphia Brand Soft) | 1 oz | 90 |
| Cream Cheese (Philadelphia Brand Whipped) | 1 oz | 100 |
| Cream Cheese with Chives (Philadelphia Brand Whipped) | 1 oz | 90 |
| Cream Cheese with Onions (Philadelphia Brand Whipped) | 1 oz | 90 |
| Cream Cheese with Smoked Salmon (Philadelphia Brand Whipped) | 1 oz | 90 |
| Edam (Kraft) | 1 oz | 100 |
| Edam (Land O' Lakes) | 1 oz | 90 |
| Fondue (Swiss Knight) | 1 oz | 60 |
| Gouda (Kraft) | 1 oz | 110 |
| Gouda (Land O' Lakes) | 1 oz | 100 |
| Havarti (Casino) | 1 oz | 120 |
| Limburger (Mohawk Valley Little Gem Size Natural) | 1 oz | 90 |
| Monterey Jack (Kraft) | 1 oz | 110 |
| Monterey Jack with Caraway Seeds (Kraft) | 1 oz | 100 |

| Protein (g) | Carbohydrates (g) | Fat (g) | Sodium (mg) | Cholesterol (mg) | Fiber (g) | Vitamin A (%) | Vitamin C (%) | Calcium (%) | Iron (%) |
|---|---|---|---|---|---|---|---|---|---|
| 1 | 4 | 8 | 90 | 25 | 0 | 6 | * | 2 | * |
| 2 | 1 | 9 | 180 | 25 | 0 | 6 | * | 2 | * |
| 1 | 4 | 8 | 75 | 20 | 0 | 4 | * | 2 | * |
| 2 | 1 | 10 | 85 | 30 | 0 | 8 | * | 2 | * |
| 2 | 1 | 8 | 150 | 30 | 0 | 8 | * | 2 | * |
| 2 | 2 | 8 | 170 | 25 | 0 | 6 | * | 2 | * |
| 2 | 2 | 8 | 170 | 30 | 0 | 8 | * | 2 | * |
| 8 | 0 | 7 | 310 | 20 | 0 | 4 | * | 25 | * |
| 8 | 0 | 7 | 310 | 20 | 0 | 4 | * | 25 | * |
| 4 | 1 | 5 | 185 | na | 0 | 4 | * | 15 | * |
| 7 | 0 | 9 | 200 | 30 | 0 | 6 | * | 20 | * |
| 7 | 1 | 8 | 230 | 30 | 0 | 4 | * | 20 | * |
| 6 | 0 | 11 | 140 | 35 | 0 | 6 | * | 20 | * |
| 6 | 0 | 8 | 250 | 25 | 0 | 6 | * | 15 | * |
| 6 | 0 | 9 | 190 | 30 | 0 | 6 | * | 20 | * |
| 7 | 1 | 8 | 180 | 30 | 0 | 6 | * | 15 | * |

| FOOD NAME | Serving Size | Calories |
|---|---|---|
| Monterey Jack with Jalapeño Peppers (Kraft) | 1 oz | 110 |
| Monterey Jack (Land O' Lakes) | 1 oz | 110 |
| Monterey Jack Hot Pepper (Land O' Lakes) | 1 oz | 110 |
| Mozzarella Fior di Latte Fresh (Polly-O) | 1 oz | 80 |
| Mozzarella Lite Reduced Fat (Polly-O) | 1 oz | 60 |
| Mozzarella Low Moisture (Kraft) | 1 oz | 90 |
| Mozzarella Low Moisture Part-Skim (Kraft) | 1 oz | 80 |
| Mozzarella Low Moisture Part-Skim (Land O' Lakes) | 1 oz | 80 |
| Mozzarella Part Skim (Polly-O) | 1 oz | 80 |
| Mozzarella Shredded Whole Milk (Polly-O) | 1 oz | 90 |
| Mozzarella Shredded Part Skim (Polly-O) | 1 oz | 80 |
| Mozzarella Shredded Lite Reduced Fat (Polly-O) | 1 oz | 60 |
| Mozzarella String (Polly-O) | 1 oz | 80 |
| Mozzarella String, and Cheddar (Polly-O) | 1 oz | 80 |
| Mozzarella String with Jalapeño Peppers (Polly-O) | 1 oz | 80 |
| Mozzarella String with Pepperoni (Polly-O) | 1 oz | 80 |
| Mozzarella String Low Moisture Part-Skim with Jalapeño Pepper (Kraft) | 1 oz | 80 |
| Mozzarella Whole Milk (Polly-O) | 1 oz | 90 |
| Muenster (Kraft) | 1 oz | 100 |

| Protein (g) | Carbohydrates (g) | Fat (g) | Sodium (mg) | Cholesterol (mg) | Fiber (g) | Vitamin A (%) | Vitamin C (%) | Calcium (%) | Iron (%) |
|---|---|---|---|---|---|---|---|---|---|
| 7 | 1 | 9 | 190 | 30 | 0 | 8 | * | 20 | * |
| 7 | <1 | 9 | 150 | 20 | 0 | 6 | * | 20 | * |
| 7 | <1 | 9 | 150 | 20 | 0 | 6 | * | 20 | * |
| 5 | 1 | 6 | 20 | 20 | 0 | 4 | * | 6 | * |
| 7 | 1 | 3 | 240 | 10 | 0 | 2 | * | 10 | * |
| 6 | 1 | 7 | 190 | 20 | 0 | 4 | * | 15 | * |
| 8 | 1 | 5 | 200 | 15 | 0 | 2 | * | 20 | * |
| 8 | 1 | 5 | 150 | 15 | 0 | 4 | * | 20 | * |
| 6 | 1 | 5 | 280 | 15 | 0 | 2 | * | 10 | * |
| 7 | 1 | 6 | 220 | 25 | 0 | 4 | * | 20 | * |
| 6 | 1 | 6 | 280 | 20 | 0 | 4 | * | 10 | * |
| 7 | 1 | 3 | 240 | 10 | 0 | 10 | * | 15 | * |
| 7 | 1 | 6 | 200 | 15 | 0 | 4 | * | 15 | * |
| 7 | 1 | 6 | 210 | 20 | 0 | 4 | * | 20 | * |
| 7 | 1 | 5 | 210 | 20 | 0 | 4 | * | 15 | * |
| 7 | 1 | 6 | 210 | 20 | 0 | 4 | * | 15 | * |
| 8 | 1 | 5 | 230 | 20 | 0 | 4 | * | 20 | * |
| 5 | 1 | 7 | 240 | 20 | 0 | 2 | * | 10 | * |
| 7 | 1 | 8 | 170 | 25 | 0 | 6 | * | 15 | * |

| FOOD NAME | Serving Size | Calories | |
|---|---|---|---|
| Muenster (Land O' Lakes) | 1 oz | 100 | |
| Neufchatel (Spreadery Cheese Snack with Classic Ranch Flavor) | 1 oz | 70 | |
| Neufchatel (Spreadery Cheese Snack with French Onion) | 1 oz | 70 | |
| Neufchatel (Spreadery Cheese Snack with Garden Vegetables) | 1 oz | 70 | |
| Neufchatel (Spreadery Cheese Snack with Garlic & Herb) | 1 oz | 70 | |
| Neufchatel (Spreadery Cheese Snack with Strawberries) | 1 oz | 70 | |
| Parmesan (Kraft) | 1 oz | 100 | |
| Parmesan (Kraft Grated) | 1 oz | 130 | |
| Parmesan (Polly-O) | 1 oz | 110 | |
| Parmesan (Polly-O Grated) | 1 oz | 130 | |
| Parmesan (Polly-O Grated with Romano) | 1 oz | 130 | |
| Pimento (Kraft Deluxe Pasteurized Process Slices) | 1 oz | 100 | |
| Provolone (Kraft) | 1 oz | 100 | |
| Provolone (Land O' Lakes) | 1 oz | 100 | |
| Ricotta (Polly-O Whole Milk) | 1 oz | 50 | |
| Ricotta (Polly-O Whole Milk No Salt) | 1 oz | 50 | |
| Ricotta (Polly-O Part Skim) | 1 oz | 45 | |
| Ricotta (Polly-O Part Skim No Salt) | 1 oz | 45 | |
| Ricotta (Polly-O Lite Reduced Fat) | 1 oz | 35 | |

| Protein (g) | Carbohydrates (g) | Fat (g) | Sodium (mg) | Cholesterol (mg) | Fiber (g) | Vitamin A (%) | Vitamin C (%) | Calcium (%) | Iron (%) |
|---|---|---|---|---|---|---|---|---|---|
| 7 | <1 | 9 | 180 | 25 | 0 | 6 | * | 20 | * |
| 2 | 1 | 7 | 190 | 20 | 0 | 4 | * | 2 | * |
| 2 | 2 | 6 | 135 | 20 | 0 | 4 | * | 2 | * |
| 2 | 2 | 6 | 220 | 20 | 0 | 8 | * | 2 | * |
| 2 | 1 | 6 | 140 | 20 | 0 | 4 | * | 2 | * |
| 2 | 0 | 5 | 270 | 15 | 0 | 4 | * | 2 | * |
| 9 | 1 | 7 | 290 | 20 | 0 | 4 | * | 30 | * |
| 12 | 1 | 9 | 430 | 30 | 0 | 4 | * | 40 | * |
| 10 | 1 | 7 | 450 | 20 | 0 | 2 | * | 30 | * |
| 12 | 1 | 9 | 430 | 30 | 0 | 4 | * | 40 | * |
| 12 | 1 | 9 | 400 | 30 | 0 | 4 | * | 40 | * |
| 6 | 1 | 8 | 440 | 25 | 0 | 6 | * | 15 | * |
| 7 | 1 | 7 | 260 | 25 | 0 | 6 | * | 20 | * |
| 7 | 1 | 8 | 250 | 20 | 0 | 4 | * | 25 | * |
| 3 | 1 | 4 | 20 | 15 | 0 | 4 | * | 8 | * |
| 3 | 1 | 4 | 10 | 15 | 0 | 4 | * | 8 | * |
| 4 | 1 | 3 | 20 | 10 | 0 | 2 | * | 10 | * |
| 4 | 1 | 3 | 10 | 10 | 0 | 2 | * | 10 | * |
| 4 | 1 | 1 | 20 | 5 | 0 | 2 | * | 10 | * |

| FOOD NAME | Serving Size | Calories |
|---|---|---|
| Ricotta (Polly-O Old Fashioned) | 1 oz | 50 |
| Romano (Kraft) | 1 oz | 100 |
| Romano (Kraft Grated) | 1 oz | 130 |
| Romano (Polly-O) | 1 oz | 110 |
| Romano (Polly-O Grated) | 1 oz | 130 |
| Romano (Polly-O Grated with Parmesan) | 1 oz | 130 |
| Roquefort | 1 oz | 110 |
| Swiss (Casino) | 1 oz | 110 |
| Swiss (Cracker Barrel) | 1 oz | 110 |
| Swiss (Kraft) | 1 oz | 110 |
| Swiss (Kraft Aged) | 1 oz | 110 |
| Swiss (Kraft Low Sodium) | 1 oz | 110 |
| Swiss (Kraft Reduced Fat Light Naturals) | 1 oz | 90 |
| Swiss, processed (Kraft Deluxe Slices) | 1 oz | 90 |
| Taco (Kraft Shredded) | 1 oz | 110 |
| **CHEESE FOOD** | | |
| American Flavored Imitation Pasteurized Process (Golden Image) | 1 oz | 90 |
| With Real Bacon (Cracker Barrel Cold Pack) | 1 oz | 90 |
| Extra Sharp Cheddar (Cracker Barrel Cold Pack) | 1 oz | 90 |
| With Garlic (Kraft Pasteurized Process) | 1 oz | 90 |
| Grated American (Kraft) | 1 oz | 130 |

| Protein (g) | Carbohydrates (g) | Fat (g) | Sodium (mg) | Cholesterol (mg) | Fiber (g) | Vitamin A (%) | Vitamin C (%) | Calcium (%) | Iron (%) |
|---|---|---|---|---|---|---|---|---|---|
| 3 | 1 | 3 | 25 | 15 | 0 | 2 | * | 10 | * |
| 8 | 1 | 7 | 250 | 20 | 0 | 4 | * | 30 | * |
| 11 | 1 | 9 | 350 | 30 | 0 | 4 | * | 35 | * |
| 9 | 1 | 8 | 340 | 30 | 0 | 4 | * | 25 | * |
| 11 | 1 | 9 | 350 | 30 | 0 | 4 | * | 35 | * |
| 12 | 1 | 9 | 400 | 30 | 0 | 4 | * | 40 | * |
| 7 | 1 | 9 | na | na | 0 | 8 | * | 8 | * |
| 8 | 1 | 8 | 35 | 30 | 0 | 6 | * | 25 | * |
| 7 | 0 | 9 | 65 | 25 | 0 | 6 | * | 20 | * |
| 8 | 1 | 8 | 40 | 25 | 0 | 6 | * | 30 | * |
| 1 | 8 | 1 | 45 | 25 | 0 | 6 | * | 30 | * |
| 8 | 1 | 8 | 10 | 25 | 0 | 6 | * | 25 | * |
| | | | | | | | | | |
| 10 | 1 | 5 | 70 | 20 | 0 | 6 | * | 35 | * |
| 7 | 1 | 7 | 420 | 25 | 0 | 6 | * | 20 | * |
| 7 | 1 | 9 | 190 | 30 | 0 | 8 | * | 20 | * |
| | | | | | | | | | |
| 7 | 2 | 6 | 360 | 5 | 0 | 10 | * | 20 | * |
| | | | | | | | | | |
| 5 | 3 | 7 | 280 | 20 | 0 | 4 | * | 15 | * |
| | | | | | | | | | |
| 5 | 3 | 7 | 240 | 20 | 0 | 6 | * | 15 | * |
| 5 | 2 | 7 | 370 | 20 | 0 | 4 | * | 15 | * |
| 8 | 8 | 7 | 740 | 25 | 0 | 6 | * | 25 | * |

| FOOD NAME | Serving Size | Calories | |
|---|---|---|---|
| Hot Mexican, shredded (Velveeta Pasteurized Process) | 1 oz | 100 | |
| Individually Wrapped Slices (Land O' Lakes) | ¾ oz | 70 | |
| Individually Wrapped Slices (Land O' Lakes) | ⅔ oz | 60 | |
| Italian Herb (Land O' Lakes) | 1 oz | 90 | |
| Jalapeño (Land O' Lakes) | 1 oz | 90 | |
| Jalapeño Singles (Kraft Pasteurized Process) | 1 oz | 90 | |
| With Jalapeño Peppers (Kraft Pasteurized Process) | 1 oz | 90 | |
| Mild Mexican (Velveeta Pasteurized Process) | 1 oz | 100 | |
| Monterey Jack Singles (Kraft Pasteurized Process) | 1 oz | 90 | |
| Onion (Land O' Lakes) | 1 oz | 90 | |
| Pasteurized Process (Nippy) | 1 oz | 90 | |
| Pasteurized Process, shredded (Velveeta) | 1 oz | 100 | |
| Pepperoni (Land O' Lakes) | 1 oz | 90 | |
| Port Wine Cheddar (Cracker Barrel Cold Pack) | 1 oz | 100 | |
| Salami (Land O' Lakes) | 1 oz | 90 | |
| Sharp Cheddar (Cracker Barrel Cold Pack) | 1 oz | 100 | |
| Sharp Singles (Kraft Pasteurized Process) | 1 oz | 100 | |

| Protein (g) | Carbohydrates (g) | Fat (g) | Sodium (mg) | Cholesterol (mg) | Fiber (g) | Vitamin A (%) | Vitamin C (%) | Calcium (%) | Iron (%) |
|---|---|---|---|---|---|---|---|---|---|
| 6 | 3 | 7 | 430 | 25 | 0 | 10 | * | 20 | * |
| 4 | 2 | 5 | 260 | 15 | 0 | 4 | * | 15 | * |
| 4 | 2 | 4 | 230 | 15 | 0 | 2 | * | 10 | * |
| 6 | 2 | 7 | 430 | 20 | 0 | 4 | * | 15 | * |
| 6 | 2 | 7 | 400 | 20 | 0 | 4 | * | 15 | * |
| 5 | 2 | 7 | 450 | 25 | 0 | 10 | * | 15 | * |
| 5 | 2 | 7 | 390 | 20 | 0 | 4 | * | 15 | * |
| 6 | 3 | 7 | 420 | 25 | 0 | 10 | * | 15 | * |
| 5 | 2 | 7 | 390 | 25 | 0 | 4 | * | 15 | * |
| 6 | 2 | 7 | 410 | 20 | 0 | 4 | * | 15 | * |
| 5 | 2 | 7 | 380 | 20 | 0 | 4 | * | 20 | * |
| 6 | 3 | 7 | 410 | 20 | 0 | 10 | * | 15 | * |
| 6 | 1 | 7 | 430 | 20 | 0 | 4 | * | 15 | * |
| 4 | 3 | 7 | 230 | 20 | 0 | 4 | * | 15 | * |
| 6 | 2 | 7 | 410 | 20 | 0 | 4 | * | 15 | * |
| 4 | 4 | 7 | 230 | 20 | 0 | 4 | * | 15 | * |
| 6 | 1 | 8 | 400 | 25 | 0 | 10 | * | 15 | * |

| FOOD NAME | Serving Size | Calories | |
|---|---|---|---|
| **CHEESE LOG** | | | |
| Port Wine Cheddar with Almonds (Cracker Barrel) | 1 oz | 90 | |
| Sharp Cheddar with Almonds (Cracker Barrel) | 1 oz | 90 | |
| Smoky Cheddar with Almonds (Cracker Barrel) | 1 oz | 90 | |
| **CHEESE SPREAD** | | | |
| American (Kraft) | 1 oz | 80 | |
| Bacon (Kraft) | 1 oz | 80 | |
| With Bacon (Squeez-a-Snak) | 1 oz | 80 | |
| Blue (Roka) | 1 oz | 70 | |
| (Cheez Whiz) | 1 oz | 80 | |
| Garlic (Squeez-a-Snak) | 1 oz | 80 | |
| (Handi-Snacks Cheez 'n Crackers) | 1 pkg | 120 | |
| (Handi-Snacks Bacon, Cheez 'n Crackers) | 1 pkg | 130 | |
| (Handi-Snacks Peanut Butter 'n Cheez Crackers) | 1 pkg | 190 | |
| Hickory Smoke Flavor (Squeez-a-Snak) | 1 oz | 80 | |
| Hot Mexican (Velveeta) | 1 oz | 80 | |
| With Jalapeño Peppers (Cheez Whiz) | 1 oz | 80 | |
| Jalapeño Pepper (Kraft) | 1 oz | 70 | |
| With Jalapeño Pepper (Squeez-a-Snak) | 1 oz | 80 | |
| Limburger (Mohawk Valley) | 1 oz | 70 | |

| Protein (g) | Carbohydrates (g) | Fat (g) | Sodium (mg) | Cholesterol (mg) | Fiber (g) | Vitamin A (%) | Vitamin C (%) | Calcium (%) | Iron (%) |
|---|---|---|---|---|---|---|---|---|---|
| 5 | 4 | 6 | 260 | 15 | 0 | 2 | * | 15 | * |
| 5 | 4 | 6 | 250 | 15 | 0 | 2 | * | 15 | * |
| 5 | 4 | 6 | 250 | 15 | 0 | 2 | * | 15 | * |
| 4 | 2 | 6 | 470 | 15 | 0 | 4 | * | 15 | * |
| 5 | 1 | 7 | 560 | 20 | 0 | 10 | * | 15 | * |
| 5 | 1 | 7 | 500 | 20 | 0 | 2 | * | 15 | * |
| 3 | 2 | 6 | 270 | 20 | 0 | 4 | * | 6 | * |
| 4 | 2 | 6 | 470 | 20 | 0 | 6 | * | 10 | * |
| 5 | 1 | 7 | 430 | 20 | 0 | 2 | * | 15 | * |
| 4 | 9 | 8 | 360 | 20 | na | 4 | * | 8 | 2 |
| 4 | 8 | 9 | 410 | 20 | na | 6 | * | 10 | 2 |
| 6 | 11 | 14 | 180 | 0 | na | * | * | * | 4 |
| 5 | 1 | 7 | 440 | 20 | 0 | 2 | * | 15 | * |
| 5 | 3 | 6 | 520 | 20 | 0 | 10 | * | 15 | * |
| 42 | 2 | 6 | 430 | 20 | 0 | 6 | * | 10 | * |
| 2 | 3 | 5 | 95 | 15 | 0 | 4 | * | 4 | * |
| 5 | 1 | 6 | 510 | 20 | 0 | 2 | * | 15 | * |
| 4 | 0 | 6 | 420 | 20 | 0 | 4 | * | 10 | * |

| FOOD NAME | Serving Size | Calories |
|---|---|---|
| Mild Mexican (Cheez Whiz) | 1 oz | 80 |
| Mild Mexican (Velveeta) | 1 oz | 80 |
| Olives & Pimento (Kraft) | 1 oz | 60 |
| Pimento (Kraft) | 1 oz | 70 |
| Pimento (Velveeta) | 1 oz | 80 |
| Pineapple (Kraft) | 1 oz | 70 |
| Sharp (Old English) | 1 oz | 80 |
| Sharp (Squeez-a-Snak Pasteurized Process) | 1 oz | 80 |
| (Velveeta) | 1 oz | 80 |
| CHERRIES | | |
| Raw, sour, pitted | 1 cup | 90 |
| Raw, sweet, pitted | 1 cup | 104 |
| Raw, sweet, whole | 10 | 49 |
| *Canned* | | |
| (Del Monte Dark Sweet with Pits) | ½ cup | 90 |
| (Del Monte Dark Sweet, Pitted) | ½ cup | 90 |
| (Del Monte Light Sweet with Pits) | ½ cup | 100 |
| CHERRY DRINK | | |
| (Hi-C) | 6 fl oz | 90 |
| (Kool-Aid) | 8 fl oz | 80 |
| (Kool-Aid Sugar Free) | 8 fl oz | 4 |
| (Kool-Aid Koolers) | 8.5 fl oz | 140 |
| (Tang Fruit Box) | 8.5 fl oz | 120 |
| CHESTNUTS | ⅓ cup | 100 |

| Protein (g) | Carbohydrates (g) | Fat (g) | Sodium (mg) | Cholesterol (mg) | Fiber (g) | Vitamin A (%) | Vitamin C (%) | Calcium (%) | Iron (%) |
|---|---|---|---|---|---|---|---|---|---|
| 4 | 2 | 6 | 430 | 20 | 0 | 4 | * | 10 | * |
| 5 | 3 | 6 | 440 | 20 | 0 | 8 | * | 15 | * |
| 2 | 2 | 5 | 160 | 15 | 0 | 4 | * | 4 | * |
| 2 | 3 | 5 | 120 | 15 | 0 | 4 | * | 4 | * |
| 5 | 3 | 6 | 400 | 20 | 0 | 15 | * | 15 | * |
| 2 | 4 | 5 | 75 | 15 | 0 | 4 | 2 | 4 | * |
| 5 | 1 | 7 | 480 | 20 | 0 | 10 | * | 15 | * |
|  |  |  |  |  |  |  |  |  |  |
| 5 | 1 | 7 | 440 | 20 | 0 | 2 | * | 15 | * |
| 5 | 3 | 6 | 430 | 20 | 0 | 6 | * | 15 | * |
|  |  |  |  |  |  |  |  |  |  |
| 2 | 23 | Tr | 3 | 0 | 0.5 | 30 | 25 | 4 | 4 |
| 2 | 26 | <1 | 3 | 0 | 1 | 4 | 25 | 4 | 4 |
| 1 | 11 | <1 | Tr | 0 | 1 | 2 | 10 | 2 | 2 |
|  |  |  |  |  |  |  |  |  |  |
| 0 | 23 | 0 | <10 | 0 | na | 4 | 6 | * | 2 |
| 0 | 24 | 0 | <10 | 0 | na | 4 | 6 | * | 2 |
| 0 | 26 | 0 | <10 | 0 | na | 2 | 4 | * | 2 |
|  |  |  |  |  |  |  |  |  |  |
| 0 | 23 | 0 | 4 | 0 | 0 | * | 100 | * | * |
| 0 | 20 | 0 | 0 | 0 | 0 | * | 10 | * | * |
| 0 | 0 | 0 | 0 | 0 | 0 | * | 10 | * | * |
| 0 | 38 | 0 | 10 | 0 | 0 | * | 10 | * | * |
| 0 | 32 | 0 | 10 | 0 | 0 | * | 100 | * | * |
| 2 | 22 | 1 | 3 | 0 | 5 | * | * | 1 | 5 |

| FOOD NAME | Serving Size | Calories | |
|---|---|---|---|
| **CHICKEN** | | | |
| Broiler-fryer, dark meat only | 4 oz | 232 | |
| Broiler-fryer, dark meat with skin | 4 oz | 287 | |
| Broiler-fryer, white meat only | 4 oz | 196 | |
| Broiler-fryer, white meat with skin | 4 oz | 252 | |
| Capon, roasted with skin | 4 oz | 260 | |
| Roaster, roasted with skin | 4 oz | 253 | |
| *Chicken Part* | | | |
| Breast, fried | 1 | 193 | |
| Drumstick, fried | 1 | 88 | |
| Liver, simmered | 4 oz | 178 | |
| Thigh, fried | 1 | 122 | |
| Wing, fried | 1 | 82 | |
| **CHICKEN, FROZEN** | | | |
| Tyson Breast Chunks | 3 oz | 240 | |
| Tyson Breast Fillets | 3 oz | 190 | |
| Tyson Breast Patties | 2.6 oz | 220 | |
| Tyson Breast Tenders | 3 oz | 220 | |
| Tyson Chick'n Cheddar | 2.6 oz | 220 | |
| Tyson Chick'n Chunks | 2.6 oz | 220 | |
| Tyson Diced Meat | 3 oz | 130 | |
| Tyson Grilled Breast Sandwich | 3.5 oz | 150 | |
| Tyson Grilled Sandwich | 3.5 oz | 200 | |
| Tyson Lemon Pepper Breast Fillet | 2.75 oz | 100 | |
| Tyson Mesquite Breast Tenders | 2.75 oz | 110 | |

| Protein (g) | Carbohydrates (g) | Fat (g) | Sodium (mg) | Cholesterol (mg) | Fiber (g) | Vitamin A (%) | Vitamin C (%) | Calcium (%) | Iron (%) |
|---|---|---|---|---|---|---|---|---|---|
| 31 | 0 | 11 | 105 | 99 | 0 | 2 | * | 2 | 8 |
| 29 | 0 | 18 | 99 | 104 | 0 | 5 | * | 2 | 9 |
| 35 | 0 | 5 | 87 | 87 | 0 | 1 | * | 2 | 7 |
| 33 | 0 | 12 | 85 | 99 | 0 | 3 | * | 2 | 7 |
| 33 | 0 | 13 | 56 | 98 | 0 | 2 | * | 2 | 9 |
| 27 | 0 | 15 | 83 | 86 | 0 | 2 | * | 1 | 8 |
| | | | | | | | | | |
| 29 | 0 | 8 | 69 | 83 | 0 | 1 | * | 1 | 7 |
| 12 | 0 | 4 | 47 | 48 | 0 | 1 | * | 1 | 5 |
| 27 | 6 | 27 | 58 | 716 | 0 | 371 | 29 | 1 | 53 |
| 15 | 1 | 6 | 52 | 58 | 0 | 2 | * | 1 | 7 |
| 9 | 1 | 5 | 28 | 29 | 0 | 2 | * | * | 3 |
| | | | | | | | | | |
| 13 | 10 | 17 | 430 | 30 | na | na | na | na | na |
| 13 | 15 | 9 | 400 | 25 | na | na | na | na | na |
| 10 | 11 | 15 | 640 | 35 | na | na | na | na | na |
| 14 | 13 | 12 | 500 | na | na | na | na | na | na |
| 11 | 11 | 15 | 310 | 40 | na | na | na | na | na |
| 10 | 11 | 15 | 500 | 35 | na | na | na | na | na |
| 24 | 1 | 3 | 40 | 70 | na | na | na | na | na |
| 17 | 2 | 8 | 400 | 44 | na | na | na | na | na |
| 15 | 25 | 5 | 470 | 32 | na | na | na | na | na |
| 14 | 4 | 3 | 380 | 40 | na | na | na | na | na |
| 17 | 4 | 3 | 420 | 45 | na | na | na | na | na |

| FOOD NAME | Serving Size | Calories |
|---|---|---|
| Tyson Microwave BBQ Sandwich | 4 oz | 230 |
| Tyson Microwave Breast Sandwich | 4.25 oz | 328 |
| Tyson Microwave Chunks | 3.5 oz | 220 |
| Tyson Oriental Breast Strips | 2.75 oz | 110 |
| Tyson Southern Fried Breast Fillets | 3 oz | 220 |
| Tyson Southern Fried Breast Patties | 2.6 oz | 220 |
| Tyson Southern Fried Chick'n Chunks | 2.6 oz | 220 |
| Weaver Breast Fillets | 4.5 oz | 270 |
| Weaver Breast Patties | 3 oz | 205 |
| Weaver Cheese Rondelet | 2.6 oz | 190 |
| Weaver Chicken Nuggets | 2.6 oz | 190 |
| Weaver Herb & Spice Mini Drums | 3 oz | 200 |
| Weaver Italian Rondelet | 2.6 oz | 190 |
| Weaver Original Rondelet | 3 oz | 190 |
| Weaver Premium Tenders | 3 oz | 170 |
| Weaver Wings, Hot | 2.7 oz | 170 |
| CHICKPEAS | ½ cup | 110 |
| (Old El Paso Garbanzo Beans) | ½ cup | 77 |
| CHILI, CANNED | | |
| (Chef Boyardee with Beans) | 7.5 oz | 330 |
| (Chef Boyardee without Beans) | 7.5 oz | 370 |
| (Heinz Hot with Beans) | 7.75 oz | 330 |
| (Old El Paso con Carne) | 1 cup | 349 |
| (Old El Paso with Beans) | 1 cup | 423 |
| CHILI BEANS  (Hunt-Wesson) | 4 oz | 100 |

| Protein (g) | Carbohydrates (g) | Fat (g) | Sodium (mg) | Cholesterol (mg) | Fiber (g) | Vitamin A (%) | Vitamin C (%) | Calcium (%) | Iron (%) |
|---|---|---|---|---|---|---|---|---|---|
| 16 | 27 | 6 | 600 | 50 | na | na | na | na | na |
| 16 | 33 | 14 | 520 | na | na | na | na | na | na |
| 10 | 11 | 15 | na | na | na | na | na | na | na |
| 14 | 6 | 3 | 250 | 40 | na | na | na | na | na |
| 14 | 15 | 11 | 630 | 25 | na | na | na | na | na |
| 11 | 9 | 15 | 460 | 35 | na | na | na | na | na |
| 10 | 11 | 15 | 540 | 35 | na | na | na | na | na |
| 20 | 18 | 13 | 520 | na | na | na | na | na | na |
| 12 | 14 | 11 | 640 | na | na | na | na | na | na |
| 11 | 12 | 11 | 520 | na | na | na | na | na | na |
| 10 | 10 | 12 | 450 | na | na | na | na | na | na |
| 13 | 13 | 11 | 320 | na | na | na | na | na | na |
| 11 | 11 | 11 | 560 | na | na | na | na | na | na |
| 13 | 13 | 10 | 610 | na | na | na | na | na | na |
| 12 | 11 | 9 | 500 | na | na | na | na | na | na |
| 17 | 1 | 11 | 670 | na | na | na | na | na | na |
| 6 | 17 | 0 | 0 | 0 | 3 | 4 | * | 3 | 7 |
| 4 | 12 | 1 | 247 | 0 | 3.2 | * | * | 3 | 8 |
| | | | | | | | | | |
| 15 | 30 | 17 | 1005 | na | na | 20 | 4 | 6 | 20 |
| 14 | 14 | 29 | 875 | na | na | 30 | 6 | 2 | 10 |
| na | 30 | 16 | 1140 | na | na | na | na | 10 | 15 |
| 18 | 12 | 21 | 907 | na | na | * | * | 7 | 51 |
| 13 | 27 | 28 | 1037 | na | na | * | * | 9 | 30 |
| 4 | 18 | 1 | 455 | na | na | * | * | 3 | 8 |

| FOOD NAME | Serving Size | Calories |
|---|---|---|
| **CHILIES, GREEN** | | |
| *Canned* | | |
| (Del Monte) | ½ cup | 20 |
| (Old El Paso Chopped) | 2 tbsp | 7 |
| (Old El Paso Whole) | 1 | 7 |
| **CHOCOLATE, BAKING** | | |
| (Baker's Milk Chocolate Chips) | 1 oz | 140 |
| (Baker's Semi-Sweet Chocolate Bar) | 1 oz | 140 |
| (Baker's Semi-Sweet Real Chocolate Chips) | ¼ cup | 200 |
| (Baker's Semi-Sweet Chocolate Flavored Chips) | ¼ cup | 200 |
| (Baker's Unsweetened Chocolate Bar) | 1 oz | 140 |
| (Baker's Big Chip Milk Chocolate Chips) | ¼ cup | 240 |
| (Baker's Big Chip Semi-Sweet Chocolate Chips) | ¼ cup | 220 |
| (German's Sweet Chocolate) | 1 oz | 140 |
| **CLAMS** | | |
| Cherrystone, raw | 5 | 65 |
| Littleneck, raw | 10 | 65 |
| Canned | 4 oz | 60 |
| **CLAM JUICE** | | |
| (Doxsee) | 4 fl oz | 10 |
| (Snow's) | 3 fl oz | 14 |
| **COCONUT** | | |
| Fresh piece | 1.6 oz | 160 |

| Protein (g) | Carbohydrates (g) | Fat (g) | Sodium (mg) | Cholesterol (mg) | Fiber (g) | Vitamin A (%) | Vitamin C (%) | Calcium (%) | Iron (%) |
|---|---|---|---|---|---|---|---|---|---|
| 0 | 5 | 0 | 690 | na | na | 4 | 80 | 6 | 4 |
| 0 | 1 | <1 | 69 | na | na | * | 22 | 4 | 3 |
| 0 | 1 | <1 | 105 | na | na | * | 21 | 6 | 3 |
| | | | | | | | | | |
| 2 | 18 | 8 | 25 | 5 | na | * | * | 4 | * |
| 1 | 17 | 9 | 0 | 0 | na | * | * | * | 6 |
| 2 | 28 | 11 | 0 | 0 | na | * | * | * | 6 |
| | | | | | | | | | |
| 2 | 30 | 9 | 30 | 0 | na | * | * | 6 | 4 |
| 3 | 9 | 15 | 0 | 0 | na | * | * | 2 | 10 |
| 3 | 30 | 13 | 40 | 10 | na | * | * | 8 | 2 |
| | | | | | | | | | |
| 2 | 31 | 13 | 0 | 0 | na | * | * | * | 6 |
| 1 | 17 | 10 | 0 | 0 | na | * | * | * | 4 |
| | | | | | | | | | |
| 11 | 2 | <1 | 50 | 30 | 0 | 2 | 10 | 4 | 30 |
| 11 | 2 | <1 | 50 | 30 | 0 | 2 | 10 | 4 | 30 |
| 9 | 3 | 1 | 76 | na | 0 | * | * | 6 | 26 |
| | | | | | | | | | |
| 0 | 2 | 0 | 140 | na | 0 | * | * | * | * |
| <1 | 2 | 0 | 110 | na | 0 | * | * | * | 2 |
| | | | | | | | | | |
| <2 | 7 | 15 | 9 | 0 | 4.1 | * | 2 | * | 4 |

| FOOD NAME | Serving Size | Calories |
|---|---|---|
| Fresh, shredded | 1 cup | 450 |
| Canned (Angel Flake) | ⅓ cup | 110 |
| Packaged (Angel Flake Bag) | ⅓ cup | 120 |
| Packaged (Angel Flake Premium Shred) | ⅓ cup | 140 |
| Packaged (Angel Flake Toasted) | ⅓ cup | 200 |
| COD | | |
| Broiled | 4 oz | 109 |
| Broiled in butter | 4 oz | 192 |
| Canned | 4 oz | 119 |
| COFFEE | 6 fl oz | 4 |
| Cafe Amaretto | 6 fl oz | 50 |
| Cafe Francais | 6 fl oz | 60 |
| Cafe Francais, Sugar Free | 6 fl oz | 35 |
| Cafe Irish Creme | 6 fl oz | 50 |
| Cafe Vienna | 6 fl oz | 60 |
| Cafe Vienna, Sugar Free | 6 fl oz | 30 |
| Double Dutch Chocolate | 6 fl oz | 50 |
| Dutch Chocolate Mint | 6 fl oz | 50 |
| Orange Cappucino | 6 fl oz | 60 |
| Orange Cappucino, Sugar Free | 6 fl oz | 30 |
| Suisse Mocha | 6 fl oz | 50 |
| Suisse Mocha, Sugar Free | 6 fl oz | 30 |
| COLLARDS  Fresh, cooked | 1 cup | 60 |
| COOKIES | | |
| Almond Windmill (Nabisco) | 3 | 140 |

| Protein (g) | Carbohydrates (g) | Fat (g) | Sodium (mg) | Cholesterol (mg) | Fiber (g) | Vitamin A (%) | Vitamin C (%) | Calcium (%) | Iron (%) |
|---|---|---|---|---|---|---|---|---|---|
| 6 | 12 | 46 | 30 | 0 | 7.2 | * | 6 | 2 | 10 |
| 1 | 10 | 9 | 5 | 0 | na | * | * | * | 2 |
| 1 | 10 | 8 | 75 | 0 | na | * | * | * | 2 |
| 1 | 12 | 9 | 85 | 0 | na | * | * | * | 2 |
| 2 | 17 | 17 | 85 | 0 | na | * | * | * | 4 |
|  |  |  |  |  |  |  |  |  |  |
| 25 | 0 | 1 | 88 | 62 | 0 | 1 | 4 | 1 | 3 |
| 32 | 0 | 6 | 124 | na | 0 | 4 | * | 4 | 7 |
| 26 | 0 | 1 | 247 | 62 | 0 | na | na | na | na |
| Tr | <1 | 0 | 4 | 0 | 0 | * | * | * | * |
| 0 | 7 | 2 | 20 | 0 | 0 | * | * | * | * |
| 0 | 6 | 3 | 25 | 0 | 0 | * | * | * | * |
| 0 | 3 | 2 | 30 | 0 | 0 | * | * | * | * |
| 0 | 8 | 2 | 15 | 0 | 0 | * | * | * | * |
| 0 | 10 | 2 | 110 | 0 | 0 | * | * | * | * |
| 0 | 3 | 2 | 30 | 0 | 0 | * | * | * | * |
| 0 | 8 | 2 | 15 | 0 | 0 | * | * | * | * |
| 0 | 8 | 2 | 80 | 0 | 0 | * | * | * | * |
| 0 | 10 | 2 | 100 | 0 | 0 | * | * | * | * |
| 0 | 3 | 2 | 60 | 0 | 0 | * | * | * | * |
| 0 | 7 | 3 | 15 | 0 | 0 | * | * | * | * |
| 0 | 3 | 2 | 15 | 0 | 0 | * | * | * | * |
| 2 | 10 | 2 | 20 | 0 | 0.6 | 296 | 240 | 35 | 8 |
|  |  |  |  |  |  |  |  |  |  |
| 2 | 21 | 5 | na | na | na | * | * | * | 4 |

| FOOD NAME | Serving Size | Calories |
|---|---|---|
| Animal Crackers (Barnum) | 11 | 130 |
| Animal Crackers (Ralston) | 15 | 130 |
| Apple Crisp (Nabisco) | 3 | 150 |
| Applesauce Raisin (Almost Home) | 2 | 140 |
| Arrowroot (Nabisco) | 6 | 130 |
| Beacon Hill Chocolate Walnut (Pepperidge Farm) | 1 | 120 |
| Biscos Sugar Wafers | 8 | 150 |
| Bordeaux (Pepperidge Farm) | 2 | 70 |
| Brownie Chocolate Nut (Pepperidge Farm) | 2 | 110 |
| Brussels (Pepperidge Farm) | 2 | 110 |
| Brussels Mint (Pepperidge Farm) | 2 | 130 |
| Butter Flavored (Nabisco) | 2 | 90 |
| Cappucino (Pepperidge Farm) | 1 | 50 |
| Capri (Pepperidge Farm) | 1 | 80 |
| Chantilly (Pepperidge Farm) | 1 | 80 |
| Chesapeake Chocolate Chunk Pecan (Pepperidge Farm) | 1 | 120 |
| Chessmen (Pepperidge Farm) | 2 | 90 |
| Cheyenne Peanut Butter Milk Chocolate Chunk (Pepperidge Farm) | 1 | 110 |
| Chips Ahoy! (Nabisco) | 3 | 160 |
| Chocolate Chip (Pepperidge Farm) | 2 | 100 |
| Chocolate Chip, Slice 'n Bake (Pillsbury) | 3 | 160 |

| Protein (g) | Carbohydrates (g) | Fat (g) | Sodium (mg) | Cholesterol (mg) | Fiber (g) | Vitamin A (%) | Vitamin C (%) | Calcium (%) | Iron (%) |
|---|---|---|---|---|---|---|---|---|---|
| 2 | 21 | 4 | na | na | na | * | * | * | 4 |
| 2 | 22 | 3 | 30 | na | na | * | * | * | 4 |
| 2 | 21 | 6 | na | na | na | * | * | * | 4 |
| 2 | 17 | 8 | na | na | na | * | * | 2 | 4 |
| 2 | 21 | 4 | na | na | na | * | * | * | 2 |
| 2 | 14 | 7 | 65 | 5 | na | * | * | * | 4 |
| 1 | 21 | 7 | 50 | na | na | * | * | * | 2 |
| 1 | 11 | 3 | 40 | 0 | na | * | * | * | * |
| 1 | 11 | 7 | 45 | <5 | na | * | * | * | 4 |
| 1 | 13 | 5 | 65 | 0 | na | * | * | * | * |
| 1 | 17 | 7 | 40 | 0 | na | * | * | * | * |
| 2 | 21 | 8 | 120 | 20 | 0 | * | * | * | 2 |
| 0 | 6 | 3 | 20 | <5 | na | * | * | * | * |
| 0 | 10 | 5 | 45 | 0 | na | * | * | * | * |
| 1 | 14 | 2 | 35 | <5 | na | * | * | * | * |
| 1 | 14 | 7 | 60 | 5 | na | * | * | * | * |
| 1 | 12 | 4 | 60 | 10 | na | * | * | * | * |
| 2 | 13 | 6 | 80 | 5 | na | * | * | * | 2 |
| 2 | 21 | 7 | 120 | na | na | * | * | * | 4 |
| 1 | 12 | 5 | 45 | 5 | na | * | * | * | * |
| 1 | 8 | 22 | 125 | na | na | * | * | * | * |

| FOOD NAME | Serving Size | Calories | |
|---|---|---|---|
| Chocolate Chip Snaps (Nabisco) | 2 | 120 | |
| Chocolate Chocolate Chip (Nabisco) | 3 | 160 | |
| Chocolate Chocolate Chip (Pepperidge Farm) | 3 | 160 | |
| Chocolate Snaps (Nabisco) | 8 | 130 | |
| Chocolate Toffee Chip (Pepperidge Farm) | 2 | 100 | |
| Chocolate Wafers (Nabisco) | 5 | 140 | |
| Cinnamon Chip (Pepperidge Farm) | 3 | 150 | |
| Coconut Macaroon (Nabisco) | 2 | 190 | |
| Coconut Macaroon Bar (Pepperidge Farm) | 1 | 210 | |
| Creme Sandwich (Nabisco) | 1 | 210 | |
| Creme Sandwich (Nabisco Cameo) | 2 | 140 | |
| Creme Sandwich (Nabisco Mayfair) | 2 | 130 | |
| Creme Sandwich (Nabisco Mayfair Tea Rose) | 3 | 160 | |
| Creme Sandwich (Nabisco Oreo Swiss) | 3 | 150 | |
| Creme Sandwich, Peanut Butter (Almost Home) | 1 | 140 | |
| Dakota Milk Chocolate Oatmeal (Pepperidge Farm) | 1 | 110 | |
| Date Nut Bar (Pepperidge Farm) | 1 | 190 | |
| Devil's Food Cakes (Nabisco) | 2 | 140 | |
| Fig Newtons (Nabisco) | 2 | 120 | |
| Fudge Chocolate Chip (Almost Home) | 2 | 130 | |
| Geneva (Pepperidge Farm) | 2 | 130 | |

| Protein (g) | Carbohydrates (g) | Fat (g) | Sodium (mg) | Cholesterol (mg) | Fiber (g) | Vitamin A (%) | Vitamin C (%) | Calcium (%) | Iron (%) |
|---|---|---|---|---|---|---|---|---|---|
| 2 | 20 | 4 | 97 | 5 | 0 | * | * | * | 2 |
| 2 | 22 | 7 | na | na | na | * | * | * | 4 |
| | | | | | | | | | |
| 2 | 15 | 7 | 50 | na | na | * | * | * | 2 |
| 2 | 22 | 4 | 171 | na | na | * | * | * | 4 |
| 1 | 12 | 5 | 75 | 5 | na | * | * | * | 2 |
| 2 | 23 | 4 | 35 | 0 | 0 | * | * | * | 6 |
| 2 | 21 | 7 | 80 | na | na | * | * | 2 | 4 |
| 2 | 23 | 10 | 107 | na | na | * | * | * | 4 |
| 2 | 28 | 11 | 80 | na | na | * | * | * | 4 |
| 2 | 28 | 11 | 80 | 0 | 0 | * | * | * | 4 |
| 2 | 21 | 5 | na | na | na | * | * | * | 2 |
| 2 | 18 | 6 | na | na | na | * | * | * | 2 |
| | | | | | | | | | |
| 2 | 23 | 7 | na | na | na | * | * | * | 4 |
| 2 | 22 | 7 | na | na | na | * | * | * | 2 |
| | | | | | | | | | |
| 3 | 20 | 6 | na | na | na | * | * | 2 | 2 |
| | | | | | | | | | |
| 1 | 15 | 6 | 70 | 5 | na | * | * | * | * |
| 2 | 30 | 7 | 90 | na | na | * | 2 | * | 4 |
| 2 | 31 | 1 | 73 | na | na | * | * | * | 4 |
| 1 | 22 | 2 | 125 | na | na | * | * | 2 | 4 |
| 2 | 20 | 5 | na | na | na | * | * | * | 4 |
| 1 | 14 | 6 | 50 | 0 | na | * | * | * | 2 |

| FOOD NAME | Serving Size | Calories |
|---|---|---|
| Gingerman (Pepperidge Farm) | 2 | 70 |
| Ginger Snaps (Nabisco) | 4 | 120 |
| Graham Crackers (Nabisco) | 4 | 120 |
| Graham Crackers (Rokeach) | 8 | 120 |
| Graham Crackers, Sugar Honey (Ralston) | 8 | 120 |
| Grahams, Chocolate (Nabisco) | 3 | 170 |
| Grahams, Party (Nabisco) | 3 | 140 |
| Hazelnut (Pepperidge Farm) | 2 | 110 |
| Heyday (Nabisco) | 1 | 120 |
| Irish Oatmeal (Pepperidge Farm) | 2 | 90 |
| Kettle | 4 | 140 |
| Lemon Nut Crunch | 2 | 110 |
| Lido (Pepperidge Farm) | 1 | 90 |
| Linzer (Pepperidge Farm) | 1 | 120 |
| Lorna Doone | 4 | 160 |
| Macaroons | 2 | 180 |
| Mallomars | 2 | 120 |
| Marshmallow Puffs (Nabisco) | 2 | 170 |
| Marshmallow Twirls | 1 | 130 |
| Milano (Pepperidge Farm) | 2 | 120 |
| Mint Milano (Pepperidge Farm) | 2 | 150 |
| Mystic Mint (Nabisco) | 2 | 180 |
| Nantucket Chocolate Chunk (Pepperidge Farm) | 1 | 120 |
| Nassau (Pepperidge Farm) | 1 | 80 |

| Protein (g) | Carbohydrates (g) | Fat (g) | Sodium (mg) | Cholesterol (mg) | Fiber (g) | Vitamin A (%) | Vitamin C (%) | Calcium (%) | Iron (%) |
|---|---|---|---|---|---|---|---|---|---|
| 1 | 10 | 3 | 50 | 5 | na | * | * | * | * |
| 2 | 22 | 3 | 140 | 0 | 0 | * | * | 2 | 8 |
| 2 | 21 | 3 | 85 | 0 | 0 | * | * | * | 4 |
| 2 | 21 | 3 | na | na | na | * | * | * | 4 |
| 2 | 22 | 3 | 140 | na | na | * | * | * | 2 |
| 2 | 21 | 8 | na | na | na | * | * | * | 6 |
| 2 | 18 | 7 | na | na | na | * | * | * | 2 |
| 1 | 15 | 6 | 75 | 0 | na | * | * | * | * |
| 2 | 13 | 7 | na | na | na | * | * | * | * |
| 1 | 13 | 5 | 80 | 5 | na | * | * | * | * |
| 2 | 21 | 5 | na | na | na | * | * | * | 4 |
| 1 | 13 | 7 | 50 | <5 | na | * | * | * | 2 |
| 1 | 10 | 5 | 30 | <5 | na | * | * | * | * |
| 2 | 20 | 4 | 55 | <5 | na | * | * | * | * |
| 2 | 20 | 8 | na | na | na | * | * | * | 4 |
| 2 | 25 | 9 | 14 | na | na | * | * | 1 | 2 |
| 1 | 17 | 5 | 50 | 0 | na | * | * | * | 2 |
| 1 | 28 | 6 | 80 | na | na | * | * | 2 | 2 |
| 0 | 20 | 5 | na | na | na | * | * | 2 | 2 |
| 1 | 15 | 6 | 45 | 5 | na | * | * | * | * |
| 1 | 17 | 7 | 60 | 5 | na | * | * | * | 2 |
| 1 | 22 | 9 | 127 | na | na | * | * | * | 4 |
| | | | | | | | | | |
| 1 | 15 | 6 | 60 | 6 | na | * | * | 2 | * |
| 1 | 9 | 5 | 45 | <5 | na | * | * | * | * |

| FOOD NAME | Serving Size | Calories |
|---|---|---|
| Nilla Wafers (Nabisco) | 7 | 130 |
| Nutter Butter (Nabisco) | 2 | 140 |
| Nutter Butter Chocolate (Nabisco) | 3 | 170 |
| Oatmeal (Drake's) | 3 | 190 |
| Oatmeal (Nabisco Bakers Bonus) | 2 | 160 |
| Oatmeal Raisin (Almost Home) | 2 | 130 |
| Oatmeal Raisin (Pepperidge Farm) | 2 | 110 |
| Orange Milano (Pepperidge Farm) | 2 | 150 |
| Oreo (Nabisco) | 3 | 150 |
| Oreo Double Stuff (Nabisco) | 2 | 140 |
| Orleans (Pepperidge Farm) | 3 | 90 |
| Orleans Sandwich (Pepperidge Farm) | 2 | 120 |
| Peanut Butter (Almost Home) | 2 | 140 |
| Peanut Butter, Slice 'n Bake (Pillsbury) | 3 | 170 |
| Peanut Butter Chip (Pepperidge Farm) | 3 | 160 |
| Peanut Butter Fudge (Nabisco) | 3 | 150 |
| Pecan Shortbread (Nabisco) | 2 | 160 |
| Pecan Shortbread (Pepperidge Farm) | 1 | 70 |
| Pinwheels, Chocolate | 1 | 140 |
| Pirouettes, Chocolate Laced (Pepperidge Farm) | 2 | 70 |
| Pirouettes, Original (Pepperidge Farm) | 2 | 70 |
| Raisin Fruit Biscuit (Nabisco) | 2 | 120 |
| Santa Fe Oatmeal Raisin (Pepperidge Farm) | 1 | 100 |

| Protein (g) | Carbohydrates (g) | Fat (g) | Sodium (mg) | Cholesterol (mg) | Fiber (g) | Vitamin A (%) | Vitamin C (%) | Calcium (%) | Iron (%) |
|---|---|---|---|---|---|---|---|---|---|
| 1 | 21 | 4 | 95 | na | na | * | * | * | 2 |
| 3 | 18 | 6 | na | na | na | * | * | * | 2 |
| 3 | 22 | 8 | na | na | na | * | * | * | 2 |
| 3 | 29 | 7 | 200 | na | na | * | * | * | 4 |
| 2 | 24 | 6 | na | na | na | * | * | * | 4 |
| 2 | 19 | 5 | na | na | na | * | * | * | 4 |
| 1 | 15 | 5 | 115 | 10 | na | * | * | * | 2 |
| 1 | 17 | 7 | 60 | 5 | na | * | * | * | 2 |
| 2 | 22 | 7 | 210 | na | na | * | * | * | 4 |
| 1 | 18 | 7 | 165 | na | na | * | * | * | 2 |
| 0 | 11 | 6 | 30 | 0 | na | * | * | * | 2 |
| 1 | 14 | 8 | 40 | 0 | na | * | * | * | * |
| 3 | 16 | 7 | na | na | na | * | * | 2 | 2 |
| 3 | 19 | 9 | 229 | na | na | * | * | * | * |
| 2 | 19 | 9 | 135 | na | na | * | * | na | na |
| 2 | 20 | 7 | na | na | na | * | * | * | 4 |
| 2 | 17 | 10 | 85 | na | na | * | * | * | 2 |
| 1 | 7 | 5 | 15 | 0 | na | * | * | * | * |
| 1 | 21 | 6 | na | na | na | * | * | * | 2 |
| | | | | | | | | | |
| 1 | 8 | 4 | 20 | <5 | na | * | * | * | * |
| 0 | 9 | 4 | 35 | <5 | na | * | * | * | * |
| 1 | 24 | 2 | na | na | na | * | * | * | 4 |
| | | | | | | | | | |
| 1 | 16 | 4 | 70 | <5 | na | * | * | * | * |

| FOOD NAME | Serving Size | Calories |
|---|---|---|
| Sausalito Milk Chocolate Macadamia (Pepperidge Farm) | 1 | 120 |
| Shortbread (Pepperidge Farm) | 2 | 150 |
| Shortcake (Nabisco Melt Away) | 2 | 14 |
| Social Tea Biscuit | 6 | 130 |
| Spiced Wafers (Nabisco) | 4 | 130 |
| Strawberry (Pepperidge Farm) | 2 | 100 |
| Striped Shortbread (Nabisco) | 3 | 150 |
| Sugar, Slice 'n Bake (Pillsbury) | 3 | 180 |
| Sugar (Pepperidge Farm) | 2 | 100 |
| Sugar Rings (Nabisco) | 2 | 140 |
| Sugar Wafers (Nabisco) | 8 | 150 |
| Tahiti (Pepperidge Farm) | 1 | 90 |
| Twiddle Sticks (Nabisco) | 3 | 160 |
| Waffle Cremes (Nabisco) | 3 | 0 |
| Zurich (Pepperidge Farm) | 1 | 60 |
| CORN | | |
| Fresh, cooked | 1 cup | 140 |
| *Canned* | | |
| (Del Monte Golden Cream Style) | ½ cup | 80 |
| (Del Monte Golden Cream Style, No Salt Added) | ½ cup | 80 |
| (Green Giant Cream Style) | ½ cup | 100 |
| (Green Giant Delicorn) | ½ cup | 80 |
| (Green Giant Mexicorn) | ½ cup | 70 |

| Protein (g) | Carbohydrates (g) | Fat (g) | Sodium (mg) | Cholesterol (mg) | Fiber (g) | Vitamin A (%) | Vitamin C (%) | Calcium (%) | Iron (%) |
|---|---|---|---|---|---|---|---|---|---|
| 1 | 14 | 7 | 65 | 5 | na | * | * | * | * |
| 1 | 17 | 8 | 85 | <5 | na | * | * | * | * |
| 2 | 16 | 7 | na | na | na | * | * | * | * |
| 2 | 21 | 4 | na | na | na | * | * | * | 4 |
| 2 | 24 | 3 | 228 | na | na | * | * | * | 4 |
| 1 | 15 | 5 | 50 | 10 | 0 | * | * | * | * |
| 1 | 19 | 7 | 80 | na | na | * | * | * | 2 |
| 1 | 23 | 9 | 210 | na | na | * | * | 2 | 2 |
| 1 | 13 | 5 | 55 | 10 | 0 | * | * | * | * |
| 2 | 21 | 5 | na | na | na | * | * | * | 4 |
| 2 | 21 | 7 | na | na | na | * | * | * | 2 |
| 0 | 9 | 6 | 25 | 5 | na | * | * | * | * |
| 0 | 21 | 8 | na | na | na | * | * | * | 2 |
| 130 | 18 | 6 | na | na | na | * | * | * | 2 |
| 1 | 10 | 2 | 30 | 0 | na | * | * | * | * |
| 6 | 21 | 1 | 14 | 0 | 3 | 15 | 20 | * | 6 |
| 2 | 18 | 1 | 355 | na | na | 2 | 8 | * | 2 |
| 2 | 20 | 1 | <10 | na | na | 2 | 10 | * | 2 |
| 2 | 24 | <1 | 480 | 0 | 2 | 2 | 4 | * | * |
| 2 | 19 | <1 | 350 | 0 | 2 | 6 | * | * | 2 |
| 2 | 18 | <1 | 580 | 0 | 3 | * | * | * | 2 |

| FOOD NAME | Serving Size | Calories |
|---|---|---|
| (Green Giant Niblets) | ½ cup | 80 |
| (Green Giant Niblets No Salt/No Sugar Added) | ½ cup | 80 |
| (Green Giant Sweet Select) | ½ cup | 60 |
| (Green Giant White) | ½ cup | 80 |
| (Green Giant Whole Kernel Golden Sweet) | ½ cup | 70 |
| (Green Giant Whole Kernel Sweet, 50% Less Salt) | ½ cup | 70 |
| *Frozen* | | |
| (Birds Eye Baby Cob) | 2.6 oz | 25 |
| (Birds Eye Big Ears on the Cob) | 1 ear | 160 |
| (Birds Eye Little Ears on the Cob) | 2 ears | 130 |
| (Birds Eye On the Cob) | 1 ear | 120 |
| (Birds Eye Petite Kernel) | 2.6 oz | 70 |
| (Birds Eye Sweet) | 3.3 oz | 80 |
| (Birds Eye Tender Sweet) | 3.3 oz | 80 |
| (Birds Eye Tender Sweet in Butter Sauce) | 3.3 oz | 90 |
| (Green Giant Niblets) | ½ cup | 80 |
| (Green Giant On the Cob, Nibblers) | 2 ears | 120 |
| (Green Giant On the Cob, Niblet Ears) | 1 ear | 120 |
| (Green Giant On the Cob, Sweet Select Ears) | 1 ear | 90 |
| (Green Giant On the Cob, Sweet Select Half Ears) | 2 ears | 90 |

| Protein (g) | Carbohydrates (g) | Fat (g) | Sodium (mg) | Cholesterol (mg) | Fiber (g) | Vitamin A (%) | Vitamin C (%) | Calcium (%) | Iron (%) |
|---|---|---|---|---|---|---|---|---|---|
| 2 | 20 | 0 | 310 | 0 | 2 | 4 | 10 | * | 2 |
| | | | | | | | | | |
| 2 | 18 | <1 | 0 | 0 | 2 | 2 | * | * | 2 |
| 2 | 15 | <1 | 280 | 0 | <1 | 2 | * | * | 2 |
| 2 | 20 | 0 | 310 | 0 | 2 | * | 15 | * | 2 |
| | | | | | | | | | |
| 2 | 18 | 0 | 360 | 0 | 2 | 2 | 6 | * | 2 |
| | | | | | | | | | |
| 2 | 16 | <1 | 180 | 0 | 2 | * | 4 | * | * |
| | | | | | | | | | |
| 2 | 4 | 0 | 10 | 0 | 2 | * | 6 | * | * |
| 5 | 37 | 1 | 0 | 0 | na | 6 | 15 | * | 6 |
| 4 | 30 | 1 | 0 | 0 | na | 6 | 15 | * | 4 |
| 4 | 29 | 1 | 0 | 0 | na | 6 | 15 | * | 4 |
| 2 | 16 | 1 | 0 | 0 | 2 | 4 | 6 | * | 2 |
| 3 | 20 | 1 | 0 | 0 | 2 | 4 | 8 | * | 2 |
| 3 | 20 | 1 | 0 | 0 | 2 | 4 | 8 | * | 2 |
| 2 | 17 | 2 | 250 | 5 | 2 | 8 | 6 | * | * |
| 2 | 17 | 1 | 40 | 0 | 2 | * | 6 | * | * |
| 4 | 27 | 1 | 10 | 0 | 2 | 2 | 8 | * | 4 |
| 4 | 27 | 1 | 10 | 0 | 2 | 2 | 8 | * | 4 |
| | | | | | | | | | |
| 3 | 19 | 2 | 10 | 0 | 2 | 4 | 4 | * | 2 |
| | | | | | | | | | |
| 3 | 19 | 2 | 10 | 0 | 2 | 4 | 4 | * | 2 |

| FOOD NAME | Serving Size | Calories |
|---|---|---|
| (Green Giant Shoepeg White) | ½ cup | 90 |
| (Green Giant Cream Style) | ½ cup | 110 |
| (Green Giant Niblets in Butter Sauce) | ½ cup | 100 |
| (Green Giant Shoepeg White in Butter Sauce) | ½ cup | 100 |
| *Frozen combinations* | | |
| (Birds Eye Broccoli, Corn and Red Peppers) | 4 oz | 60 |
| CORN CHIPS | | |
| Flavor Tree | 1 oz | 150 |
| Bugles | 1 oz | 150 |
| Bugles Nacho Cheese | 1 oz | 160 |
| Cheetos | 1 oz | 160 |
| Cheez Doodles, Crunchy | 1 oz | 160 |
| Cheez Doodles, Puffed | 1 oz | 160 |
| Diggers (Nabisco) | 1 oz | 150 |
| Korkers | 1 oz | 160 |
| Sticks (Flavor Tree) | 1 oz | 160 |
| Doo Dads | 1 oz | 140 |
| Doritos | 1 oz | 140 |
| Doritos Taco-Flavored | 1 oz | 140 |
| Tortilla (Nabisco) | 1 oz | 150 |
| Tortilla (Old El Paso) | 1 oz | 170 |
| Tortilla Nacho Cheese (Lite-Line) | 1 oz | 130 |
| Tortilla Nacho Cheese (Nabisco) | 1 oz | 150 |

| Protein (g) | Carbohydrates (g) | Fat (g) | Sodium (mg) | Cholesterol (mg) | Fiber (g) | Vitamin A (%) | Vitamin C (%) | Calcium (%) | Iron (%) |
|---|---|---|---|---|---|---|---|---|---|
| 3 | 19 | 1 | 60 | 0 | 2 | * | 10 | * | * |
| 3 | 25 | 1 | 370 | 0 | 2.5 | 2 | 8 | * | * |
| 3 | 19 | 2 | 310 | 5 | 2 | * | 4 | * | 2 |
| 2 | 20 | 2 | 280 | 5 | 2 | * | 8 | * | 10 |
| 3 | 14 | 1 | 15 | 0 | 3 | 35 | 60 | 2 | 4 |
| 2 | 17 | 8 | 260 | na | na | * | * | 4 | 2 |
| 2 | 18 | 8 | 335 | na | na | * | * | * | 4 |
| 2 | 16 | 10 | 285 | na | na | * | * | * | 4 |
| 2 | 15 | 10 | 260 | na | na | * | * | * | 4 |
| 2 | 16 | 10 | na | na | na | 4 | 4 | 2 | 4 |
| 2 | 16 | 10 | na | na | na | 6 | 6 | 2 | 4 |
| 2 | 17 | 9 | na | na | na | * | * | * | * |
| 2 | 16 | 10 | na | na | na | * | * | 2 | 2 |
| 2 | 15 | 10 | 220 | na | na | * | * | 2 | 2 |
| 3 | 17 | 7 | 380 | na | na | * | * | 2 | 4 |
| 2 | 19 | 7 | 230 | 0 | na | * | * | 2 | 2 |
| 2 | 18 | 7 | 185 | na | na | 2 | * | 2 | 2 |
| 2 | 19 | 7 | na | na | na | * | * | 4 | 2 |
| 3 | 17 | 10 | 111 | 0 | na | * | * | 4 | 4 |
| 2 | 19 | 5 | 165 | na | na | * | * | 4 | 2 |
| 2 | 17 | 8 | na | na | na | * | * | 4 | 2 |

| FOOD NAME | Serving Size | Calories |
|---|---|---|
| Tortilla Nacho Cheese (Wise) | 1 oz | 150 |
| Tortilla Sour Cream and Onion (Nabisco) | 1 oz | 150 |
| COUSCOUS  Cooked | ½ cup | 100 |
| COWPEAS  Cooked | 1 cup | 190 |
| CRABMEAT | | |
| Canned | 3 oz | 90 |
| Fresh, cooked | 1 cup | 144 |
| CRACKERS | | |
| Arrowroot Biscuit | 6 | 130 |
| Bacon 'n Dip (Nabisco) | 17 | 150 |
| Butter Flavored Thins (Nabisco) | 4 | 70 |
| Buttery Flavored Sesame Snack (Nabisco) | 1 oz | 150 |
| Cheddar Snacks (Ralston) | 18 | 130 |
| Cheddar Triangles (Nabisco) | 1 oz | 150 |
| Cheese Nips (Nabisco) | 1 oz | 140 |
| Cheese Peanut Butter Sandwich (Nabisco) | 1 oz | 140 |
| Cheese Snacks (Ralston) | 25 | 140 |
| Cheese Tid-Bits (Nabisco) | 1 oz | 150 |
| Chicken in a Biskit (Nabisco) | 1 oz | 150 |
| Chippers (Nabisco) | 1 oz | 150 |
| Cracked Wheat (Pepperidge Farm) | 3 | 100 |
| Crown Pilot (Nabisco) | 1 oz | 150 |
| Dip in a Chip (Nabisco) | 1 oz | 150 |
| Dixies (Nabisco) | 1 oz | 140 |
| English Water Biscuits (Pepperidge Farm) | 4 | 70 |

| Protein (g) | Carbohydrates (g) | Fat (g) | Sodium (mg) | Cholesterol (mg) | Fiber (g) | Vitamin A (%) | Vitamin C (%) | Calcium (%) | Iron (%) |
|---|---|---|---|---|---|---|---|---|---|
| 4 | 17 | 8 | na | na | na | 2 | * | 6 | 2 |
| 3 | 18 | 7 | na | na | na | * | * | 4 | 2 |
| 4 | 20 | 0 | na | 0 | na | na | na | na | na |
| 18 | 35 | 1 | 20 | 0 | 3.2 | * | * | 4 | 20 |
| | | | | | | | | | |
| 20 | 1 | 2 | 850 | na | 0 | 20 | * | 4 | 4 |
| 27 | 1 | 3 | 325 | 115 | 0 | 67 | 5 | 7 | 7 |
| | | | | | | | | | |
| 2 | 21 | 4 | 100 | 0 | 0 | * | * | * | 2 |
| 2 | 16 | 8 | na | na | na | * | * | 2 | 4 |
| 1 | 10 | 3 | 115 | <5 | 0 | * | * | * | * |
| 3 | 17 | 8 | na | na | na | * | * | 2 | 4 |
| 3 | 20 | 5 | 320 | na | na | * | * | 2 | 4 |
| 3 | 16 | 8 | na | na | na | * | * | 4 | 2 |
| 3 | 18 | 6 | 130 | <2 | na | * | * | 2 | 4 |
| 3 | 17 | 6 | 300 | 0 | na | * | * | 4 | 4 |
| 3 | 18 | 7 | 330 | na | na | * | * | 2 | 4 |
| 2 | 16 | 9 | 400 | 4 | na | * | * | 4 | 4 |
| 2 | 16 | 9 | 260 | na | na | * | * | * | 4 |
| 2 | 17 | 8 | na | na | na | * | * | 2 | 4 |
| 2 | 14 | 4 | 180 | 0 | 0 | * | * | * | * |
| 3 | 26 | 4 | na | na | na | * | * | * | 6 |
| 2 | 16 | 8 | na | na | na | * | * | 2 | 4 |
| 2 | 17 | 7 | na | na | na | * | * | * | 4 |
| 2 | 13 | 1 | 100 | 0 | na | * | * | * | * |

| FOOD NAME | Serving Size | Calories |
|---|---|---|
| Escort (Nabisco) | 7 | 150 |
| Flutters Garden Herb (Pepperidge Farm) | ¾ oz | 100 |
| Flutters Golden Sesame (Pepperidge Farm) | ¾ oz | 110 |
| Flutters Original Butter (Pepperidge Farm) | ¾ oz | 100 |
| Flutters Toasted Wheat (Pepperidge Farm) | ¾ oz | 110 |
| French Onion | 12 | 150 |
| Goldfish Cheddar Cheese (Pepperidge Farm) | 1 oz | 120 |
| Goldfish Cheese Thins (Pepperidge Farm) | 4 | 50 |
| Goldfish Low Salt Cheddar Cheese (Pepperidge Farm) | 1 oz | 120 |
| Goldfish Original (Pepperidge Farm) | 1 oz | 130 |
| Goldfish Parmesan Cheese (Pepperidge Farm) | 1 oz | 120 |
| Goldfish Pizza Flavored (Pepperidge Farm) | 1 oz | 130 |
| Goldfish Pretzel (Pepperidge Farm) | 1 oz | 110 |
| Graham | 2 | 55 |
| Hearty Wheat (Pepperidge Farm) | 4 | 100 |
| Meal Mates (Nabisco) | 1 oz | 130 |
| Melba Toast (Old London) | 3 | 50 |
| Melba Toast, Bacon (Old London) | 5 | 60 |

| Protein (g) | Carbohydrates (g) | Fat (g) | Sodium (mg) | Cholesterol (mg) | Fiber (g) | Vitamin A (%) | Vitamin C (%) | Calcium (%) | Iron (%) |
|---|---|---|---|---|---|---|---|---|---|
| 2 | 18 | 8 | 240 | na | na | * | * | * | 4 |
| 2 | 14 | 4 | 190 | 0 | na | * | * | * | * |
| 2 | 13 | 5 | 150 | 0 | na | * | * | * | * |
| 2 | 15 | 4 | 150 | 5 | na | * | * | * | * |
| 2 | 13 | 5 | 170 | 0 | na | * | * | * | * |
| 2 | 18 | 7 | 280 | 0 | 0 | * | * | 4 | 4 |
| 4 | 19 | 4 | 230 | 5 | na | * | * | 4 | 2 |
| 1 | 8 | 2 | 160 | 0 | na | * | * | * | * |
| 4 | 19 | 4 | 130 | 5 | na | * | * | 4 | 2 |
| 3 | 18 | 5 | 190 | 0 | na | * | * | * | * |
| 4 | 19 | 4 | 330 | <5 | na | * | * | 6 | * |
| 4 | 19 | 5 | 220 | <5 | na | * | 2 | * | 4 |
| 3 | 20 | 3 | 160 | 0 | na | * | 2 | * | 2 |
| 1 | 10 | 1 | 96 | 0 | 1 | * | * | 1 | 3 |
| 2 | 13 | 5 | 140 | 0 | na | * | * | * | 2 |
| 3 | 19 | 5 | na | na | na | * | * | 6 | 4 |
| 2 | 10 | 0 | 0 | 0 | 2 | * | * | * | 2 |
| 2 | 9 | 2 | 126 | 0 | 1 | * | * | * | 2 |

| FOOD NAME | Serving Size | Calories | |
|---|---|---|---|
| Melba Toast, Cheese (Old London) | 5 | 60 | |
| Melba Toast, Garlic (Old London) | 5 | 50 | |
| Melba Toast, Onion (Old London) | 5 | 50 | |
| Melba Toast, Pumpernickel (Old London) | 3 | 50 | |
| Melba Toast, Rye (Old London) | 3 | 50 | |
| Melba Toast, Sesame (Old London) | 5 | 55 | |
| Melba Toast, White (Old London) | 5 | 50 | |
| Melba Toast, Whole Grain (Old London) | 3 | 60 | |
| Milk (Nabisco) | 2 | 110 | |
| Oysterettes | 36 | 120 | |
| Rich & Crisp (Ralston) | 10 | 140 | |
| Ritz (Nabisco) | 9 | 150 | |
| RyKrisp, natural | 2 | 50 | |
| RyKrisp, seasoned | 2 | 60 | |
| RyKrisp, sesame | 2 | 60 | |
| Saltines (Nabisco) | 10 | 122 | |
| Sea Rounds (Nabisco) | 2 | 90 | |
| Sesame | 4 | 80 | |
| Sesame Wheats! (Nabisco) | 9 | 150 | |
| *Snack Mix* | | | |
| Classic (Pepperidge Farm) | 1 oz | 140 | |
| Lightly Smoked (Pepperidge Farm) | 1 oz | 150 | |
| Spicy (Pepperidge Farm) | 1 oz | 140 | |
| *Snack Sticks* | | | |
| Pretzel (Pepperidge Farm) | 8 | 120 | |

| Protein (g) | Carbohydrates (g) | Fat (g) | Sodium (mg) | Cholesterol (mg) | Fiber (g) | Vitamin A (%) | Vitamin C (%) | Calcium (%) | Iron (%) |
|---|---|---|---|---|---|---|---|---|---|
| 2 | 9 | 2 | na | 0 | na | * | * | * | 2 |
| 2 | 9 | 1 | 132 | 0 | 0.6 | * | * | * | 2 |
| 2 | 9 | 1 | 120 | 0 | 0.7 | * | * | * | 2 |
| 2 | 10 | 0 | 150 | 0 | 0.8 | * | * | * | 2 |
| 2 | 10 | 0 | 130 | 0 | 0.8 | * | * | * | 2 |
| 2 | 8 | 2 | 150 | 0 | 0.9 | * | * | 2 | 4 |
| 2 | 10 | <1 | 111 | 0 | 0.8 | na | na | na | na |
| 2 | 10 | 1 | 116 | 0 | 0.9 | * | * | * | 2 |
| 2 | 16 | 4 | 140 | <2 | 0 | * | * | 4 | 4 |
| 3 | 20 | 3 | 440 | na | na | * | * | * | 6 |
| 2 | 19 | 6 | 300 | na | na | * | * | 2 | 4 |
| 2 | 18 | 8 | 270 | na | na | * | * | 4 | 4 |
| 1 | 10 | 0 | 110 | na | na | * | * | * | 2 |
| 1 | 9 | 1 | 220 | na | na | * | * | * | 2 |
| 1 | 10 | 2 | 220 | na | na | * | * | * | 2 |
| 2 | 20 | 2 | 312 | <2 | 1 | * | * | 1 | 7 |
| 2 | 15 | 2 | na | na | na | * | * | 2 | 6 |
| 2 | 12 | 4 | 140 | 0 | 0 | * | * | * | 2 |
| 2 | 16 | 9 | 250 | na | na | * | * | 4 | 6 |
| | | | | | | | | | |
| 4 | 14 | 8 | 360 | 0 | na | * | * | 4 | 4 |
| 4 | 13 | 9 | 350 | 0 | na | * | * | 4 | 2 |
| 4 | 14 | 8 | 340 | <5 | na | * | * | 2 | * |
| | | | | | | | | | |
| 3 | 23 | 3 | 430 | 0 | na | * | * | * | * |

| FOOD NAME | Serving Size | Calories |
|---|---|---|
| Pumpernickel (Pepperidge Farm) | 8 | 140 |
| Sesame (Pepperidge Farm) | 8 | 140 |
| Three Cheese (Pepperidge Farm) | 8 | 130 |
| Snacks Ahoy (Nabisco) | 15 | 140 |
| Sociables (Nabisco) | 14 | 150 |
| Swiss Cheese (Nabisco) | 15 | 150 |
| Triscuits (Nabisco) | 7 | 140 |
| Twigs (Nabisco) | 1 oz | 140 |
| Uneeda Biscuits (Nabisco) | 6 | 130 |
| Vegetable Thins (Nabisco) | 13 | 150 |
| Waverly Wafers (Nabisco) | 8 | 140 |
| Wheat, Toasted (Pepperidge Farm) | 4 | 80 |
| Wheat Snacks (Ralston) | 15 | 130 |
| Wheat Thins (Nabisco) | 16 | 140 |
| Wheatsworth (Nabisco) | 9 | 130 |
| Zwieback | 4 | 120 |
| CRANBERRIES  Raw | 1 cup | 100 |
| CRANBERRY DRINK | | |
| Cranberry Juice Cocktail (Ocean Spray) | 6 fl oz | 110 |
| Cranberry Juice Cocktail, Low Calorie (Ocean Spray) | 6 fl oz | 35 |
| Cranberry Juice Cocktail, frozen (Ocean Spray) | 6 fl oz | 110 |
| Cranberry Juice Cocktail, frozen (Welch's) | 6 fl oz | 100 |

| Protein (g) | Carbohydrates (g) | Fat (g) | Sodium (mg) | Cholesterol (mg) | Fiber (g) | Vitamin A (%) | Vitamin C (%) | Calcium (%) | Iron (%) |
|---|---|---|---|---|---|---|---|---|---|
| 3 | 20 | 6 | 330 | 0 | na | * | * | * | 4 |
| 4 | 19 | 5 | 280 | 0 | na | * | * | 6 | 4 |
| 4 | 19 | 5 | 400 | 0 | na | * | * | 4 | * |
| 2 | 17 | 7 | na | na | na | * | * | * | 2 |
| 3 | 18 | 7 | 330 | na | na | * | * | 4 | 6 |
| 3 | 17 | 8 | 330 | <2 | 0 | * | * | 4 | 4 |
| 3 | 21 | 5 | 180 | na | na | * | * | * | 4 |
| 3 | 16 | 7 | na | na | na | * | * | 6 | 6 |
| 3 | 22 | 4 | 230 | na | na | * | * | * | 8 |
| 2 | 17 | 8 | 300 | <2 | 0 | * | * | 4 | 4 |
| 2 | 21 | 6 | na | na | na | * | * | 4 | 4 |
| 2 | 12 | 3 | 140 | 0 | 1 | * | * | * | * |
| 2 | 19 | 6 | 200 | na | na | * | * | * | 4 |
| 2 | 19 | 6 | 240 | <2 | 0 | * | * | * | 4 |
| 3 | 16 | 6 | 330 | <2 | 0 | * | * | 2 | 6 |
| 3 | 21 | 3 | 80 | <2 | 0 | * | * | * | 4 |
| 2 | 26 | Tr | 2 | 0 | 1.2 | * | 15 | 2 | 2 |
| 0 | 26 | 0 | <10 | 0 | 0 | * | 100 | * | * |
| 0 | 9 | 0 | <10 | 0 | 0 | * | 100 | * | * |
| 0 | 28 | 0 | <10 | 0 | 0 | * | 100 | * | * |
| 0 | 26 | 0 | na | 0 | 0 | * | 45 | * | * |

| FOOD NAME | Serving Size | Calories |
|---|---|---|
| Cranberry Apple (Ocean Spray) | 6 fl oz | 130 |
| Cranberry Apple, Low Calorie (Ocean Spray) | 6 fl oz | 30 |
| Cranberry Apple, frozen (Ocean Spray) | 6 fl oz | 120 |
| Cranberry Apple, frozen (Welch's) | 6 fl oz | 120 |
| Cranberry Apricot (Ocean Spray) | 6 fl oz | 110 |
| Cranberry Grape (Ocean Spray) | 6 fl oz | 110 |
| Cranberry Grape, frozen (Welch's) | 6 fl oz | 110 |
| Cranberry Orange, frozen (Ocean Spray) | 6 fl oz | 100 |
| CREAM | | |
| Half and Half | 1 cup | 315 |
| Half and Half | 1 tbsp | 20 |
| Light, Coffee or Table | 1 cup | 469 |
| Light, Coffee or Table | 1 tbsp | 29 |
| Whipping, Heavy | 1 cup | 821 |
| Whipping, Heavy | 1 tbsp | 52 |
| Whipping, Light | 1 cup | 699 |
| Whipping, Light | 1 tbsp | 44 |
| CREAMER, NONDAIRY | | |
| Coffee-mate | 1 tsp | 11 |
| Cremora | 1 tsp | 12 |
| CROISSANT  (Pepperidge Farm) | 1 | 170 |
| CROUTONS | | |
| Cheddar & Romano Cheese (Pepperidge Farm) | ½ oz | 60 |

| Protein (g) | Carbohydrates (g) | Fat (g) | Sodium (mg) | Cholesterol (mg) | Fiber (g) | Vitamin A (%) | Vitamin C (%) | Calcium (%) | Iron (%) |
|---|---|---|---|---|---|---|---|---|---|
| 0 | 32 | 0 | <10 | 0 | 0 | * | 100 | * | * |
| | | | | | | | | | |
| 0 | 7 | 0 | <10 | 0 | 0 | * | 100 | * | * |
| 0 | 29 | 0 | <10 | 0 | 0 | * | 100 | * | * |
| 0 | 30 | 0 | 0 | 0 | 0 | * | 45 | * | * |
| 0 | 26 | 0 | <10 | 0 | 0 | * | * | * | * |
| 0 | 26 | 0 | <10 | 0 | 0 | * | 100 | * | * |
| 0 | 27 | 0 | 0 | 0 | 0 | * | 45 | * | * |
| 0 | 25 | 0 | <10 | 0 | 0 | * | 100 | * | * |
| | | | | | | | | | |
| 7 | 10 | 28 | 98 | 89 | 0 | 25 | 4 | 25 | * |
| Tr | <1 | <2 | 6 | 6 | 0 | 2 | * | 2 | * |
| 7 | 9 | 46 | 95 | 159 | 0 | 40 | 4 | 25 | * |
| Tr | <1 | 3 | 6 | 10 | 0 | 2 | * | 2 | * |
| 5 | 7 | 88 | 89 | 326 | 0 | 70 | 4 | 20 | * |
| Tr | Tr | 6 | 6 | 21 | 0 | 4 | * | 2 | * |
| 5 | 7 | 74 | 82 | 265 | 0 | 60 | 4 | 20 | * |
| Tr | Tr | 5 | 5 | 17 | 0 | 4 | * | 2 | * |
| | | | | | | | | | |
| 0 | 1 | 1 | 4 | 0 | 0 | * | * | * | * |
| 0 | 1 | 1 | 5 | 0 | 0 | * | * | * | * |
| 4 | 22 | 7 | 250 | 0 | Tr | 6 | * | 6 | 6 |
| | | | | | | | | | |
| | | | | | | | | | |
| 2 | 10 | 2 | 200 | 0 | na | * | * | 2 | 4 |

| FOOD NAME | Serving Size | Calories |
|---|---|---|
| Cheese & Garlic (Pepperidge Farm) | ½ oz | 70 |
| Onion & Garlic (Pepperidge Farm) | ½ oz | 70 |
| Seasoned (Pepperidge Farm) | ½ oz | 70 |
| Sour Cream & Chive (Pepperidge Farm) | ½ oz | 70 |
| CUCUMBER  Raw | 1 cup | 16 |
| CURRANTS | ½ cup | 200 |
| DANISH | | |
| Apple (Pepperidge Farm) | 1 | 220 |
| Apple (Sara Lee) | 1 | 120 |
| Cheese (Awrey's) | 1 | 280 |
| Cheese (Pepperidge Farm) | 1 | 240 |
| Cinnamon Raisin (Awrey's) | 1 | 290 |
| Cinnamon Raisin (Pepperidge Farm) | 1 | 250 |
| Raspberry (Pepperidge Farm) | 1 | 220 |
| DATES  Pitted, chopped | 1 cup | 490 |
| DIET BAR | | |
| Chocolate (Figurines) | 1 | 100 |
| Chocolate Caramel (Figurines) | 1 | 100 |
| Chocolate Peanut Butter (Figurines) | 1 | 100 |
| Granola & Apple (Nature Valley) | 1 | 140 |
| Granola & Date (Nature Valley) | 1 | 140 |
| Granola & Raspberry (Nature Valley) | 1 | 150 |
| Granola Almond (Nature Valley) | 1 | 110 |
| Granola Cinnamon (Nature Valley) | 1 | 110 |

| Protein (g) | Carbohydrates (g) | Fat (g) | Sodium (mg) | Cholesterol (mg) | Fiber (g) | Vitamin A (%) | Vitamin C (%) | Calcium (%) | Iron (%) |
|---|---|---|---|---|---|---|---|---|---|
| 2 | 9 | 3 | 180 | 0 | na | * | * | 2 | 2 |
| 2 | 9 | 3 | 160 | 0 | na | * | * | * | 2 |
| 2 | 9 | 3 | 180 | 0 | na | * | * | 2 | 2 |
| 2 | 9 | 3 | 170 | 0 | na | * | * | 2 | 2 |
| 2 | 4 | Tr | 6 | 0 | 1 | 6 | 20 | 2 | 6 |
| 2 | 53 | 0 | <10 | 0 | 2 | * | 4 | 6 | 10 |
| 2 | 35 | 8 | 130 | na | na | * | * | 4 | 4 |
| 2 | 15 | 6 | 120 | na | na | * | * | na | na |
| 3 | 34 | 15 | 350 | 5 | 1 | * | * | na | na |
| 3 | 25 | 14 | 230 | na | na | * | * | 4 | 6 |
| 3 | 41 | 12 | 280 | 15 | 1 | * | * | na | na |
| 3 | 35 | 11 | 170 | na | na | * | * | 4 | 4 |
| 3 | 31 | 9 | 140 | na | na | 4 | * | 4 | 8 |
| 10 | 130 | 1 | 2 | 0 | 8 | 2 | * | 10 | 30 |
| 2 | 11 | 5 | 50 | 0 | 1 | 10 | 15 | 6 | 15 |
| 2 | 11 | 6 | 65 | 0 | 1 | 10 | 15 | 6 | 10 |
| 3 | 10 | 6 | 50 | 0 | 1 | 10 | 15 | 6 | 15 |
| 2 | 25 | 4 | 150 | na | na | * | * | * | 4 |
| 2 | 25 | 4 | 130 | na | na | * | * | 2 | 4 |
| 2 | 25 | 5 | 160 | na | na | * | * | * | 2 |
| 2 | 16 | 4 | 80 | na | na | * | * | * | 4 |
| 2 | 16 | 4 | 65 | na | na | * | * | * | 4 |

| FOOD NAME | Serving Size | Calories |
|---|---|---|
| Granola Coconut (Nature Valley) | 1 | 120 |
| Granola Oats 'n Honey (Nature Valley) | 1 | 110 |
| S'mores (Figurines) | 1 | 100 |
| Vanilla (Figurines) | 1 | 100 |
| **DIET DRINK** | | |
| Berry Blend (Crystal Light) | 8 fl oz | 4 |
| Citrus Blend (Crystal Light) | 8 fl oz | 4 |
| Decaffeinated Iced Tea (Crystal Light) | 8 fl oz | 4 |
| Fruit Punch (Crystal Light) | 8 fl oz | 4 |
| Iced Tea (Crystal Light) | 8 fl oz | 4 |
| Lemonade (Crystal Light) | 8 fl oz | 4 |
| Lemon-Lime (Crystal Light) | 8 fl oz | 4 |
| Pink Lemonade (Country Time) | 8 fl oz | 4 |
| **DIPS** | | |
| Avocado (Kraft) | 2 tbsp | 50 |
| Bacon & Horseradish (Kraft) | 2 tbsp | 60 |
| Bacon & Horseradish (Kraft Premium) | 2 tbsp | 50 |
| Bacon & Onion (Kraft Premium) | 2 tbsp | 60 |
| Blue Cheese (Kraft Premium) | 2 tbsp | 50 |
| Clam (Kraft) | 2 tbsp | 60 |
| Clam (Kraft Premium) | 2 tbsp | 45 |
| Creamy Cucumber (Kraft Premium) | 2 tbsp | 50 |
| Creamy Onion (Kraft Premium) | 2 tbsp | 45 |
| French Onion (Kraft) | 2 tbsp | 60 |
| French Onion (Kraft Premium) | 2 tbsp | 45 |

| Protein (g) | Carbohydrates (g) | Fat (g) | Sodium (mg) | Cholesterol (mg) | Fiber (g) | Vitamin A (%) | Vitamin C (%) | Calcium (%) | Iron (%) |
|---|---|---|---|---|---|---|---|---|---|
| 2 | 15 | 6 | 65 | na | na | * | * | * | 4 |
| 2 | 16 | 4 | 65 | na | na | * | * | * | 4 |
| 2 | 11 | 5 | 55 | 0 | 1 | 10 | 15 | 25 | 25 |
| 2 | 11 | 6 | 55 | 0 | 1 | 10 | 15 | 25 | 25 |
| | | | | | | | | | |
| 0 | 0 | 0 | 0 | 0 | 0 | * | 10 | * | * |
| 0 | 0 | 0 | 0 | 0 | 0 | * | 10 | * | * |
| 0 | 0 | 0 | 0 | 0 | 0 | * | 10 | * | * |
| 0 | 0 | 0 | 0 | 0 | 0 | * | 10 | * | * |
| 0 | 0 | 0 | 0 | 0 | 0 | * | 10 | * | * |
| 0 | 0 | 0 | 0 | 0 | 0 | * | 10 | * | * |
| 0 | 0 | 0 | 0 | 0 | 0 | * | 10 | * | * |
| 0 | 0 | 0 | 0 | 0 | 0 | * | 10 | * | * |
| | | | | | | | | | |
| 1 | 3 | 4 | 210 | 0 | na | * | * | * | * |
| 1 | 3 | 5 | 200 | 0 | na | * | * | * | * |
| 1 | 2 | 5 | 270 | 15 | na | 2 | * | 2 | * |
| 1 | 2 | 5 | 170 | 15 | na | 2 | * | 2 | * |
| 1 | 2 | 4 | 210 | 10 | na | 2 | * | 4 | * |
| 1 | 3 | 4 | 240 | 10 | na | * | * | * | * |
| 1 | 2 | 4 | 210 | 20 | na | 2 | * | 2 | * |
| 1 | 2 | 4 | 130 | 10 | na | 2 | * | 2 | * |
| 1 | 2 | 4 | 160 | 10 | na | 2 | * | 2 | * |
| 1 | 3 | 4 | 240 | 0 | na | 4 | * | * | * |
| 1 | 2 | 4 | 150 | 10 | na | * | * | 2 | * |

| FOOD NAME | Serving Size | Calories |
|---|---|---|
| Green Onion (Kraft) | 2 tbsp | 60 |
| Jalapeño Pepper (Kraft) | 2 tbsp | 50 |
| Jalapeño Cheese (Kraft Premium) | 2 tbsp | 50 |
| Nacho Cheese (Kraft Premium) | 2 tbsp | 55 |
| DONUT | | |
| Plain | 1 | 100 |
| Cinnamon (Hostess) | 1 | 110 |
| Glazed (Hostess) | 1 | 230 |
| Krunch (Hostess) | 1 | 110 |
| Powdered Sugar (Hostess) | 1 | 110 |
| DUCK | | |
| Roasted with skin | 4 oz | 382 |
| Roasted without skin | 4 oz | 228 |
| EEL  Cooked | 4 oz | 268 |
| EGG | | |
| Large, whole | 1 | 80 |
| Large, white only | 1 | 17 |
| Large, yolk only | 1 | 60 |
| Hard-boiled | 1 | 79 |
| Poached | 1 | 79 |
| Scrambled with milk | 1 | 79 |
| EGG SUBSTITUTE | | |
| (Morningstar Farm Scramblers) | ¼ cup | 60 |
| EGGPLANT  Boiled | 1 cup | 38 |
| ENDIVE  Raw, cut | 1 cup | 10 |

| Protein (g) | Carbohydrates (g) | Fat (g) | Sodium (mg) | Cholesterol (mg) | Fiber (g) | Vitamin A (%) | Vitamin C (%) | Calcium (%) | Iron (%) |
|---|---|---|---|---|---|---|---|---|---|
| 1 | 3 | 4 | 170 | 0 | na | * | * | * | * |
| 1 | 3 | 4 | 160 | 0 | na | * | 4 | * | * |
| 1 | 3 | 4 | 160 | 15 | na | 2 | * | 4 | * |
| 2 | 2 | 4 | 200 | 10 | na | 2 | 2 | 4 | * |
| 1 | 13 | 5 | 125 | 5 | na | * | * | 1 | 2 |
| 1 | 15 | 6 | 140 | 6 | na | * | * | 2 | 2 |
| 2 | 30 | 12 | 200 | 11 | na | 1 | * | 2 | 2 |
| 1 | 16 | 4 | 130 | 4 | na | * | * | 2 | 2 |
| 1 | 17 | 4 | 118 | 5 | na | * | * | * | 2 |
| 22 | 0 | 32 | 67 | 67 | 0 | 5 | * | 1 | 17 |
| 27 | 0 | 13 | 74 | 101 | 0 | 2 | * | 1 | 17 |
| 27 | 0 | 17 | 74 | 183 | 0 | na | na | na | na |
| 6 | <1 | 5 | 63 | 213 | 0 | 10 | * | 2 | 6 |
| <4 | Tr | 0 | 55 | 0 | 0 | * | * | * | * |
| <3 | Tr | 5 | 7 | 213 | 0 | 10 | * | 2 | 4 |
| 6 | <1 | 5 | 62 | 213 | 0 | 5 | * | 3 | 6 |
| 6 | <1 | 5 | 140 | 212 | 0 | 5 | * | 3 | 6 |
| 6 | 1 | 7 | na | 220 | 0 | 6 | * | 5 | 5 |
| 6 | 3 | 3 | 126 | 0 | 0 | 10 | * | 4 | 11 |
| 2 | 8 | 0 | 2 | 0 | 1 | * | 10 | 2 | 7 |
| <1 | 2 | Tr | 7 | 0 | 0.4 | 35 | 8 | 4 | 4 |

| FOOD NAME | Serving Size | Calories | |
|---|---|---|---|
| FAST FOOD | | | |
| *Arby's* | | | |
| Bac 'n Cheddar Deluxe | 1 | 532 | |
| Bacon Platter | 1 | 869 | |
| Baked Potato, Broccoli & Cheddar | 1 | 417 | |
| Baked Potato, Deluxe | 1 | 621 | |
| Baked Potato, Plain | 1 | 240 | |
| Beef 'n Cheddar | 1 | 451 | |
| Biscuit, Bacon | 1 | 318 | |
| Biscuit, Plain | 1 | 280 | |
| Biscuit, Sausage | 1 | 460 | |
| Blueberry Muffin | 1 | 200 | |
| Chicken Breast Sandwich | 1 | 489 | |
| Chicken Cordon Bleu | 1 | 658 | |
| Chicken Fajita Pita | 1 | 256 | |
| Croissant, Ham and Cheese | 1 | 345 | |
| Croissant, Mushroom and Cheese | 1 | 493 | |
| Croissant, Sausage and Egg | 1 | 519 | |
| Croissant, Plain | 1 | 260 | |
| Curly Fries | 1 | 337 | |
| Egg Platter | 1 | 460 | |
| Fish Fillet Sandwich | 1 | 537 | |
| French Dip Roast Beef Sandwich | 1 | 345 | |
| French Dip 'n Swiss Roast Beef Sandwich | 1 | 425 | |
| French Fries, large | 1 order | 492 | |

| Protein (g) | Carbohydrates (g) | Fat (g) | Sodium (mg) | Cholesterol (mg) | Fiber (g) | Vitamin A (%) | Vitamin C (%) | Calcium (%) | Iron (%) |
|---|---|---|---|---|---|---|---|---|---|
| 29 | 35 | 33 | 1672 | 83 | na | * | 2 | 15 | 25 |
| 17 | 49 | 32 | 1051 | 366 | na | 8 | 6 | 6 | 20 |
| 10 | 55 | 18 | 361 | 22 | na | 6 | 75 | 10 | 15 |
| 17 | 59 | 36 | 605 | 58 | na | 10 | 55 | 15 | 15 |
| 6 | 50 | 2 | 58 | 0 | na | * | 55 | * | 15 |
| 25 | 43 | 20 | 955 | 52 | na | 4 | * | 2 | 20 |
| 7 | 35 | 18 | 904 | 8 | na | * | * | 10 | 15 |
| 6 | 34 | 15 | 730 | 0 | na | * | * | 10 | 15 |
| 12 | 35 | 32 | 1000 | 60 | na | * | * | 10 | 20 |
| 3 | 34 | 6 | 269 | 22 | na | * | * | 4 | 6 |
| 23 | 48 | 26 | 1019 | 45 | na | * | 8 | 8 | 20 |
| 31 | 50 | 37 | 1824 | 65 | na | * | * | 15 | 20 |
| 15 | 32 | 9 | 787 | 33 | na | na | na | na | na |
| 16 | 29 | 21 | 939 | 90 | na | * | * | 15 | 15 |
| 13 | 34 | 38 | 935 | 116 | na | * | * | 20 | 15 |
| 17 | 29 | 39 | 632 | 271 | na | 4 | * | 6 | 20 |
| 6 | 28 | 16 | 300 | 49 | na | * | * | 4 | 15 |
| 4 | 43 | 18 | 167 | 0 | na | * | * | 2 | 8 |
| 15 | 45 | 24 | 591 | 346 | na | 8 | 6 | 6 | 20 |
| 21 | 47 | 29 | 994 | 79 | na | * | * | 8 | 20 |
| 24 | 34 | 12 | 678 | 5 | na | * | * | 2 | 15 |
| 30 | 36 | 18 | 1078 | 87 | na | 4 | * | 25 | 15 |
| 4 | 60 | 26 | 228 | 0 | na | * | 12 | * | 12 |

| FOOD NAME | Serving Size | Calories |
|---|---|---|
| French Fries, medium | 1 order | 394 |
| French Fries, small | 1 order | 246 |
| Grilled Chicken Barbecue | 1 | 378 |
| Grilled Chicken Deluxe | 1 | 426 |
| Ham Platter | 1 | 518 |
| Light Roast Beef Deluxe | 1 | 296 |
| Light Roast Chicken Deluxe | 1 | 253 |
| Light Roast Turkey Deluxe | 1 | 249 |
| Milk, 2% low-fat | 8 fl oz | 121 |
| Orange Juice | 6 fl oz | 82 |
| Philly Beef 'n Swiss | 1 | 498 |
| Potato Cakes | 1 order | 204 |
| Roast Beef, Giant | 1 | 530 |
| Roast Beef, Junior | 1 | 218 |
| Roast Beef, Regular | 1 | 353 |
| Roast Beef, Super | 1 | 529 |
| Roast Chicken Club | 1 | 513 |
| Roast Chicken Deluxe | 1 | 373 |
| Salad, Chef | 1 | 217 |
| Salad, Garden | 1 | 109 |
| Salad, Roast Chicken | 1 | 172 |
| Salad, Side | 1 | 25 |
| Sausage Platter | 1 | 640 |
| Shake, Chocolate | 1 | 451 |
| Shake, Jamocha | 1 | 368 |

| Protein (g) | Carbohydrates (g) | Fat (g) | Sodium (mg) | Cholesterol (mg) | Fiber (g) | Vitamin A (%) | Vitamin C (%) | Calcium (%) | Iron (%) |
|---|---|---|---|---|---|---|---|---|---|
| 3 | 48 | 21 | 182 | 0 | na | * | 10 | * | 10 |
| 2 | 30 | 13 | 114 | 0 | na | * | 6 | * | 6 |
| 21 | 44 | 14 | 1059 | 44 | na | * | * | 10 | 20 |
| 21 | 39 | 21 | 877 | 44 | na | * | * | 10 | 20 |
| 24 | 45 | 26 | 1177 | 374 | na | 8 | 6 | 6 | 20 |
| 18 | 33 | 10 | 826 | 42 | na | 6 | 2 | * | 20 |
| 17 | 33 | 5 | 874 | 39 | na | 6 | 2 | * | 20 |
| 19 | 33 | 4 | 1172 | 30 | na | 6 | 2 | * | 20 |
| 8 | 12 | 4 | 122 | 18 | na | 10 | 4 | 30 | * |
| 1 | 20 | 0 | 2 | 0 | na | * | 119 | * | * |
| 25 | 37 | 26 | 1194 | 91 | na | 6 | 4 | 30 | 20 |
| 2 | 20 | 12 | 397 | 0 | na | * | 15 | * | 8 |
| 36 | 41 | 27 | 908 | 78 | na | * | * | 6 | 35 |
| 13 | 21 | 11 | 345 | 23 | na | * | * | 2 | 10 |
| 22 | 32 | 15 | 588 | 39 | na | * | * | 4 | 20 |
| 33 | 46 | 28 | 798 | 47 | na | 6 | 2 | 6 | 25 |
| 31 | 40 | 29 | 1423 | 75 | na | * | * | 15 | 20 |
| 17 | 37 | 19 | 913 | 2 | na | * | * | 4 | 20 |
| 20 | 11 | 11 | 706 | 172 | na | 40 | 40 | 10 | 15 |
| 7 | 10 | 5 | 134 | 12 | na | 35 | 35 | 10 | 10 |
| 15 | 12 | 7 | 562 | 45 | na | na | na | na | na |
| 2 | 4 | 0 | 30 | 0 | na | 20 | 6 | 4 | 4 |
| 21 | 46 | 41 | 861 | 406 | na | 8 | 6 | 8 | 20 |
| 10 | 76 | 12 | 341 | 36 | na | 6 | * | 25 | 4 |
| 9 | 59 | 10 | 262 | 35 | na | 6 | * | 25 | * |

| FOOD NAME | Serving Size | Calories |
|---|---|---|
| Shake, Vanilla | 1 | 511 |
| Soup, Beef with Vegetables and Barley | 6 fl oz | 96 |
| Soup, Boston Clam Chowder | 6 fl oz | 207 |
| Soup, Cream of Broccoli | 6 fl oz | 180 |
| Soup, French Onion | 6 fl oz | 67 |
| Sub Deluxe | 1 | 482 |
| Turkey Deluxe | 1 | 399 |
| Turnover, Apple | 1 | 303 |
| Turnover, Blueberry | 1 | 320 |
| Turnover, Cherry | 1 | 280 |
| *Burger King* | | |
| Apple Pie | 1 | 311 |
| BK Broiler Chicken Sandwich | 1 | 267 |
| Bacon Double Cheeseburger | 1 | 515 |
| Bacon Double Cheeseburger Deluxe | 1 | 592 |
| Burger Buddies | 1 | 349 |
| Cheese, Processed American | 1 | 92 |
| Cheeseburger | 1 | 318 |
| Cheeseburger Deluxe | 1 | 390 |
| Chicken Sandwich, Fried | 1 | 685 |
| Chicken Tenders | 6 pc | 236 |
| Croissan'wich with Bacon, Egg and Cheese | 1 | 361 |
| Croissan'wich with Egg and Cheese | 1 | 315 |
| Croissan'wich with Ham, Egg and Cheese | 1 | 346 |
| Croissan'wich with Sausage, Egg and Cheese | 1 | 534 |

| Protein (g) | Carbohydrates (g) | Fat (g) | Sodium (mg) | Cholesterol (mg) | Fiber (g) | Vitamin A (%) | Vitamin C (%) | Calcium (%) | Iron (%) |
|---|---|---|---|---|---|---|---|---|---|
| 12 | 73 | 19 | 351 | 33 | na | 6 | * | 25 | * |
| 5 | 14 | 3 | 996 | 10 | na | 30 | 8 | 2 | 8 |
| 10 | 18 | 11 | 1157 | 28 | na | 10 | 6 | 20 | 10 |
| 8 | 19 | 8 | 1113 | 3 | na | 10 | 15 | 30 | 4 |
| 2 | 19 | 8 | 1113 | 0 | na | 2 | 4 | 2 | 4 |
| 24 | 38 | 26 | 1530 | 50 | na | * | 4 | 15 | 20 |
| 27 | 35 | 20 | 1047 | 39 | na | 6 | 8 | 8 | 15 |
| 4 | 27 | 18 | 178 | 0 | na | 2 | 2 | * | 4 |
| 3 | 32 | 19 | 240 | 0 | na | * | 10 | * | 4 |
| 5 | 25 | 18 | 200 | 0 | na | 0 | 8 | * | 4 |
| | | | | | | | | | |
| 3 | 44 | 14 | 412 | 4 | na | * | 8 | * | 7 |
| 22 | 28 | 8 | 728 | 45 | na | 4 | 6 | 5 | 14 |
| 32 | 26 | 31 | 748 | 105 | na | 8 | * | 18 | 21 |
| 33 | 28 | 39 | 804 | 111 | na | 12 | 5 | 18 | 21 |
| 18 | 31 | 17 | 717 | 52 | na | 9 | 8 | 11 | 19 |
| 5 | 1 | 7 | 312 | 25 | na | 8 | * | 14 | * |
| 17 | 28 | 15 | 661 | 50 | na | 7 | 5 | 11 | 15 |
| 18 | 29 | 23 | 652 | 56 | na | 10 | 9 | 11 | 15 |
| 26 | 56 | 40 | 1417 | 82 | na | 3 | 0 | 8 | 19 |
| 16 | 14 | 13 | 541 | 46 | na | * | * | * | 4 |
| 15 | 19 | 24 | 719 | 227 | na | 10 | * | 14 | 10 |
| 13 | 19 | 20 | 607 | 222 | na | 10 | * | 14 | 10 |
| 19 | 19 | 21 | 962 | 241 | na | 10 | * | 15 | 11 |
| 21 | 22 | 40 | 985 | 268 | na | 10 | * | 15 | 16 |

| FOOD NAME | Serving Size | Calories |
|---|---|---|
| Croissant, Plain | 1 | 180 |
| Double Cheeseburger | 1 | 483 |
| French Fries, medium | 1 order | 372 |
| French Toast Sticks | 1 order | 538 |
| Frozen Yogurt, Breyers Vanilla | 1 | 120 |
| Frozen Yogurt, Breyers Chocolate | 1 | 130 |
| Hamburger | 1 | 272 |
| Hamburger Deluxe | 1 | 344 |
| Milk, whole | 8 fl oz | 157 |
| Milk, 2% low-fat | 8 fl oz | 121 |
| Mini Muffins, Blueberry | 1 order | 292 |
| Ocean Catch Fish Filet | 1 | 495 |
| Onion Rings | 1 order | 339 |
| Orange Juice | 6 fl oz | 82 |
| Salad, Chef | 1 | 178 |
| Salad, Chunky Chicken | 1 | 142 |
| Salad, Garden | 1 | 95 |
| Salad, Side | 1 | 25 |
| Sausage Breakfast Buddy | 1 | 255 |
| Shake, Chocolate, large | 1 | 472 |
| Shake, Chocolate, large with syrup | 1 | 598 |
| Shake, Strawberry, large with syrup | 1 | 569 |
| Shake, Vanilla, regular | 1 | 345 |
| Shake, Vanilla, large | 1 | 483 |
| Snickers Ice Cream Bar | 1 | 220 |

| Protein (g) | Carbohydrates (g) | Fat (g) | Sodium (mg) | Cholesterol (mg) | Fiber (g) | Vitamin A (%) | Vitamin C (%) | Calcium (%) | Iron (%) |
|---|---|---|---|---|---|---|---|---|---|
| 4 | 18 | 10 | 285 | 4 | na | * | * | 3 | 6 |
| 30 | 29 | 27 | 851 | 100 | na | 11 | 5 | 18 | 21 |
| 5 | 43 | 20 | 238 | 0 | na | * | 5 | * | 7 |
| 10 | 53 | 32 | 537 | 80 | na | * | * | 8 | 16 |
| 2 | 20 | 3 | 40 | 10 | na | 2 | * | 8 | * |
| 3 | 21 | 3 | 40 | 10 | na | 2 | * | 8 | * |
| 15 | 28 | 11 | 505 | 37 | na | 3 | 5 | 4 | 15 |
| 15 | 28 | 19 | 496 | 43 | na | 5 | 9 | 4 | 15 |
| 8 | 11 | 9 | 119 | 35 | na | 7 | 6 | 29 | * |
| 8 | 12 | 5 | 122 | 18 | na | 10 | 4 | 30 | * |
| 4 | 37 | 14 | 244 | 72 | na | * | * | 4 | 7 |
| 20 | 49 | 25 | 879 | 57 | na | * | 4 | 6 | 14 |
| 5 | 38 | 19 | 628 | 0 | na | 15 | * | 11 | 3 |
| 1 | 20 | 0 | 2 | 0 | na | 3 | 100 | * | * |
| 17 | 7 | 9 | 568 | 103 | na | 95 | 25 | 16 | 9 |
| 20 | 8 | 4 | 443 | 49 | na | 92 | 34 | 4 | 7 |
| 6 | 8 | 5 | 125 | 15 | na | 100 | 58 | 15 | 6 |
| 1 | 5 | 0 | 27 | 0 | na | 88 | 20 | 3 | 3 |
| 11 | 15 | 16 | 492 | 127 | na | 5 | * | 8 | 10 |
| 13 | 71 | 15 | 286 | 45 | na | 10 | 6 | 45 | 6 |
| 14 | 103 | 14 | 357 | 44 | na | * | * | 42 | 2 |
| 12 | 99 | 14 | 319 | 44 | na | * | 2 | 43 | * |
| 9 | 53 | 11 | 220 | 34 | na | * | * | 32 | * |
| 13 | 74 | 15 | 308 | 47 | na | * | * | 44 | * |
| 5 | 20 | 14 | 65 | 15 | na | 2 | * | 6 | 2 |

| FOOD NAME | Serving Size | Calories | |
|---|---|---|---|
| Tater Tenders | 1 order | 213 | |
| Whopper | 1 | 614 | |
| Whopper with Cheese | 1 | 706 | |
| Whopper, Double | 1 | 844 | |
| Whopper, Double, with Cheese | 1 | 935 | |
| *Carl's Jr.* | | | |
| Bacon Strips | 2 | 45 | |
| Baked Potato, Bacon & Cheese | 1 | 730 | |
| Baked Potato, Broccoli & Cheese | 1 | 590 | |
| Baked Potato, Cheese | 1 | 690 | |
| Baked Potato, Fiesta | 1 | 720 | |
| Baked Potato, Lite | 1 | 290 | |
| Baked Potato, Sour Cream & Chive | 1 | 470 | |
| Breakfast Burrito | 1 | 430 | |
| Carl's Catch Fish Sandwich | 1 | 560 | |
| Charbroiler BBQ Chicken Sandwich | 1 | 310 | |
| Charbroiler Chicken Club Sandwich | 1 | 570 | |
| Chocolate Chip Cookie | 1 | 330 | |
| Cinnamon Roll | 1 | 460 | |
| Country Fried Steak Sandwich | 1 | 720 | |
| Danish | 1 | 520 | |
| Dog, All Star Chili | 1 | 720 | |
| Dog, All Star Hot | 1 | 540 | |
| Double Western Bacon Cheeseburger | 1 | 1030 | |
| English Muffin, with margarine | 1 | 190 | |

| Protein (g) | Carbohydrates (g) | Fat (g) | Sodium (mg) | Cholesterol (mg) | Fiber (g) | Vitamin A (%) | Vitamin C (%) | Calcium (%) | Iron (%) |
|---|---|---|---|---|---|---|---|---|---|
| 2 | 25 | 12 | 318 | 0 | na | 12 | 9 | * | 2 |
| 27 | 45 | 36 | 865 | 90 | na | 11 | 20 | 8 | 27 |
| 32 | 47 | 44 | 1177 | 115 | na | 19 | 20 | 22 | 27 |
| 46 | 45 | 53 | 933 | 169 | na | 11 | 20 | 9 | 40 |
| 51 | 47 | 61 | 1245 | 194 | na | 19 | 20 | 24 | 40 |
| | | | | | | | | | |
| 3 | 0 | 4 | 150 | 5 | na | * | 6 | * | * |
| 26 | 60 | 43 | 1670 | 45 | na | 15 | 85 | 20 | 20 |
| 18 | 60 | 31 | 830 | 25 | na | 20 | 90 | 30 | 30 |
| 23 | 70 | 36 | 1160 | 40 | na | 30 | 75 | 45 | 10 |
| 31 | 64 | 38 | 1470 | 15 | na | 45 | 100 | 30 | 30 |
| 9 | 60 | 1 | 60 | 0 | na | * | 50 | 4 | 15 |
| 11 | 64 | 19 | 180 | 20 | na | 30 | 2 | 10 | 15 |
| 22 | 29 | 26 | 740 | 285 | na | 30 | * | 35 | 25 |
| 17 | 54 | 30 | 1220 | 5 | na | * | * | 20 | 20 |
| 25 | 34 | 6 | 680 | 30 | na | 30 | * | 10 | 10 |
| 35 | 42 | 29 | 1160 | 60 | na | 4 | 2 | 35 | 20 |
| 4 | 41 | 17 | 170 | 5 | na | 4 | * | 4 | 10 |
| 7 | 70 | 18 | 230 | 0 | na | * | * | * | 10 |
| 20 | 61 | 43 | 1420 | 50 | na | 5 | 2 | 20 | 20 |
| 7 | 73 | 16 | 230 | 0 | na | * | * | * | 10 |
| 24 | 51 | 47 | 1530 | 15 | na | * | 2 | 12 | 20 |
| 16 | 41 | 35 | 1130 | 5 | na | * | * | 10 | 15 |
| 56 | 58 | 63 | 1810 | 145 | na | 10 | 10 | 50 | 35 |
| 6 | 30 | 5 | 280 | 0 | na | 20 | * | 10 | 8 |

| FOOD NAME | Serving Size | Calories | |
|---|---|---|---|
| French Fries, Criss-Cut | 1 order | 330 | |
| French Fries, large | 1 order | 546 | |
| French Fries, regular | 1 order | 420 | |
| French Fries, small | 1 order | 281 | |
| French Toast Dips | 1 order | 490 | |
| Fudge Brownie | 1 | 430 | |
| Fudge Brownie Mousse Cake | 1 | 400 | |
| Hamburger, Carl's Original | 1 | 460 | |
| Hamburger, Famous Star | 1 | 610 | |
| Hamburger, Happy Star | 1 | 320 | |
| Hamburger, Super Star | 1 | 820 | |
| Hash Brown Nuggets | 1 order | 270 | |
| Hot Cakes, with margarine | 1 order | 510 | |
| Jr. Crisp Burritos | 3 | 420 | |
| Milk, 1% low-fat | 10 fl oz | 138 | |
| Muffin, Blueberry | 1 | 340 | |
| Muffin, Bran | 1 | 310 | |
| Onion Rings | 1 order | 520 | |
| Orange Juice | 8 fl oz | 90 | |
| Raspberry Cheesecake | 1 sl | 310 | |
| Roast Beef Club Sandwich | 1 | 620 | |
| Roast Beef Deluxe Sandwich | 1 | 540 | |
| Salad, Charbroiler Chicken | 1 | 200 | |
| Salad, Garden | 1 | 50 | |
| Santa Fe Chicken Sandwich | 1 | 540 | |

| Protein (g) | Carbohydrates (g) | Fat (g) | Sodium (mg) | Cholesterol (mg) | Fiber (g) | Vitamin A (%) | Vitamin C (%) | Calcium (%) | Iron (%) |
|---|---|---|---|---|---|---|---|---|---|
| 4 | 27 | 22 | 890 | 0 | na | * | * | * | 10 |
| 5 | 70 | 26 | 260 | 0 | na | * | 13 | * | 8 |
| 4 | 54 | 20 | 200 | 0 | na | * | 10 | * | 6 |
| 3 | 36 | 13 | 134 | 0 | na | * | 7 | * | 4 |
| 8 | 55 | 26 | 620 | 40 | na | 10 | * | 6 | 15 |
| 6 | 64 | 19 | 210 | 0 | na | * | * | * | 10 |
| 5 | 42 | 23 | 85 | 110 | na | * | * | 8 | 8 |
| 25 | 46 | 20 | 810 | 50 | na | 6 | 6 | 20 | 10 |
| 26 | 42 | 38 | 890 | 50 | na | 10 | 6 | 30 | 20 |
| 17 | 33 | 14 | 590 | 35 | na | 2 | 2 | 15 | 15 |
| 43 | 41 | 53 | 1210 | 105 | na | 15 | 10 | 35 | 35 |
| 3 | 27 | 17 | 410 | 5 | na | 2 | * | 2 | 4 |
| 11 | 61 | 24 | 950 | 10 | na | 30 | * | 25 | 10 |
| 15 | 39 | 21 | 600 | 195 | na | 18 | * | 12 | 18 |
| 11 | 15 | 2 | 160 | 12 | na | 12 | 5 | 35 | * |
| 5 | 61 | 9 | 300 | 45 | na | 4 | * | 4 | 20 |
| 6 | 52 | 7 | 370 | 60 | na | * | * | * | 10 |
| 9 | 63 | 26 | 960 | 0 | na | * | 4 | 4 | 20 |
| 2 | 21 | 1 | 2 | 0 | na | 4 | 120 | 2 | 2 |
| 7 | 32 | 17 | 200 | 60 | na | 10 | * | 15 | 4 |
| 30 | 48 | 34 | 1950 | 45 | na | 15 | 4 | 35 | 25 |
| 28 | 46 | 26 | 1340 | 40 | na | 15 | 10 | 40 | 20 |
| 24 | 8 | 8 | 300 | 70 | na | 100 | 8 | 15 | 10 |
| 3 | 4 | 3 | 75 | 5 | na | 80 | 2 | 8 | 2 |
| 30 | 75 | 13 | 1180 | 40 | na | 6 | 10 | 25 | 20 |

| FOOD NAME | Serving Size | Calories | |
|---|---|---|---|
| Sausage | 1 patty | 190 | |
| Shake, large | 1 | 459 | |
| Shake, regular | 1 | 350 | |
| Shake, small | 1 | 268 | |
| Sunrise Sandwich | 1 | 300 | |
| Sunrise Sandwich with Bacon | 1 | 345 | |
| Sunrise Sandwich with Sausage | 1 | 490 | |
| Taco Sauce | 1 pkt | 8 | |
| Western Bacon Cheeseburger | 1 | 730 | |
| Zucchini, breaded and fried | 1 order | 390 | |
| *Dairy Queen* | | | |
| BBQ Beef Sandwich | 1 | 225 | |
| Banana Split | 1 | 510 | |
| Buster Bar | 1 | 450 | |
| Chicken Fillet Sandwich | 1 | 430 | |
| Chicken Fillet Sandwich with Cheese | 1 | 480 | |
| Cone, Chocolate, large | 1 | 350 | |
| Cone, Chocolate, regular | 1 | 230 | |
| Cone, Vanilla, large | 1 | 340 | |
| Cone, Vanilla, regular | 1 | 230 | |
| Cone, Vanilla, small | 1 | 140 | |
| DQ Homestyle Ultimate Burger | 1 | 700 | |
| DQ Sandwich | 1 | 140 | |
| Dilly Bar | 1 | 210 | |
| Dipped Cone, Chocolate, large | 1 | 525 | |

| Protein (g) | Carbohydrates (g) | Fat (g) | Sodium (mg) | Cholesterol (mg) | Fiber (g) | Vitamin A (%) | Vitamin C (%) | Calcium (%) | Iron (%) |
|---|---|---|---|---|---|---|---|---|---|
| 8 | 0 | 18 | 520 | 30 | na | * | * | * | 6 |
| 14 | 79 | 9 | 300 | 19 | na | * | * | 59 | 13 |
| 11 | 61 | 7 | 230 | 15 | na | * | * | 45 | 10 |
| 8 | 46 | 5 | 175 | 11 | na | * | * | 35 | 8 |
| 15 | 31 | 13 | 550 | 160 | na | 20 | * | 15 | 10 |
| 18 | 31 | 17 | 700 | 165 | na | 20 | 6 | 15 | 10 |
| 23 | 31 | 31 | 1070 | 190 | na | 20 | * | 15 | 16 |
| 0 | 2 | 0 | 160 | 0 | na | * | * | * | * |
| 34 | 59 | 39 | 1490 | 90 | na | 8 | 6 | 40 | 30 |
| 7 | 38 | 23 | 1040 | 0 | na | 20 | * | 4 | 10 |
| | | | | | | | | | |
| 12 | 34 | 4 | 700 | 20 | na | 8 | * | 10 | 20 |
| 9 | 93 | 11 | 250 | 30 | na | * | * | 30 | 20 |
| 11 | 40 | 29 | 220 | 15 | na | 2 | * | 30 | 8 |
| 24 | 37 | 20 | 760 | 55 | na | * | * | 4 | 10 |
| 27 | 38 | 25 | 980 | 70 | na | 8 | * | 10 | 10 |
| 8 | 54 | 11 | 170 | 30 | na | 10 | * | 25 | 6 |
| 6 | 36 | 7 | 115 | 20 | na | 6 | * | 15 | 4 |
| 9 | 53 | 10 | 140 | 30 | na | 6 | * | 20 | 6 |
| 6 | 36 | 7 | 95 | 20 | na | 4 | * | 15 | 4 |
| 4 | 22 | 4 | 60 | 15 | na | 2 | * | 10 | 2 |
| 43 | 30 | 47 | 1110 | 140 | na | 20 | 15 | 20 | 40 |
| 3 | 24 | 4 | 135 | 5 | na | * | * | 6 | 4 |
| 3 | 21 | 13 | 50 | 10 | na | * | * | 25 | 4 |
| 9 | 61 | 24 | 145 | 30 | na | 6 | * | 45 | 8 |

| FOOD NAME | Serving Size | Calories |
|---|---|---|
| Dipped Cone, Chocolate, regular | 1 | 330 |
| Dipped Cone, Chocolate, small | 1 | 190 |
| Fish Fillet Sandwich | 1 | 370 |
| Fish Fillet Sandwich with Cheese | 1 | 420 |
| French Fries, large | 1 order | 390 |
| French Fries, regular | 1 order | 300 |
| French Fries, small | 1 order | 210 |
| Grilled Chicken Fillet Sandwich | 1 | 300 |
| Hamburger | 1 | 310 |
| Hamburger with Cheese | 1 | 365 |
| Hamburger, Double | 1 | 460 |
| Hamburger, Double with Cheese | 1 | 570 |
| Heath Blizzard, regular | 1 | 820 |
| Heath Blizzard, small | 1 | 560 |
| Hot Dog | 1 | 280 |
| Hot Dog with Cheese | 1 | 330 |
| Hot Dog with Chili | 1 | 320 |
| Mr. Misty Float | 1 | 390 |
| Mr. Misty Freeze | 1 | 500 |
| Onion Rings, regular | 1 order | 240 |
| Peanut Buster Parfait | 1 | 710 |
| Salad, Garden | 1 | 200 |
| Salad, Side | 1 | 25 |
| Shake, Chocolate, regular | 1 | 540 |
| Shake, Vanilla, large | 1 | 600 |

| Protein (g) | Carbohydrates (g) | Fat (g) | Sodium (mg) | Cholesterol (mg) | Fiber (g) | Vitamin A (%) | Vitamin C (%) | Calcium (%) | Iron (%) |
|---|---|---|---|---|---|---|---|---|---|
| 6 | 40 | 16 | 100 | 20 | na | 4 | * | 30 | 6 |
| 4 | 25 | 10 | 60 | 10 | na | 2 | * | 20 | 4 |
| 16 | 39 | 16 | 630 | 45 | na | * | * | 4 | 10 |
| 19 | 43 | 21 | 850 | 60 | na | 8 | * | 10 | 10 |
| 5 | 52 | 18 | 200 | 0 | na | * | 15 | * | 8 |
| 4 | 40 | 14 | 160 | 0 | na | * | 10 | * | 6 |
| 3 | 29 | 10 | 115 | 0 | na | * | 8 | * | 4 |
| 25 | 33 | 8 | 800 | 50 | na | 2 | 4 | 6 | 20 |
| 17 | 29 | 13 | 580 | 45 | na | * | * | 4 | 20 |
| 20 | 30 | 18 | 800 | 60 | na | 8 | * | 15 | 20 |
| 31 | 29 | 25 | 630 | 95 | na | * | * | 4 | 30 |
| 37 | 31 | 34 | 1070 | 120 | na | 15 | * | 20 | 30 |
| 16 | 114 | 36 | 410 | 60 | na | 8 | * | 40 | 10 |
| 11 | 79 | 23 | 280 | 40 | na | 6 | * | 30 | 8 |
| 9 | 23 | 16 | 700 | 25 | na | * | * | 4 | 8 |
| 12 | 24 | 21 | 920 | 35 | na | 8 | * | 10 | 8 |
| 11 | 26 | 19 | 720 | 30 | na | * | * | 4 | 8 |
| 5 | 74 | 7 | 95 | 20 | na | 4 | * | 20 | 4 |
| 9 | 91 | 12 | 140 | 30 | na | 8 | * | 30 | 8 |
| 4 | 29 | 12 | 135 | 0 | na | * | * | * | 6 |
| 16 | 94 | 32 | 410 | 30 | na | 6 | * | 25 | 20 |
| 13 | 7 | 59 | 240 | 185 | na | 60 | 35 | 25 | 10 |
| 1 | 4 | 0 | 15 | 0 | na | 50 | 25 | 2 | 4 |
| 12 | 94 | 14 | 290 | 45 | na | 8 | * | 40 | 8 |
| 13 | 101 | 16 | 260 | 50 | na | 10 | * | 45 | 8 |

| FOOD NAME | Serving Size | Calories | |
|---|---|---|---|
| Shake, Vanilla, regular | 1 | 520 | |
| Strawberry Blizzard, regular | 1 | 740 | |
| Strawberry Blizzard, small | 1 | 500 | |
| Strawberry Breeze (Yogurt), regular | 1 | 590 | |
| Strawberry Breeze (Yogurt), small | 1 | 400 | |
| Sundae, Chocolate, regular | 1 | 300 | |
| Super Dog, Quarter Pound | 1 | 590 | |
| Yogurt Cone, large | 1 | 260 | |
| Yogurt Cone, regular | 1 | 180 | |
| Yogurt, Cup, large | 1 | 230 | |
| Yogurt, Cup, regular | 1 | 170 | |
| Yogurt Strawberry Sundae, regular | 1 | 200 | |
| *Domino's Pizza* | | | |
| Cheese Pizza | 2 sl | 376 | |
| Deluxe Pizza | 2 sl | 498 | |
| Ham Pizza | 2 sl | 417 | |
| Pepperoni Pizza | 2 sl | 460 | |
| Sausage and Mushroom Pizza | 2 sl | 430 | |
| Veggie Pizza | 2 sl | 498 | |
| *Dunkin' Donuts* | | | |
| Apple Filled Cinnamon Donut | 1 | 190 | |
| Apple 'n Spice Muffin | 1 | 300 | |
| Bagel, Cinnamon 'n Raisin | 1 | 250 | |
| Bagel, Egg | 1 | 250 | |
| Bagel, Onion | 1 | 230 | |

| Protein (g) | Carbohydrates (g) | Fat (g) | Sodium (mg) | Cholesterol (mg) | Fiber (g) | Vitamin A (%) | Vitamin C (%) | Calcium (%) | Iron (%) |
|---|---|---|---|---|---|---|---|---|---|
| 12 | 88 | 14 | 230 | 45 | na | 8 | * | 40 | 8 |
| 13 | 92 | 16 | 230 | 50 | na | 8 | 40 | 35 | 10 |
| 9 | 64 | 12 | 160 | 35 | na | 6 | 25 | 25 | 6 |
| 12 | 90 | 1 | 170 | 5 | na | * | 40 | 50 | 10 |
| 9 | 63 | 0 | 115 | 5 | na | * | 25 | 35 | 6 |
| 6 | 54 | 7 | 140 | 20 | na | 4 | * | 15 | 6 |
| 20 | 41 | 38 | 1360 | 60 | na | * | * | 10 | 15 |
| 9 | 56 | 0 | 115 | 0 | na | * | * | 35 | 6 |
| 6 | 38 | 0 | 80 | 0 | na | * | * | 20 | 4 |
| 8 | 49 | 0 | 100 | 0 | na | * | * | 30 | 6 |
| 6 | 35 | 0 | 70 | 0 | na | * | * | 25 | 4 |
| 6 | 43 | 0 | 80 | 0 | na | * | 20 | 25 | 4 |
|  |  |  |  |  |  |  |  |  |  |
| 22 | 56 | 10 | 483 | 19 | na | 7 | 2 | 17 | 13 |
| 27 | 59 | 20 | 954 | 40 | na | 9 | 4 | 23 | 23 |
| 23 | 58 | 11 | 805 | 26 | na | 4 | 2 | 19 | 19 |
| 24 | 56 | 17 | 825 | 28 | na | 7 | 2 | 19 | 15 |
| 24 | 55 | 16 | 552 | 28 | na | 8 | 2 | 20 | 17 |
| 31 | 60 | 18 | 1035 | 36 | na | 10 | 4 | 39 | 26 |
|  |  |  |  |  |  |  |  |  |  |
| 4 | 25 | 9 | 220 | 0 | na | na | na | na | na |
| 6 | 52 | 8 | 360 | 25 | na | na | na | na | na |
| 8 | 49 | 2 | 370 | 0 | na | * | * | 2 | 15 |
| 9 | 47 | 2 | 380 | 15 | na | * | * | 2 | 15 |
| 9 | 46 | 1 | 480 | 0 | na | * | * | 2 | 15 |

| FOOD NAME | Serving Size | Calories |
|---|---|---|
| Bagel, Plain | 1 | 240 |
| Banana Nut Muffin | 1 | 310 |
| Blueberry Filled Donut | 1 | 210 |
| Blueberry Muffin | 1 | 280 |
| Bran Muffin with Raisins | 1 | 310 |
| Chocolate Chunk Cookie | 1 | 200 |
| Chocolate Chunk Cookie with Nuts | 1 | 210 |
| Corn Muffin | 1 | 340 |
| Cranberry Nut Muffin | 1 | 290 |
| Croissant, Almond | 1 | 420 |
| Croissant, Chocolate | 1 | 440 |
| Croissant, Plain | 1 | 310 |
| Dunkin' Donut, Plain | 1 | 240 |
| Glazed Buttermilk Ring | 1 | 290 |
| Glazed French Cruller | 1 | 140 |
| Glazed Whole Wheat Ring | 1 | 330 |
| Honey Dipped Cruller | 1 | 260 |
| Jelly Filled Donut | 1 | 220 |
| Lemon Filled Donut | 1 | 260 |
| Oat Bran Muffin | 1 | 330 |
| *Hardee's* | | |
| Apple Turnover | 1 | 270 |
| Bacon Cheeseburger | 1 | 610 |
| Big Deluxe Burger | 1 | 500 |
| Big Twin | 1 | 450 |

| Protein (g) | Carbohydrates (g) | Fat (g) | Sodium (mg) | Cholesterol (mg) | Fiber (g) | Vitamin A (%) | Vitamin C (%) | Calcium (%) | Iron (%) |
|---|---|---|---|---|---|---|---|---|---|
| 9 | 47 | 1 | 450 | 0 | na | * | * | 2 | 15 |
| 7 | 49 | 10 | 410 | 30 | na | na | na | na | na |
| 4 | 29 | 8 | 240 | 0 | na | na | na | na | na |
| 6 | 46 | 8 | 340 | 30 | na | na | na | na | na |
| 6 | 51 | 9 | 560 | 15 | na | na | na | na | na |
| 3 | 25 | 10 | 110 | 30 | na | na | na | na | na |
| 3 | 23 | 11 | 100 | 30 | na | na | na | na | na |
| 7 | 51 | 12 | 560 | 40 | na | na | na | na | na |
| 6 | 44 | 9 | 360 | 25 | na | na | na | na | na |
| 8 | 38 | 27 | 280 | 0 | na | na | na | na | na |
| 7 | 38 | 29 | 220 | 0 | na | na | na | na | na |
| 7 | 27 | 19 | 240 | 0 | na | na | na | na | na |
| 4 | 26 | 14 | 370 | 0 | na | na | na | na | na |
| 4 | 37 | 14 | 370 | 10 | na | na | na | na | na |
| 2 | 16 | 8 | 130 | 30 | na | na | na | na | na |
| 4 | 39 | 18 | 380 | 5 | na | na | na | na | na |
| 4 | 36 | 11 | 330 | 0 | na | na | na | na | na |
| 4 | 31 | 9 | 330 | 0 | na | na | na | na | na |
| 4 | 33 | 12 | 280 | 0 | na | na | na | na | na |
| 7 | 50 | 11 | 450 | 0 | na | na | na | na | na |
| | | | | | | | | | |
| 3 | 38 | 12 | 250 | 0 | na | na | na | * | 4 |
| 34 | 31 | 39 | 1030 | 80 | na | na | na | 20 | 30 |
| 27 | 22 | 30 | 760 | 70 | na | na | na | 20 | 30 |
| 23 | 34 | 25 | 580 | 55 | na | na | na | 20 | 20 |

| FOOD NAME | Serving Size | Calories | |
|---|---|---|---|
| Biscuit 'n Gravy | 1 | 440 | |
| Biscuit, Bacon | 1 | 360 | |
| Biscuit, Bacon & Egg | 1 | 410 | |
| Biscuit, Bacon, Egg & Cheese | 1 | 460 | |
| Biscuit, Ham | 1 | 320 | |
| Biscuit, Ham & Egg | 1 | 370 | |
| Biscuit, Ham, Egg & Cheese | 1 | 420 | |
| Biscuit, Rise 'n Shine | 1 | 320 | |
| Biscuit, Sausage | 1 | 440 | |
| Biscuit, Sausage & Egg | 1 | 490 | |
| Cheeseburger | 1 | 320 | |
| Chicken Fillet | 1 | 370 | |
| Cool Twist Cone, chocolate | 1 | 200 | |
| Cool Twist Cone, vanilla | 1 | 190 | |
| Crispy Curls | 1 order | 300 | |
| Fisherman's Fillet | 1 | 500 | |
| French Fries, Big Fry | 5½ oz | 500 | |
| French Fries, large | 4 oz | 360 | |
| French Fries, regular | 2½ oz | 230 | |
| Fried Chicken Breast | 1 | 412 | |
| Fried Chicken Breast and Wing | 1 | 604 | |
| Fried Chicken Leg | 1 | 140 | |
| Fried Chicken Leg and Thigh | 1 | 436 | |
| Fried Chicken Thigh | 1 | 296 | |
| Fried Chicken Wing | 1 | 192 | |

| Protein (g) | Carbohydrates (g) | Fat (g) | Sodium (mg) | Cholesterol (mg) | Fiber (g) | Vitamin A (%) | Vitamin C (%) | Calcium (%) | Iron (%) |
|---|---|---|---|---|---|---|---|---|---|
| 9 | 45 | 24 | 1250 | 15 | na | na | na | 15 | 10 |
| 10 | 34 | 21 | 950 | 10 | na | na | na | 10 | 10 |
| 15 | 35 | 24 | 990 | 155 | na | na | na | 15 | 20 |
| 17 | 35 | 28 | 1220 | 165 | na | na | na | 20 | 20 |
| 10 | 34 | 16 | 1000 | 15 | na | na | na | 10 | 10 |
| 15 | 35 | 19 | 1050 | 160 | na | na | na | 15 | 20 |
| 18 | 35 | 23 | 1270 | 170 | na | na | na | 20 | 20 |
| 5 | 34 | 18 | 740 | 0 | na | na | na | 12 | 10 |
| 13 | 34 | 28 | 1100 | 25 | na | na | na | 15 | 15 |
| 18 | 35 | 31 | 1150 | 179 | na | na | na | 15 | 20 |
| 16 | 33 | 14 | 710 | 30 | na | na | na | 20 | 20 |
| 19 | 44 | 13 | 1060 | 55 | na | na | na | 10 | 15 |
| 4 | 31 | 6 | 65 | 20 | na | na | na | 10 | 10 |
| 5 | 28 | 6 | 100 | 15 | na | na | na | 10 | * |
| 4 | 36 | 16 | 840 | 0 | na | na | na | 2 | 8 |
| 23 | 49 | 24 | 1030 | 70 | na | na | na | 20 | 20 |
| 6 | 66 | 23 | 180 | 0 | na | na | na | 2 | 10 |
| 4 | 48 | 17 | 135 | 0 | na | na | na | * | 8 |
| 3 | 30 | 11 | 85 | 0 | na | na | na | * | 6 |
| 33 | 17 | 24 | 609 | 0 | na | na | na | na | na |
| 44 | 25 | 37 | 894 | 165 | na | na | na | na | na |
| 12 | 6 | 8 | 190 | 40 | na | na | na | na | na |
| 30 | 17 | 28 | 596 | 125 | na | na | na | na | na |
| 18 | 12 | 20 | 406 | 85 | na | na | na | na | na |
| 11 | 9 | 13 | 285 | 47 | na | na | na | na | na |

| FOOD NAME | Serving Size | Calories |
|---|---|---|
| Grilled Chicken Sandwich | 1 | 310 |
| Hamburger | 1 | 270 |
| Hash Rounds | 1 order | 230 |
| Hot Dog | 1 | 300 |
| Hot Ham 'n Cheese | 1 | 330 |
| Muffin, Blueberry | 1 | 400 |
| Muffin, Oat Bran Raisin | 1 | 440 |
| Pancakes | 3 | 280 |
| Quarter Pound Cheeseburger | 1 | 500 |
| Real Lean Deluxe | 1 | 340 |
| Roast Beef, big | 1 | 360 |
| Roast Beef, regular | 1 | 310 |
| Roast Beef Sandwich (RR) | 1 | 350 |
| Roast Beef Sandwich with Cheese (RR) | 1 | 403 |
| Roast Beef Sandwich, large (RR) | 1 | 373 |
| Salad, Chef | 1 | 240 |
| Salad, Garden | 1 | 210 |
| Salad, Grilled Chicken | 1 | 280 |
| Salad, Side | 1 | 20 |
| Shake, Chocolate | 1 | 460 |
| Shake, Strawberry | 1 | 440 |
| Shake, Vanilla | 1 | 400 |
| Turkey Club | 1 | 390 |
| Yogurt, Chocolate, Frozen Soft Serve | 1 | 170 |
| Yogurt, Vanilla, Frozen Soft Serve | 1 | 160 |

| Protein (g) | Carbohydrates (g) | Fat (g) | Sodium (mg) | Cholesterol (mg) | Fiber (g) | Vitamin A (%) | Vitamin C (%) | Calcium (%) | Iron (%) |
|---|---|---|---|---|---|---|---|---|---|
| 24 | 34 | 9 | 890 | 60 | na | na | na | 15 | 15 |
| 13 | 33 | 10 | 490 | 20 | na | na | na | 10 | 15 |
| 3 | 24 | 14 | 560 | 0 | na | na | na | * | 6 |
| 11 | 25 | 17 | 710 | 25 | na | na | na | 8 | 15 |
| 23 | 32 | 12 | 1420 | 65 | na | na | na | 30 | 15 |
| 6 | 51 | 19 | 320 | 80 | na | na | na | 4 | 6 |
| 8 | 62 | 18 | 350 | 55 | na | na | na | 8 | * |
| 8 | 56 | 2 | 890 | 15 | na | na | na | 6 | 20 |
| 29 | 34 | 29 | 1060 | 70 | na | na | na | 25 | 30 |
| 23 | 35 | 13 | 650 | 80 | na | na | na | 10 | 25 |
| 24 | 33 | 15 | 1150 | 65 | na | na | na | 10 | 30 |
| 20 | 32 | 12 | 930 | 0 | na | na | na | 10 | 25 |
| 26 | 37 | 11 | 732 | 58 | na | na | na | na | na |
| 29 | 37 | 15 | 954 | 70 | na | na | na | na | na |
| 35 | 31 | 12 | 840 | 82 | na | na | na | na | na |
| 22 | 5 | 15 | 930 | 115 | na | na | na | 30 | 10 |
| 14 | 3 | 14 | 270 | 105 | na | na | na | 30 | 6 |
| 26 | 4 | 15 | 640 | 145 | na | na | na | 30 | 10 |
| 2 | 1 | 0 | 15 | 0 | na | na | na | 2 | 2 |
| 11 | 85 | 8 | 340 | 45 | na | na | na | 50 | 6 |
| 11 | 82 | 8 | 300 | 40 | na | na | na | 50 | * |
| 13 | 66 | 9 | 320 | 50 | na | na | na | 50 | * |
| 29 | 32 | 16 | 1280 | 70 | na | na | na | 15 | 15 |
| 6 | 27 | 4 | 75 | 10 | na | na | na | 15 | 8 |
| 6 | 27 | 4 | 75 | 10 | na | na | na | 15 | 4 |

| FOOD NAME | Serving Size | Calories | |
|---|---|---|---|
| Yogurt, Chocolate Nutrasweet | 1 | 120 | |
| Yogurt, Vanilla Nutrasweet | 1 | 110 | |
| *Jack in the Box* | | | |
| Bacon Cheeseburger | 1 | 705 | |
| Breakfast Jack | 1 | 307 | |
| Cheeseburger | 1 | 315 | |
| Cheesecake | 1 sl | 309 | |
| Chicken Fajita Pita | 1 | 292 | |
| Chicken Strips | 4 pc | 285 | |
| Chicken Strips | 6 pc | 451 | |
| Chicken Supreme | 1 | 641 | |
| Coffee | 8 fl oz | 2 | |
| Crescent, Sausage | 1 | 584 | |
| Crescent, Supreme | 1 | 547 | |
| Double Cheeseburger | 1 | 467 | |
| Double Fudge Cake | 1 sl | 288 | |
| Egg Rolls | 3 | 437 | |
| Egg Rolls | 5 | 753 | |
| Fish Supreme | 1 | 510 | |
| French Fries, Jumbo | 1 order | 396 | |
| French Fries, regular | 1 order | 351 | |
| French Fries, small | 1 order | 219 | |
| Fries, Seasoned Curly | 1 order | 358 | |
| Grilled Chicken Fillet | 1 | 408 | |
| Grilled Sourdough Burger | 1 | 712 | |

| Protein (g) | Carbohydrates (g) | Fat (g) | Sodium (mg) | Cholesterol (mg) | Fiber (g) | Vitamin A (%) | Vitamin C (%) | Calcium (%) | Iron (%) |
|---|---|---|---|---|---|---|---|---|---|
| 6 | 22 | 0 | 75 | 0 | na | na | na | 20 | * |
| 5 | 21 | 1 | 75 | 0 | na | na | na | 15 | 2 |
| | | | | | | | | | |
| 35 | 41 | 45 | 1240 | 113 | na | 7 | 13 | 25 | 28 |
| 18 | 30 | 13 | 871 | 203 | na | 9 | * | 17 | 17 |
| 15 | 33 | 14 | 746 | 41 | na | 4 | * | 25 | 15 |
| 8 | 29 | 18 | 208 | 63 | na | * | * | 11 | 3 |
| 24 | 29 | 8 | 703 | 34 | na | 10 | * | 25 | 15 |
| 25 | 18 | 13 | 695 | 52 | na | * | * | * | 4 |
| 39 | 28 | 20 | 1100 | 82 | na | * | * | * | 6 |
| 27 | 47 | 39 | 1470 | 85 | na | 8 | 10 | 24 | 16 |
| 0 | 0 | 0 | 26 | 0 | 0 | * | * | * | * |
| 22 | 28 | 43 | 1012 | 187 | na | 11 | * | 17 | 16 |
| 20 | 27 | 40 | 1053 | 178 | na | 11 | * | 15 | 15 |
| 21 | 33 | 27 | 842 | 72 | na | 8 | * | 40 | 15 |
| 4 | 49 | 9 | 259 | 20 | na | 4 | * | 4 | 10 |
| 3 | 54 | 24 | 957 | 29 | na | * | 6 | 8 | 20 |
| 5 | 92 | 41 | 1640 | 49 | na | * | 11 | 15 | 34 |
| 24 | 44 | 27 | 1040 | 55 | na | * | 9 | 16 | 15 |
| 5 | 51 | 19 | 219 | 0 | na | * | 49 | * | 8 |
| 4 | 45 | 17 | 194 | 0 | na | * | 43 | * | 7 |
| 3 | 28 | 11 | 121 | 0 | na | * | 27 | * | 4 |
| 5 | 39 | 20 | 1030 | 0 | na | * | 9 | 3 | 9 |
| 31 | 33 | 17 | 1130 | 64 | na | 4 | 13 | 17 | 12 |
| 32 | 34 | 50 | 1140 | 109 | na | 14 | * | 19 | 24 |

| FOOD NAME | Serving Size | Calories |
|---|---|---|
| Ham and Turkey Melt | 1 | 592 |
| Hamburger | 1 | 267 |
| Hash Browns | 1 order | 156 |
| Hot Apple Turnover | 1 | 348 |
| Iced Tea | 12 fl oz | 3 |
| Jumbo Jack | 1 | 584 |
| Jumbo Jack with Cheese | 1 | 677 |
| Milk Shake, Chocolate | 1 | 330 |
| Milk Shake, Strawberry | 1 | 320 |
| Milk Shake, Vanilla | 1 | 320 |
| Milk, 2% low-fat | 8 fl oz | 122 |
| Onion Rings | 1 order | 380 |
| Old Fashion Patty Melt | 1 | 713 |
| Orange Juice | 6 fl oz | 80 |
| Pancake Platter | 1 | 612 |
| Salad, Chef | 1 | 325 |
| Salad, Side | 1 | 51 |
| Salad, Taco | 1 | 503 |
| Scrambled Egg Platter | 1 | 559 |
| Scrambled Egg Pocket | 1 | 431 |
| Sesame Breadsticks | 1 order | 70 |
| Sirloin Cheesesteak | 1 | 621 |
| Taco | 1 | 187 |
| Taco, Super | 1 | 281 |
| Taquitos | 5 pc | 362 |

| Protein (g) | Carbohydrates (g) | Fat (g) | Sodium (mg) | Cholesterol (mg) | Fiber (g) | Vitamin A (%) | Vitamin C (%) | Calcium (%) | Iron (%) |
|---|---|---|---|---|---|---|---|---|---|
| 27 | 40 | 36 | 1120 | 79 | na | 30 | * | 43 | 14 |
| 13 | 28 | 11 | 556 | 26 | na | * | * | 15 | 10 |
| 1 | 14 | 11 | 312 | 0 | na | * | 12 | * | 2 |
| 3 | 42 | 19 | 316 | 7 | na | * | 4 | * | 10 |
| 0 | 0 | 0 | 5 | 0 | 0 | * | * | * | * |
| 26 | 42 | 34 | 733 | 73 | na | * | * | 14 | 17 |
| 32 | 46 | 40 | 1090 | 102 | na | * | * | 27 | 21 |
| 11 | 55 | 7 | 270 | 25 | na | * | * | 35 | 4 |
| 10 | 55 | 7 | 240 | 25 | na | * | * | 35 | 2 |
| 10 | 57 | 6 | 230 | 25 | na | * | * | 35 | * |
| 8 | 12 | 5 | 122 | 18 | na | 10 | 4 | 30 | * |
| 5 | 38 | 23 | 451 | 0 | na | * | 5 | 3 | 12 |
| 33 | 42 | 46 | 1360 | 92 | na | 11 | 6 | 21 | 21 |
| 1 | 20 | 0 | 0 | 0 | na | 8 | 160 | 2 | 2 |
| 15 | 87 | 22 | 888 | 99 | na | 8 | 10 | 10 | 10 |
| 30 | 10 | 18 | 900 | 142 | na | 73 | 46 | 44 | 8 |
| 7 | 0 | 3 | 84 | 0 | na | * | * | 6 | * |
| 34 | 28 | 31 | 1600 | 92 | na | 27 | 15 | 41 | 21 |
| 18 | 50 | 32 | 1060 | 378 | na | 14 | 16 | 15 | 27 |
| 29 | 31 | 21 | 1060 | 354 | na | 21 | * | 21 | 20 |
| 2 | 12 | 2 | 110 | 0 | na | * | * | * | * |
| 36 | 51 | 30 | 1450 | 79 | na | 17 | * | 29 | 32 |
| 7 | 15 | 11 | 414 | 18 | na | * | * | 11 | 7 |
| 12 | 22 | 17 | 718 | 29 | na | 12 | 4 | 16 | 12 |
| 15 | 42 | 15 | 462 | 24 | na | * | 3 | 15 | 15 |

| FOOD NAME | Serving Size | Calories | |
|---|---|---|---|
| Tortilla Chips | 1 order | 139 | |
| Ultimate Cheeseburger | 1 | 942 | |
| *KFC (Kentucky Fried Chicken)* | | | |
| Baked Beans | 1 | 133 | |
| Buttermilk Biscuit | 1 | 235 | |
| Chicken Littles Sandwich | 1 | 169 | |
| Chocolate Pudding | 1 | 156 | |
| Coleslaw | 1 | 119 | |
| Colonel's Chicken Sandwich | 1 | 482 | |
| Colonel's Deluxe Chicken Sandwich | 1 | 547 | |
| Corn on the Cob | 1 | 176 | |
| Extra Tasty Crispy Center Breast | 1 | 342 | |
| Extra Tasty Crispy Drumstick | 1 | 204 | |
| Extra Tasty Crispy Side Breast | 1 | 343 | |
| Extra Tasty Crispy Thigh | 1 | 406 | |
| Extra Tasty Crispy Wing | 1 | 254 | |
| French Fries | 1 order | 244 | |
| Hot Wings | 6 pc | 376 | |
| Kentucky Nuggets | 6 pc | 276 | |
| Mashed Potatoes and Gravy | 1 order | 71 | |
| Original Recipe Center Breast | 1 | 283 | |
| Original Recipe Drumstick | 1 | 146 | |
| Original Recipe Side Breast | 1 | 267 | |
| Original Recipe Thigh | 1 | 294 | |
| Original Recipe Wing | 1 | 178 | |

| Protein (g) | Carbohydrates (g) | Fat (g) | Sodium (mg) | Cholesterol (mg) | Fiber (g) | Vitamin A (%) | Vitamin C (%) | Calcium (%) | Iron (%) |
|---|---|---|---|---|---|---|---|---|---|
| 2 | 18 | 6 | 134 | 0 | na | * | * | * | * |
| 47 | 33 | 69 | 1176 | 127 | na | 15 | * | 60 | 35 |
| | | | | | | | | | |
| 6 | na | 2 | 492 | 1 | na | na | na | na | na |
| 4 | 28 | 12 | 655 | 1 | na | * | * | 10 | 9 |
| 6 | 14 | 10 | 331 | 18 | na | * | * | 2 | 10 |
| 2 | 20 | 7 | 127 | 2 | na | * | * | 6 | 3 |
| 2 | 13 | 7 | 197 | 5 | na | 6 | 36 | 3 | * |
| 21 | 39 | 27 | 1060 | 47 | na | * | * | 5 | 7 |
| 25 | na | 32 | 1362 | 64 | na | na | na | na | na |
| 5 | 32 | 3 | 0 | 0 | na | 5 | 4 | * | 4 |
| 33 | 12 | 20 | 790 | 114 | na | * | * | 3 | 5 |
| 14 | 6 | 14 | 324 | 71 | na | * | * | 1 | 4 |
| 22 | 14 | 22 | 748 | 81 | na | * | * | 3 | 5 |
| 20 | 14 | 30 | 688 | 129 | na | 3 | * | 5 | 7 |
| 12 | 9 | 19 | 422 | 67 | na | * | * | 2 | 4 |
| 3 | 31 | 12 | 139 | 2 | na | * | 26 | * | 3 |
| 22 | 17 | 24 | 677 | 148 | na | * | * | na | na |
| 17 | 13 | 17 | 840 | 71 | na | * | * | 1 | 4 |
| 2 | 12 | 2 | 339 | 0 | na | * | * | 2 | 2 |
| 28 | 9 | 15 | 672 | 93 | na | * | * | 4 | 5 |
| 13 | 4 | 8 | 275 | 67 | na | * | * | 2 | 6 |
| 19 | 11 | 16 | 735 | 77 | na | * | * | 7 | 7 |
| 18 | 11 | 20 | 619 | 123 | na | 2 | * | 7 | 7 |
| 12 | 6 | 12 | 372 | 64 | na | * | * | 5 | 7 |

| FOOD NAME | Serving Size | Calories |
|---|---|---|
| Parfait, Apple Shortcake | 1 | 276 |
| Parfait, Chocolate Creme | 1 | 360 |
| Parfait, Fudge Brownie | 1 | 331 |
| Parfait, Lemon Cream | 1 | 513 |
| Parfait, Strawberry Shortcake | 1 | 230 |
| Potato Salad | 1 | 177 |
| Vanilla Pudding | 1 | 159 |
| *Longjohn Silver's* | | |
| Apple Pie | 1 sl | 320 |
| Cherry Pie | 1 sl | 360 |
| Chicken Plank | 1 pc | 130 |
| Chicken Sandwich, Baked | 1 | 320 |
| Chicken Sandwich, Batter-Dipped | 2 pc | 440 |
| Chowder, Seafood | 1 | 140 |
| Clams, Breaded | 1 order | 240 |
| Club Crackers | 1 pkt | 35 |
| Corn Cobbette | ½ ear | 140 |
| Dijon Herb Sauce | 1 pkt | 90 |
| Fish, Battered | 1 pc | 210 |
| Fish, Homestyle | 1 pc | 125 |
| Fish Sandwich, Batter-Dipped | 1 | 380 |
| Fryes | 1 order | 170 |
| Green Beans | 1 order | 30 |
| Honey-Mustard Sauce | 1 pkt | 45 |
| Hushpuppy | 1 pc | 70 |

| Protein (g) | Carbohydrates (g) | Fat (g) | Sodium (mg) | Cholesterol (mg) | Fiber (g) | Vitamin A (%) | Vitamin C (%) | Calcium (%) | Iron (%) |
|---|---|---|---|---|---|---|---|---|---|
| 2 | 44 | 10 | 248 | 23 | na | * | 83 | 3 | 3 |
| 4 | 44 | 19 | 231 | 3 | na | * | * | 5 | 7 |
| 3 | 55 | 11 | 299 | 40 | na | * | * | 4 | 6 |
| 8 | 74 | 20 | 232 | 9 | na | 4 | 8 | 22 | 3 |
| 2 | 36 | 9 | 162 | 20 | na | 1 | 30 | 3 | 3 |
| 2 | na | 12 | 497 | 14 | na | na | na | na | na |
| 2 | 21 | 7 | 130 | 1 | na | * | * | 6 | 1 |
| | | | | | | | | | |
| 3 | 45 | 13 | 420 | 0 | na | * | 8 | * | 6 |
| 4 | 55 | 13 | 200 | 5 | na | 8 | 15 | * | 6 |
| 9 | 10 | 6 | 490 | 45 | na | * | 2 | * | 4 |
| 33 | 29 | 8 | 900 | 70 | na | 2 | * | 15 | 10 |
| 25 | 47 | 17 | 1280 | 95 | na | * | 6 | 15 | 15 |
| 11 | 10 | 6 | 590 | 20 | na | 15 | * | 20 | 10 |
| 7 | 26 | 12 | 410 | 4 | na | * | * | 4 | 6 |
| 0 | 5 | 2 | 85 | 0 | na | * | * | * | * |
| 3 | 18 | 8 | 0 | 0 | na | 6 | 15 | * | 2 |
| 0 | 6 | 7 | 220 | 5 | na | * | * | * | * |
| 12 | 13 | 12 | 570 | 30 | na | * | * | * | 4 |
| 7 | 9 | 7 | 200 | 20 | na | 2 | * | * | 45 |
| 19 | 40 | 16 | 860 | 30 | na | * | 4 | 15 | 15 |
| 3 | 26 | 6 | 55 | 0 | na | * | 20 | * | 10 |
| 1 | 6 | 0 | 540 | 0 | na | * | 6 | 2 | 4 |
| 0 | 10 | 0 | 125 | 0 | na | * | * | * | * |
| 2 | 10 | 2 | 25 | 4 | na | * | * | 4 | 4 |

| FOOD NAME | Serving Size | Calories |
|---|---|---|
| Lemon Pie | 1 sl | 340 |
| Milk, 2% low-fat | 8 fl oz | 121 |
| Rice Pilaf | 1 order | 210 |
| Salad, Ocean Chef | 1 | 150 |
| Salad, Seafood | 1 | 230 |
| Salad, Side | 1 | 25 |
| Salad, Small | 1 | 11 |
| Seafood Gumbo | 1 order | 120 |
| Seafood Sauce | 1 pkt | 35 |
| Shrimp, Battered | 1 pc | 60 |
| Shrimp, Homestyle | 1 pc | 45 |
| Sweet 'n Sour Sauce | 1 pkt | 40 |
| Tartar Sauce | 1 pkt | 70 |
| *McDonald's* | | |
| Apple Juice | 6 fl oz | 91 |
| Apple Pie | 1 pc | 260 |
| Big Mac | 1 | 500 |
| Biscuit with Spread | 1 | 260 |
| Biscuit with Bacon, Egg & Cheese | 1 | 430 |
| Biscuit with Sausage | 1 | 420 |
| Biscuit with Sausage & Egg | 1 | 500 |
| Breakfast Burrito | 1 | 280 |
| Carrot Sticks | 1 bag | 37 |
| Celery Sticks | 1 bag | 14 |
| Cheerios | ¾ cup | 80 |

| Protein (g) | Carbohydrates (g) | Fat (g) | Sodium (mg) | Cholesterol (mg) | Fiber (g) | Vitamin A (%) | Vitamin C (%) | Calcium (%) | Iron (%) |
|---|---|---|---|---|---|---|---|---|---|
| 7 | 60 | 9 | 120 | 45 | na | * | * | 15 | 4 |
| 8 | 12 | 4 | 122 | 18 | na | 10 | 4 | 30 | * |
| 5 | 43 | 2 | 570 | 0 | na | * | * | 4 | 6 |
| 15 | 13 | 5 | 860 | 40 | na | 70 | 35 | 20 | 20 |
| 16 | 31 | 5 | 580 | 90 | na | 60 | 30 | 15 | 25 |
| 1 | 5 | 0 | 15 | 0 | na | 40 | 25 | 2 | 4 |
| 0 | 2 | 0 | 5 | 0 | na | 15 | 15 | * | * |
| 9 | 4 | 8 | 740 | 25 | na | * | 10 | 10 | 10 |
| 0 | 6 | 0 | 380 | 0 | na | 4 | * | 2 | 2 |
| 4 | 4 | 4 | 180 | 15 | na | * | * | * | * |
| 2 | 4 | 3 | 70 | 15 | na | * | * | * | * |
| 0 | 10 | 0 | 95 | 0 | na | * | * | * | * |
| 0 | 10 | 3 | 70 | 0 | na | * | * | 2 | * |
| | | | | | | | | | |
| 0 | 50 | 0 | 5 | 0 | na | * | 2 | * | 4 |
| 2 | 30 | 15 | 240 | 6 | na | * | 20 | * | 4 |
| 25 | 42 | 26 | 890 | 100 | na | 6 | 2 | 25 | 20 |
| 5 | 32 | 13 | 730 | 1 | na | * | * | 8 | 8 |
| 15 | 33 | 26 | 1190 | 248 | na | 10 | * | 20 | 15 |
| 12 | 32 | 28 | 1040 | 44 | na | * | * | 8 | 10 |
| 19 | 33 | 33 | 1210 | 270 | na | 6 | * | 10 | 20 |
| 12 | 21 | 17 | 580 | 135 | na | 10 | 10 | 10 | 8 |
| 0 | 9 | 0 | 40 | 0 | na | 100 | 10 | 2 | 2 |
| 0 | 3 | 0 | 100 | 0 | na | * | 10 | 2 | * |
| 3 | 14 | 1 | 210 | 0 | na | 15 | 15 | 2 | 30 |

| FOOD NAME | Serving Size | Calories |
|---|---|---|
| Cheeseburger | 1 | 305 |
| Chicken Fajitas | 1 order | 185 |
| Chicken McNuggets | 6 pc | 270 |
| Chocolate Chip Cookies | 1 box | 330 |
| Danish, Apple | 1 | 390 |
| Danish, Cinnamon | 1 | 440 |
| Danish, Raspberry | 1 | 410 |
| English Muffin with margarine | 1 | 170 |
| Filet-O-Fish | 1 | 370 |
| French Fries, large | 1 order | 400 |
| French Fries, medium | 1 order | 320 |
| French Fries, small | 1 order | 220 |
| Frozen Yogurt Cone, Low-Fat Vanilla | 1 | 105 |
| Frozen Yogurt Sundae, Low-Fat | | |
|   Hot Fudge | 1 | 240 |
| Grapefruit Juice | 6 fl oz | 80 |
| Grilled Chicken Breast Sandwich | 1 | 252 |
| Hamburger | 1 | 255 |
| Hashbrown Potatoes | 1 order | 130 |
| Hotcakes with syrup and margarine | 1 order | 410 |
| McChicken | 1 | 415 |
| McDonaldland Cookies | 1 box | 290 |
| McLean Deluxe | 1 | 320 |
| McLean Deluxe with Cheese | 1 | 370 |
| McMuffin, Egg | 1 | 280 |

| Protein (g) | Carbohydrates (g) | Fat (g) | Sodium (mg) | Cholesterol (mg) | Fiber (g) | Vitamin A (%) | Vitamin C (%) | Calcium (%) | Iron (%) |
|---|---|---|---|---|---|---|---|---|---|
| 15 | 30 | 13 | 710 | 50 | na | 8 | 4 | 20 | 15 |
| 11 | 20 | 8 | 310 | 35 | na | 2 | 8 | 8 | 4 |
| 20 | 17 | 15 | 580 | 56 | na | * | * | * | 6 |
| 4 | 42 | 16 | 280 | 4 | na | * | * | 2 | 10 |
| 6 | 51 | 17 | 370 | 25 | na | * | 25 | * | 8 |
| 6 | 58 | 21 | 430 | 34 | na | * | 6 | 4 | 10 |
| 6 | 62 | 16 | 310 | 26 | na | * | 6 | * | 8 |
| 5 | 26 | 5 | 230 | 0 | na | 2 | * | 15 | 8 |
| 14 | 38 | 18 | 930 | 50 | na | 2 | * | 15 | 10 |
| 6 | 46 | 22 | 200 | 0 | na | * | 25 | * | 6 |
| 4 | 36 | 17 | 150 | 0 | na | * | 20 | * | 4 |
| 3 | 26 | 12 | 110 | 0 | na | * | 15 | * | 2 |
| 4 | 22 | 1 | 80 | 3 | na | 2 | * | 10 | * |
| 7 | 50 | 3 | 170 | 6 | na | 4 | * | 25 | 2 |
| 1 | 19 | 0 | 0 | 0 | na | * | 100 | * | * |
| 24 | 30 | 44 | 740 | 50 | na | 8 | 8 | 15 | 15 |
| 12 | 30 | 9 | 490 | 37 | na | 4 | 4 | 10 | 15 |
| 1 | 15 | 7 | 330 | 0 | na | * | 2 | * | * |
| 8 | 74 | 9 | 640 | 8 | na | 4 | * | 10 | 10 |
| 19 | 39 | 20 | 770 | 42 | na | 2 | 4 | 15 | 15 |
| 4 | 47 | 9 | 300 | 0 | na | * | * | * | 10 |
| 22 | 35 | 10 | 670 | 60 | na | 10 | 10 | 15 | 20 |
| 24 | 35 | 14 | 890 | 75 | na | 15 | 10 | 20 | 20 |
| 18 | 28 | 11 | 710 | 224 | na | 10 | * | 25 | 15 |

| FOOD NAME | Serving Size | Calories |
|---|---|---|
| McMuffin, Sausage | 1 | 345 |
| McMuffin, Sausage with Egg | 1 | 415 |
| McRib Sandwich | 1 | 445 |
| Milk Shake, Low-Fat Chocolate | 1 | 320 |
| Milk Shake, Low-Fat Strawberry | 1 | 320 |
| Milk Shake, Low-Fat Vanilla | 1 | 290 |
| Milk, 1% low-fat | 8 fl oz | 110 |
| Muffin, Apple Bran Fat-Free | 1 | 180 |
| Muffin, Blueberry Fat-Free | 1 | 170 |
| Orange Drink | 12 fl oz | 130 |
| Orange Juice | 6 fl oz | 80 |
| Orange Sorbet Ice Cone | 1 | 106 |
| Pork Sausage | 1 order | 180 |
| Quarter Pounder | 1 | 410 |
| Quarter Pounder with Cheese | 1 | 510 |
| Salad, Chef | 1 | 170 |
| Salad, Chunky Chicken | 1 | 150 |
| Salad, Garden | 1 | 50 |
| Salad, Side | 1 | 30 |
| Sausage | 1 order | 160 |
| Wheaties | ¾ cup | 90 |
| *Pizza Hut* | | |
| Pan Pizza, Cheese | 2 sl | 492 |
| Pan Pizza, Pepperoni | 2 sl | 540 |
| Pan Pizza, Super Supreme | 2 sl | 563 |

| Protein (g) | Carbohydrates (g) | Fat (g) | Sodium (mg) | Cholesterol (mg) | Fiber (g) | Vitamin A (%) | Vitamin C (%) | Calcium (%) | Iron (%) |
|---|---|---|---|---|---|---|---|---|---|
| 15 | 27 | 20 | 770 | 57 | na | 4 | * | 20 | 15 |
| 21 | 27 | 25 | 915 | 256 | na | 10 | * | 25 | 20 |
| 24 | 48 | 22 | 972 | 75 | na | na | na | na | na |
| 11 | 66 | 2 | 240 | 10 | na | 6 | * | 35 | * |
| 11 | 67 | 1 | 170 | 10 | na | 6 | * | 35 | * |
| 11 | 60 | 1 | 170 | 10 | na | 6 | * | 35 | * |
| 9 | 12 | 2 | 130 | 10 | na | 10 | 4 | 30 | * |
| 5 | 40 | 0 | 200 | 0 | na | * | * | 4 | 6 |
| 3 | 40 | 0 | 220 | 0 | na | * | 2 | 8 | 4 |
| 0 | 33 | 0 | 10 | 0 | na | * | * | * | * |
| 1 | 19 | 0 | 0 | 0 | na | * | 120 | * | * |
| 0 | 27 | 0 | 25 | 0 | na | * | 30 | * | * |
| 8 | 0 | 16 | 350 | 48 | na | * | * | * | 4 |
| 23 | 34 | 20 | 650 | 85 | na | 4 | 6 | 15 | 20 |
| 28 | 34 | 28 | 1090 | 115 | na | 15 | 6 | 30 | 20 |
| 17 | 8 | 9 | 400 | 111 | na | 35 | 8 | 15 | 8 |
| 25 | 7 | 4 | 230 | 78 | na | 100 | 45 | 4 | 6 |
| 4 | 6 | 2 | 70 | 65 | na | 90 | 35 | 4 | 8 |
| 2 | 4 | 1 | 35 | 35 | na | 80 | 20 | 2 | 4 |
| 7 | 0 | 15 | 310 | 43 | na | * | * | * | 4 |
| 2 | 19 | 1 | 220 | 0 | na | 20 | 20 | 2 | 20 |
|  |  |  |  |  |  |  |  |  |  |
| 30 | 57 | 18 | 940 | 34 | na | 9 | 12 | 63 | 30 |
| 29 | 62 | 22 | 1127 | 42 | na | 10 | 14 | 52 | 35 |
| 33 | 53 | 26 | 1447 | 55 | na | 12 | 18 | 54 | 37 |

| FOOD NAME | Serving Size | Calories |
|---|---|---|
| Pan Pizza, Supreme | 2 sl | 589 |
| Personal Pan Pizza, Supreme | 1 | 647 |
| Personal Pan Pizza, Pepperoni | 1 | 675 |
| Thin 'n Crispy Pizza, Cheese | 2 sl | 398 |
| Thin 'n Crispy Pizza, Pepperoni | 2 sl | 413 |
| Thin 'n Crispy Pizza, Super Supreme | 2 sl | 463 |
| Thin 'n Crispy Pizza, Supreme | 2 sl | 459 |
| Traditional Hand-Tossed Pizza, Cheese | 2 sl | 518 |
| Traditional Hand-Tossed Pizza, Pepperoni | 2 sl | 500 |
| Traditional Hand-Tossed Pizza, Super Supreme | 2 sl | 556 |
| Traditional Hand-Tossed Pizza, Supreme | 2 sl | 540 |
| *Subway* | | |
| Salad, Chef, small | 1 | 189 |
| Salad, Garden, large | 1 | 46 |
| Salad, Ham, small | 1 | 170 |
| Salad, Roast Beef, small | 1 | 185 |
| Salad, Seafood and Crab, small | 1 | 198 |
| Salad, Tuna, small | 1 | 212 |
| Salad, Turkey, small | 1 | 167 |
| Sandwich, Ham | 6 inch | 360 |
| Sandwich, Meatball | 6 inch | 429 |
| Sandwich, Roast Beef | 6 inch | 375 |
| Sandwich, Seafood and Crab | 6 inch | 388 |
| Sandwich, Steak | 6 inch | 423 |

| Protein (g) | Carbohydrates (g) | Fat (g) | Sodium (mg) | Cholesterol (mg) | Fiber (g) | Vitamin A (%) | Vitamin C (%) | Calcium (%) | Iron (%) |
|---|---|---|---|---|---|---|---|---|---|
| 32 | 53 | 30 | 1363 | 48 | na | 12 | 16 | 50 | 28 |
| 33 | 76 | 28 | 1313 | 49 | na | 12 | 18 | 52 | 37 |
| 37 | 76 | 29 | 1335 | 53 | na | 12 | 17 | 73 | 32 |
| 28 | 37 | 17 | 867 | 33 | na | 7 | 8 | 66 | 18 |
| 26 | 36 | 20 | 986 | 46 | na | 7 | 10 | 45 | 18 |
| 29 | 44 | 21 | 1336 | 56 | na | 10 | 14 | 46 | 27 |
| 28 | 41 | 22 | 1328 | 42 | na | 10 | 16 | 43 | 33 |
| 34 | 55 | 20 | 1276 | 55 | na | 10 | 16 | 75 | 30 |
| 28 | 50 | 23 | 1267 | 50 | na | 10 | 12 | 44 | 28 |
| | | | | | | | | | |
| 33 | 54 | 25 | 1648 | 54 | na | 11 | 20 | 44 | 38 |
| 32 | 50 | 26 | 1470 | 55 | na | 11 | 20 | 48 | 45 |
| | | | | | | | | | |
| 19 | 6 | 10 | 479 | na | na | 10 | 42 | 12 | * |
| 2 | 10 | 0 | 634 | 0 | na | 10 | 84 | 4 | 6 |
| 14 | 6 | 10 | 479 | na | na | 10 | 42 | 12 | * |
| 18 | 6 | 10 | 479 | na | na | 10 | 42 | 12 | * |
| 12 | 13 | 11 | 946 | na | na | 10 | 42 | 12 | 7 |
| 20 | 8 | 12 | 545 | na | na | 10 | 42 | 13 | 9 |
| 15 | 4 | 9 | 479 | na | na | 10 | 42 | 12 | * |
| 20 | 45 | 11 | 839 | na | na | 10 | 42 | 12 | * |
| 26 | 45 | 16 | 876 | na | na | 10 | 42 | 13 | 21 |
| 24 | 45 | 11 | 839 | na | na | 10 | 42 | 12 | * |
| 18 | 52 | 12 | 1306 | na | na | 10 | 42 | 12 | 13 |
| 28 | 46 | 14 | 883 | na | na | 10 | 42 | 13 | 22 |

| FOOD NAME | Serving Size | Calories |
|---|---|---|
| Sandwich, Subway Club | 6 inch | 379 |
| Sandwich, Tuna | 6 inch | 402 |
| Sandwich, Turkey | 6 inch | 357 |
| *Taco Bell* | | |
| Burrito, Bean with Red Sauce | 1 | 447 |
| Burrito, Beef with Red Sauce | 1 | 493 |
| Burrito, Chicken, Plain | 1 | 334 |
| Burrito, Combination | 1 | 407 |
| Burrito, Fiesta | 1 | 226 |
| Burrito Supreme with Red Sauce | 1 | 503 |
| Chilito | 1 | 383 |
| Enchirito with Red Sauce | 1 | 382 |
| Guacamole | ¾ oz | 34 |
| Hot Taco Sauce | 1 oz | 3 |
| Jalapeño Peppers | 1 order | 20 |
| Mexican Pizza | 1 | 575 |
| Meximelt, Beef | 1 | 266 |
| Meximelt, Chicken | 1 | 257 |
| Nachos | 1 order | 346 |
| Nachos Bellgrande | 1 order | 649 |
| Nachos Supreme | 1 order | 367 |
| Pico de Gallo | 1 order | 8 |
| Pintos 'n Cheese with Red Sauce | 1 | 190 |
| Salad, Chicken | 1 | 125 |
| Salsa | ⅓ fl oz | 18 |

| Protein (g) | Carbohydrates (g) | Fat (g) | Sodium (mg) | Cholesterol (mg) | Fiber (g) | Vitamin A (%) | Vitamin C (%) | Calcium (%) | Iron (%) |
|---|---|---|---|---|---|---|---|---|---|
| 25 | 45 | 11 | 839 | na | na | 10 | 42 | 12 | * |
| 26 | 45 | 13 | 905 | na | na | 10 | 42 | 13 | 15 |
| 21 | 46 | 10 | 839 | na | na | * | 42 | 12 | * |
|  |  |  |  |  |  |  |  |  |  |
| 15 | 63 | 14 | 1148 | 9 | na | 7 | 88 | 19 | 21 |
| 25 | 48 | 21 | 1311 | 57 | na | 10 | 3 | 15 | 23 |
| 17 | 38 | 12 | 880 | 52 | na | 9 | 19 | 11 | 43 |
| 18 | 46 | 16 | 1136 | 33 | na | 9 | 45 | 15 | 19 |
| 8 | 29 | 9 | 652 | 9 | na | 5 | 57 | 15 | 15 |
| 20 | 55 | 22 | 1181 | 33 | na | 18 | 43 | 19 | 22 |
| 18 | 36 | 18 | 893 | 47 | na | 17 | * | 27 | 14 |
| 20 | 31 | 20 | 1243 | 54 | na | 19 | 47 | 27 | 16 |
| 0 | 3 | 2 | 113 | 0 | na | 2 | 5 | 1 | 1 |
| 0 | 0 | 0 | 82 | 0 | na | 3 | * | 1 | * |
| 1 | 4 | 0 | 1370 | 0 | na | 5 | 4 | 4 | 2 |
| 21 | 40 | 37 | 1031 | 52 | na | 20 | 51 | 26 | 21 |
| 13 | 19 | 15 | 689 | 38 | na | 16 | 3 | 25 | 11 |
| 14 | 19 | 15 | 779 | 48 | na | 10 | 4 | 20 | 22 |
| 7 | 37 | 18 | 399 | 9 | na | 11 | 3 | 19 | 24 |
| 22 | 61 | 35 | 997 | 36 | na | 23 | 96 | 30 | 19 |
| 12 | 41 | 27 | 471 | 18 | na | 14 | 50 | 26 | 2 |
| 0 | 1 | 0 | 88 | 1 | na | 11 | 3 | 1 | 1 |
| 9 | 19 | 9 | 642 | 16 | na | 9 | 86 | 16 | 8 |
| 8 | 5 | 8 | 252 | 32 | na | 16 | 17 | 9 | 17 |
| 1 | 4 | 0 | 376 | 0 | na | 5 | 0 | 4 | 3 |

| FOOD NAME | Serving Size | Calories |
|---|---|---|
| Taco, Beef Hard Shell | 1 | 183 |
| Taco Bellgrande | 1 | 335 |
| Taco, Chicken Hard Shell | 1 | 171 |
| Taco, Fiesta Beef | 1 | 127 |
| Taco, Fiesta Soft | 1 | 147 |
| Taco Salad, with shell | 1 | 905 |
| Taco Salad, without shell | 1 | 484 |
| Taco, Soft, Beef | 1 | 225 |
| Taco, Soft, Chicken | 1 | 213 |
| Taco, Soft, Steak | 1 | 218 |
| Taco Supreme | 1 | 230 |
| Taco Supreme, Soft | 1 | 272 |
| Tostada, Beef with Red Sauce | 1 | 243 |
| Tostada, Chicken with Red Sauce | 1 | 264 |
| Tostada, Fiesta | 1 | 167 |
| *TCBY* | | |
| Nonfat Frozen Yogurt, giant | 31.6 oz | 869 |
| Nonfat Frozen Yogurt, kiddie | 3.2 oz | 88 |
| Nonfat Frozen Yogurt, large | 10.5 oz | 289 |
| Nonfat Frozen Yogurt, regular | 8.2 oz | 226 |
| Nonfat Frozen Yogurt, small | 5.9 oz | 162 |
| Nonfat Frozen Yogurt, super | 15.2 oz | 418 |
| Regular Frozen Yogurt, giant | 31.6 oz | 1027 |
| Regular Frozen Yogurt, kiddie | 3.2 oz | 104 |
| Regular Frozen Yogurt, large | 10.5 oz | 342 |

| Protein (g) | Carbohydrates (g) | Fat (g) | Sodium (mg) | Cholesterol (mg) | Fiber (g) | Vitamin A (%) | Vitamin C (%) | Calcium (%) | Iron (%) |
|---|---|---|---|---|---|---|---|---|---|
| 10 | 11 | 11 | 276 | 32 | na | 7 | 2 | 8 | 6 |
| 18 | 18 | 23 | 472 | 56 | na | 17 | 9 | 18 | 11 |
| 12 | 11 | 9 | 337 | 52 | na | 6 | 5 | 8 | 31 |
| 6 | 10 | 7 | 139 | 16 | na | 5 | 1 | 6 | 4 |
| 7 | 15 | 7 | 361 | 16 | na | 3 | 1 | 5 | 6 |
| 34 | 55 | 61 | 910 | 80 | na | 33 | 125 | 32 | 33 |
| 28 | 22 | 31 | 680 | 80 | na | 33 | 124 | 29 | 22 |
| 12 | 18 | 12 | 554 | 32 | na | 4 | 2 | 12 | 13 |
| 14 | 19 | 10 | 615 | 52 | na | 4 | 4 | 8 | 35 |
| 14 | 18 | 11 | 456 | 14 | na | 3 | 2 | 11 | 16 |
| 11 | 12 | 15 | 276 | 32 | na | 11 | 5 | 11 | 6 |
| 13 | 19 | 16 | 554 | 32 | na | 9 | 5 | 14 | 13 |
| 9 | 27 | 11 | 596 | 16 | na | 13 | 75 | 18 | 9 |
| 12 | 20 | 15 | 454 | 37 | na | 18 | 36 | 18 | 19 |
| 6 | 17 | 7 | 324 | 9 | na | 8 | 45 | 11 | 5 |
|  |  |  |  |  |  |  |  |  |  |
| 32 | 182 | 0 | 356 | 0 | na | * | * | 63 | * |
| 3 | 18 | 0 | 36 | 0 | na | * | * | 6 | * |
| 10 | 60 | 0 | 118 | 0 | na | * | * | 21 | * |
| 8 | 47 | 0 | 92 | 0 | na | * | * | 16 | * |
| 6 | 34 | 0 | 66 | 0 | na | * | * | 12 | * |
| 15 | 87 | 0 | 171 | 0 | na | * | * | 30 | * |
| 32 | 182 | 24 | 474 | 79 | na | * | * | 47 | 32 |
| 3 | 18 | 2 | 48 | 8 | na | * | * | 5 | 3 |
| 10 | 60 | 8 | 156 | 26 | na | * | * | 16 | 11 |

| FOOD NAME | Serving Size | Calories | |
|---|---|---|---|
| Regular Frozen Yogurt, regular | 8.2 oz | 267 | |
| Regular Frozen Yogurt, small | 5.9 oz | 192 | |
| Regular Frozen Yogurt, super | 15.2 oz | 494 | |
| Sugar-Free Frozen Yogurt, giant | 31.6 oz | 632 | |
| Sugar-Free Frozen Yogurt, kiddie | 3.2 oz | 64 | |
| Sugar-Free Frozen Yogurt, large | 10.5 oz | 210 | |
| Sugar-Free Frozen Yogurt, regular | 8.2 oz | 164 | |
| Sugar-Free Frozen Yogurt, small | 5.9 oz | 118 | |
| Sugar-Free Frozen Yogurt, super | 15.2 oz | 304 | |
| *Wendy's* | | | |
| Applesauce | 1 oz | 22 | |
| Baked Potato, Plain | 1 | 270 | |
| Baked Potato, Stuffed with Bacon and Cheese | 1 | 520 | |
| Baked Potato, Stuffed with Broccoli and Cheese | 1 | 400 | |
| Baked Potato, Stuffed with Cheese | 1 | 420 | |
| Baked Potato, Stuffed with Chili and Cheese | 1 | 500 | |
| Big Classic | 1 | 570 | |
| Big Classic with Cheese | 1 | 640 | |
| Big Classic, Double | 1 | 750 | |
| Big Classic, Double with Cheese | 1 | 820 | |
| Broccoli, fresh | ½ cup | 12 | |
| Cantaloupe, fresh | 2 oz | 20 | |

| Protein (g) | Carbohydrates (g) | Fat (g) | Sodium (mg) | Cholesterol (mg) | Fiber (g) | Vitamin A (%) | Vitamin C (%) | Calcium (%) | Iron (%) |
|---|---|---|---|---|---|---|---|---|---|
| 8 | 47 | 6 | 126 | 20 | na | * | * | 12 | 8 |
| 6 | 34 | 4 | 90 | 15 | na | * | * | 9 | 6 |
| 15 | 87 | 11 | 228 | 38 | na | * | * | 23 | 15 |
| 32 | 142 | 0 | 316 | 0 | na | 32 | * | 63 | * |
| 3 | 14 | 0 | 32 | 0 | na | 3 | * | 6 | * |
| 10 | 47 | 0 | 105 | 0 | na | 11 | * | 21 | * |
| 8 | 37 | 0 | 82 | 0 | na | 8 | * | 16 | * |
| 6 | 27 | 0 | 59 | 0 | na | 6 | * | 12 | * |
| 15 | 68 | 0 | 152 | 0 | na | 15 | * | 30 | * |
| | | | | | | | | | |
| 0 | 6 | 0 | 0 | 0 | na | * | * | * | * |
| 6 | 63 | 0 | 20 | 0 | na | * | 50 | 2 | 20 |
| | | | | | | | | | |
| 20 | 70 | 18 | 1460 | 20 | na | 10 | 60 | 8 | 25 |
| | | | | | | | | | |
| 8 | 58 | 16 | 455 | 0 | na | 14 | 60 | 10 | 15 |
| 8 | 66 | 15 | 310 | 10 | na | 10 | 50 | 6 | 20 |
| | | | | | | | | | |
| 15 | 71 | 18 | 630 | 25 | na | 15 | 60 | 8 | 28 |
| 27 | 47 | 33 | 1085 | 90 | na | 10 | 20 | 15 | 35 |
| 31 | 47 | 39 | 1345 | 105 | na | 16 | 20 | 27 | 35 |
| 46 | 47 | 45 | 1295 | 155 | na | 10 | 20 | 15 | 55 |
| 50 | 47 | 51 | 1555 | 170 | na | 16 | 20 | 27 | 55 |
| 1 | 2 | 0 | 10 | 0 | na | 6 | 65 | 2 | 2 |
| 0 | 5 | 0 | 5 | 0 | na | 20 | 30 | 0 | 0 |

## FOOD NAME

| FOOD NAME | Serving Size | Calories |
|---|---|---|
| Carrots, fresh | ¼ cup | 12 |
| Cauliflower, fresh | ½ cup | 14 |
| Cheeseburger | 1 | 410 |
| Cheeseburger, Double | 1 | 590 |
| Chicken Club Sandwich | 1 | 506 |
| Chicken Salad | 2 oz | 120 |
| Chicken Sandwich, fried | 1 | 430 |
| Chili | 9 oz | 220 |
| Chocolate Chip Cookie | 1 | 275 |
| Chocolate Milk | 8 fl oz | 160 |
| Chocolate Pudding | ¼ cup | 90 |
| Coleslaw | 2 oz | 70 |
| Cottage Cheese | ½ cup | 108 |
| Crispy Chicken Nuggets | 6 pc | 280 |
| Cucumber, fresh | 4 sl | 2 |
| Eggs, hard-cooked | 1 tbsp | 30 |
| Fettucini | 2 oz | 190 |
| Fish Filet Sandwich | 1 | 460 |
| French Fries, Biggie | 1 order | 449 |
| French Fries, large | 1 order | 312 |
| French Fries, small | 1 order | 240 |
| Frosty Dairy Dessert, large | 1 | 680 |
| Frosty Dairy Dessert, medium | 1 | 520 |
| Frosty Dairy Dessert, small | 1 | 400 |
| Green Peppers, fresh | ¼ cup | 10 |

| Protein (g) | Carbohydrates (g) | Fat (g) | Sodium (mg) | Cholesterol (mg) | Fiber (g) | Vitamin A (%) | Vitamin C (%) | Calcium (%) | Iron (%) |
|---|---|---|---|---|---|---|---|---|---|
| 0 | 2 | 0 | 10 | 0 | na | 80 | 4 | 0 | 0 |
| 1 | 3 | 0 | 10 | 0 | na | * | 70 | 2 | 2 |
| 28 | 30 | 21 | 760 | 80 | na | 6 | * | 22 | 30 |
| 47 | 30 | 33 | 970 | 145 | na | 6 | * | 22 | 50 |
| 30 | 42 | 25 | 930 | 70 | na | 2 | 15 | 10 | 80 |
| 7 | 4 | 8 | 215 | 0 | na | * | 4 | * | 2 |
| 26 | 41 | 19 | 725 | 60 | na | 2 | 8 | 10 | 80 |
| 21 | 23 | 7 | 750 | 45 | na | 15 | 15 | 8 | 35 |
| 3 | 40 | 13 | 256 | 15 | na | 2 | * | 2 | 8 |
| 7 | 24 | 5 | 140 | 15 | na | 15 | 4 | 25 | 4 |
| 0 | 12 | 4 | 70 | 0 | na | * | * | 15 | 2 |
| 0 | 8 | 5 | 130 | 5 | na | 4 | 25 | 2 | * |
| 13 | 3 | 4 | 425 | 15 | na | 6 | * | 6 | * |
| 14 | 12 | 20 | 600 | 50 | na | * | * | 4 | 4 |
| 0 | 0 | 0 | 0 | 0 | na | * | * | * | * |
| 3 | 0 | 2 | 25 | 90 | na | 4 | * | * | * |
| 4 | 27 | 3 | 3 | 10 | na | * | * | * | 6 |
| 18 | 42 | 25 | 780 | 55 | na | 2 | 2 | 10 | 15 |
| 6 | 62 | 22 | 271 | 0 | na | * | 19 | * | 7 |
| 4 | 43 | 16 | 189 | 0 | na | * | 13 | * | 5 |
| 3 | 33 | 12 | 145 | 0 | na | * | 10 | * | 4 |
| 14 | 100 | 24 | 374 | 85 | na | 17 | * | 51 | 10 |
| 10 | 77 | 18 | 286 | 65 | na | 13 | * | 39 | 9 |
| 8 | 59 | 14 | 220 | 50 | na | 10 | * | 30 | 6 |
| 0 | 2 | 0 | 0 | 0 | na | 4 | 60 | * | * |

| FOOD NAME | Serving Size | Calories |
|---|---|---|
| Grilled Chicken Sandwich | 1 | 320 |
| Hamburger | 1 | 340 |
| Hamburger, with Everything | 1 | 420 |
| Hamburger, Double | 1 | 520 |
| Honeydew Melon | 2 oz | 20 |
| Junior Bacon Cheeseburger | 1 | 430 |
| Junior Cheeseburger | 1 | 310 |
| Junior Hamburger | 1 | 260 |
| Junior Swiss Deluxe | 1 | 360 |
| Lemonade | 8 fl oz | 90 |
| Lettuce, Romaine | 1 cup | 9 |
| Milk, 2% low-fat | 8 fl oz | 110 |
| Pasta Medley | 2 oz | 60 |
| Pasta Salad | ¼ cup | 35 |
| Potato Salad | ¼ cup | 125 |
| Salad, Chef | 1 | 180 |
| Salad, Garden | 1 | 70 |
| Salad, Taco | 1 | 660 |
| Seafood Salad | 2 oz | 110 |
| Spanish Rice | 2 oz | 70 |
| Strawberries, fresh | 2 oz | 17 |
| Tuna Salad | 2 oz | 100 |
| FILBERTS  Shelled | 1 cup | 800 |
| FLOUNDER | | |
| Baked or broiled with butter | 3 oz | 170 |

| Protein (g) | Carbohydrates (g) | Fat (g) | Sodium (mg) | Cholesterol (mg) | Fiber (g) | Vitamin A (%) | Vitamin C (%) | Calcium (%) | Iron (%) |
|---|---|---|---|---|---|---|---|---|---|
| 24 | 37 | 9 | 715 | 60 | na | 2 | 8 | 10 | 20 |
| 24 | 30 | 15 | 500 | 65 | na | * | * | 10 | 30 |
| 25 | 35 | 21 | 890 | 70 | na | 5 | 15 | 10 | 30 |
| 43 | 30 | 27 | 710 | 130 | na | * | * | 10 | 50 |
| 0 | 5 | 0 | 5 | 0 | na | * | 25 | * | * |
| 22 | 32 | 25 | 835 | 50 | na | 2 | 15 | 10 | 20 |
| 18 | 33 | 13 | 770 | 34 | na | 2 | 4 | 10 | 20 |
| 15 | 33 | 9 | 570 | 34 | na | 2 | 4 | 10 | 20 |
| 18 | 34 | 18 | 765 | 40 | na | 4 | 10 | 20 | 20 |
| 0 | 24 | 0 | 0 | 0 | na | * | 15 | * | 2 |
| 0 | 1 | 0 | 5 | 0 | na | 20 | 4 | 2 | 4 |
| 8 | 11 | 4 | 115 | 20 | na | 10 | 4 | 30 | * |
| 2 | 9 | 2 | 5 | 0 | na | 6 | 15 | * | 4 |
| 2 | 6 | 0 | 120 | 0 | na | * | * | * | 2 |
| 0 | 6 | 11 | 90 | 10 | na | * | 10 | * | 2 |
| 15 | 10 | 9 | 140 | 120 | na | 110 | 110 | 25 | 15 |
| 4 | 9 | 2 | 60 | 0 | na | 110 | 70 | 10 | 8 |
| 40 | 46 | 37 | 1110 | 35 | na | 80 | 80 | 80 | 35 |
| 4 | 7 | 7 | 455 | 0 | na | * | 2 | 20 | 2 |
| 2 | 13 | 1 | 440 | 0 | na | 6 | * | 4 | 10 |
| 0 | 4 | 0 | 0 | 0 | na | * | 50 | * | * |
| 8 | 4 | 6 | 290 | 0 | na | * | 4 | * | 2 |
| 15 | 18 | 18 | 1 | 0 | 1.1 | * | * | 30 | 25 |
| | | | | | | | | | |
| 21 | 0 | 7 | 201 | 7 | 0 | * | 4 | 10 | 2 |

| FOOD NAME | Serving Size | Calories | |
|---|---|---|---|
| **FLOUR** | | | |
| Cornmeal | 1 oz | 100 | |
| Rye, Medium | 1 cup | 374 | |
| Rye and Wheat | 1 cup | 400 | |
| White, All-Purpose | 1 cup | 400 | |
| White, Self-Rising | 1 cup | 440 | |
| White, Unbleached | 1 cup | 400 | |
| Whole Wheat | 1 cup | 400 | |
| **FRANKFURTER** | | | |
| Eckrich | 1 | 120 | |
| Eckrich Beef | 1 | 110 | |
| Eckrich Cheese | 1 | 190 | |
| Hormel 12 oz | 1 | 110 | |
| Kahn's | 1 | 140 | |
| Louis Rich | 1 | 100 | |
| Oscar Mayer | 1 | 145 | |
| Oscar Mayer Beef | 1 | 145 | |
| Oscar Mayer Beef with Cheddar | 1 | 130 | |
| Oscar Mayer Beef Little | 1 | 30 | |
| Oscar Mayer Beef Light | 1 | 135 | |
| Oscar Mayer Bun-Length Beef | 1 | 185 | |
| Oscar Mayer Bun-Length ¼ Pound Beef | 1 | 360 | |
| Oscar Mayer Wiener | 1 | 145 | |
| Oscar Mayer Wiener, Bun-Length | 1 | 185 | |
| Oscar Mayer Wiener, Light | 1 | 130 | |

| Protein (g) | Carbohydrates (g) | Fat (g) | Sodium (mg) | Cholesterol (mg) | Fiber (g) | Vitamin A (%) | Vitamin C (%) | Calcium (%) | Iron (%) |
|---|---|---|---|---|---|---|---|---|---|
| 2 | 22 | 0 | na | 0 | 0.2 | * | * | * | 4 |
| 9 | 82 | <2 | 3 | 0 | 14.9 | * | * | 2 | 15 |
| 11 | 86 | 1 | 0 | 0 | na | * | * | 2 | 20 |
| 13 | 95 | 1 | 2 | 0 | 3.4 | * | * | 2 | 25 |
| 12 | 93 | 1 | 1300 | 0 | 0.3 | * | * | 30 | 25 |
| 12 | 86 | 1 | 0 | 0 | 3.4 | * | * | 2 | 25 |
| 16 | 87 | 2 | 1 | 0 | 15.1 | * | * | 2 | 25 |
| | | | | | | | | | |
| na | 2 | 11 | 360 | 16 | 0 | * | 6 | * | 2 |
| na | 2 | 10 | 380 | na | 0 | * | 10 | * | 2 |
| na | 3 | 17 | 650 | na | 0 | * | 20 | 2 | 4 |
| 4 | 1 | 10 | 378 | na | 0 | * | na | * | na |
| 5 | 1 | 13 | 500 | na | 0 | * | na | * | na |
| 6 | 1 | 8 | 472 | na | 0 | * | * | 5 | 4 |
| 5 | 1 | 13 | 455 | 30 | 0 | * | 18 | * | 3 |
| 5 | 1 | 13 | 455 | 30 | 0 | * | 18 | * | 3 |
| 6 | 1 | 11 | 520 | 30 | 0 | * | na | na | na |
| 1 | <1 | 3 | 90 | 5 | 0 | * | na | * | na |
| 7 | 1 | 11 | 595 | 25 | 0 | * | na | * | na |
| 6 | 1 | 17 | 565 | 35 | 0 | * | na | * | na |
| 13 | 1 | 34 | 1140 | 65 | 0 | * | na | * | na |
| 5 | 1 | 13 | 445 | 30 | 0 | * | na | * | na |
| 6 | 1 | 17 | 565 | 35 | 0 | * | na | * | na |
| 7 | 1 | 11 | 625 | 30 | 0 | * | na | * | na |

| FOOD NAME | Serving Size | Calories |
|---|---|---|
| Oscar Mayer Wiener, Little | 1 | 30 |
| **FRENCH TOAST** | | |
| Frozen, with Sausage (Swanson) | 5.5 oz | 380 |
| Frozen, Cinnamon Swirl with Sausage (Swanson) | 5.5 oz | 390 |
| Frozen, Mini with Sausage (Swanson) | 2.5 oz | 190 |
| Frozen, Oatmeal with Lite Links (Swanson) | 4.65 oz | 310 |
| **FROSTING** | | |
| Butter Fudge Supreme (Pillsbury) | ½ can | 140 |
| Caramel Pecan Supreme (Pillsbury) | ½ can | 150 |
| Chocolate Chip Supreme (Pillsbury) | ½ can | 150 |
| Chocolate Fudge Supreme (Pillsbury) | ½ can | 150 |
| Coconut Almond Supreme (Pillsbury) | ½ can | 150 |
| Coconut Pecan Supreme (Pillsbury) | ½ can | 160 |
| Cream Cheese Supreme (Pillsbury) | ½ can | 160 |
| Double Dutch Supreme (Pillsbury) | ½ can | 140 |
| Funfetti Chocolate Fudge | ½ can | 140 |
| Funfetti Pink Vanilla | ½ can | 150 |
| Funfetti Sunshine Vanilla | ½ can | 150 |
| Funfetti Vanilla | ½ can | 150 |
| Lemon Supreme (Pillsbury) | ½ can | 160 |
| Lovin' Lites Chocolate Fudge | ½ can | 130 |
| Lovin' Lites Milk Chocolate | ½ can | 130 |
| Lovin' Lites Vanilla | ½ can | 130 |
| Milk Chocolate with Fudge Swirl | | |
| Supreme (Pillsbury) | ½ can | 150 |

| Protein (g) | Carbohydrates (g) | Fat (g) | Sodium (mg) | Cholesterol (mg) | Fiber (g) | Vitamin A (%) | Vitamin C (%) | Calcium (%) | Iron (%) |
|---|---|---|---|---|---|---|---|---|---|
| 1 | <1 | 3 | 90 | 5 | 0 | * | na | * | na |
| | | | | | | | | | |
| 12 | 35 | 21 | 550 | na | na | * | * | 10 | 15 |
| 12 | 37 | 21 | 530 | na | na | * | * | 10 | 15 |
| 6 | 6 | 22 | 320 | na | na | 2 | * | 4 | 8 |
| 13 | 35 | 13 | 500 | na | na | * | * | 8 | 10 |
| | | | | | | | | | |
| 1 | 22 | 6 | 50 | 0 | na | * | * | * | * |
| 0 | 20 | 8 | 70 | 0 | 0 | * | * | * | * |
| 0 | 27 | 4 | 70 | 0 | * | * | * | * | * |
| 0 | 22 | 6 | 85 | 0 | na | * | * | * | * |
| 1 | 17 | 9 | 60 | 0 | 0 | * | * | * | * |
| 0 | 17 | 10 | 60 | 0 | 0 | * | * | * | * |
| 0 | 26 | 6 | 75 | 0 | 0 | * | * | * | * |
| 1 | 22 | 6 | 50 | 0 | na | * | * | * | * |
| 0 | 23 | 6 | 80 | 0 | na | * | * | * | * |
| 0 | 25 | 6 | 70 | 0 | 0 | * | * | * | * |
| 0 | 25 | 6 | 75 | 0 | 0 | * | * | * | * |
| 0 | 25 | 6 | 75 | 0 | 0 | * | * | * | * |
| 0 | 25 | 6 | 80 | 0 | 0 | * | * | * | * |
| <1 | 28 | 2 | 95 | 0 | 1 | * | * | * | * |
| <1 | 28 | 2 | 95 | 0 | 1 | * | * | * | * |
| 0 | 29 | 2 | 70 | 0 | 0 | * | * | * | * |
| | | | | | | | | | |
| 0 | 23 | 6 | 65 | 0 | na | * | * | * | * |

| FOOD NAME | Serving Size | Calories |
|---|---|---|
| Milk Chocolate Supreme (Pillsbury) | ½ can | 150 |
| Strawberry Supreme (Pillsbury) | ½ can | 160 |
| Vanilla Supreme (Pillsbury) | ½ can | 160 |
| Vanilla with Fudge Swirl Supreme (Pillsbury) | ½ can | 150 |
| **FROZEN BREAKFAST** | | |
| *Healthy Choice* | | |
| Apple Spice Muffin | 1 | 190 |
| Banana Nut Muffin | 1 | 180 |
| Blueberry Muffin | 1 | 190 |
| Cholesterol Free Egg Product | ¼ cup | 30 |
| English Muffin Sandwich | 1 | 200 |
| Turkey Sausage Omelet on | | |
|   English Muffin | 1 | 210 |
| Western Style Omelet on English Muffin | 1 | 200 |
| *Swanson* | | |
| Belgian Waffles and Sausage | 2.85 oz | 280 |
| Belgian Waffles and Strawberries in Sausage | 3.5 oz | 210 |
| Egg, Beefsteak & Cheese on a Muffin | 4.9 oz | 360 |
| Egg, Canadian Bacon & Cheese on a Biscuit | 5.2 oz | 420 |
| Egg, Canadian Bacon & Cheese on a Muffin | 4.1 oz | 290 |
| Egg, Sausage & Cheese on a Biscuit | 5.5 oz | 460 |
| French Toast (Cinnamon Swirl) with Sausage | 5.5 oz | 390 |
| French Toast with Sausage | 5.5 oz | 380 |
| Ham & Cheese on a Bagel | 3 oz | 240 |
| Mini French Toast with Sausage | 2.5 oz | 190 |

| Protein (g) | Carbohydrates (g) | Fat (g) | Sodium (mg) | Cholesterol (mg) | Fiber (g) | Vitamin A (%) | Vitamin C (%) | Calcium (%) | Iron (%) |
|---|---|---|---|---|---|---|---|---|---|
| 0 | 23 | 6 | 65 | 0 | na | * | * | * | * |
| 0 | 25 | 6 | 80 | 0 | 0 | * | * | * | * |
| 0 | 25 | 6 | 75 | 0 | 0 | * | * | * | * |
| 0 | 25 | 6 | 75 | 0 | 0 | * | * | * | * |
| | | | | | | | | | |
| 3 | 40 | 4 | 90 | 0 | na | <2 | 8 | 10 | 10 |
| 3 | 32 | 6 | 80 | 0 | na | <2 | <2 | 10 | 10 |
| 3 | 39 | 4 | 110 | 0 | na | <2 | 6 | 10 | 8 |
| 5 | 1 | <1 | 90 | 0 | na | 10 | <2 | 2 | 4 |
| 16 | 30 | 3 | 510 | 20 | na | 6 | 6 | 15 | 20 |
| | | | | | | | | | |
| 16 | 30 | 4 | 470 | 20 | na | 6 | <2 | 20 | 20 |
| 16 | 29 | 3 | 480 | 15 | na | 10 | 6 | 20 | 20 |
| | | | | | | | | | |
| 7 | 21 | 19 | 420 | na | na | * | 2 | 4 | 6 |
| 3 | 31 | 8 | 240 | na | na | * | 4 | 4 | 6 |
| 17 | 27 | 20 | 730 | na | na | 4 | * | 10 | 15 |
| 16 | 37 | 22 | 1845 | na | na | * | 2 | 25 | 25 |
| 15 | 25 | 15 | 770 | na | na | 2 | * | 15 | 15 |
| 18 | 35 | 28 | 1310 | na | na | 4 | * | 20 | 10 |
| 12 | 37 | 21 | 530 | na | na | * | * | 10 | 15 |
| 12 | 35 | 21 | 550 | na | na | * | * | 10 | 15 |
| 12 | 28 | 8 | 600 | na | na | 6 | 6 | 10 | 10 |
| 6 | 22 | 9 | 320 | na | na | 2 | * | 4 | 8 |

| FOOD NAME | Serving Size | Calories |
|---|---|---|
| Omelets with Cheese Sauce and Ham | 7 oz | 390 |
| Pancakes with Bacon | 4.5 oz | 400 |
| Pancakes with Sausage | 6 oz | 460 |
| Reduced Cholesterol Eggs with | | |
|    Mini Oatbran Muffins | 4.75 oz | 250 |
| Sausage on a Biscuit | 4.7 oz | 410 |
| Scrambled Eggs with Cheese and | | |
|    Cinnamon Pancakes | 3.4 oz | 290 |
| Scrambled Eggs, Home Fries | 4.6 oz | 260 |
| Scrambled Eggs & Bacon with Home Fries | 5.6 oz | 340 |
| Scrambled Eggs & Sausage | | |
|    with Hash Browns | 6.5 oz | 430 |
| Silver Dollar Pancakes and Sausage | 3.75 oz | 310 |
| Waffle with Bacon | 2.2 oz | 230 |
| Whole Wheat Pancakes with Lite Links | 5.5 oz | 350 |
| FROZEN DINNERS | | |
| *Le Menu* | | |
| Chicken Parmigiana | 11.75 oz | 410 |
| Chopped Sirloin Beef | 12.25 oz | 430 |
| Ham Steak | 10 oz | 300 |
| Manicotti with Three Cheeses | 11.75 oz | 390 |
| Pepper Steak | 11.5 oz | 370 |
| Salisbury Steak | 10.5 oz | 370 |
| Sliced Breast of Turkey with | | |
|    Mushroom Gravy | 10.5 oz | 300 |

| Protein (g) | Carbohydrates (g) | Fat (g) | Sodium (mg) | Cholesterol (mg) | Fiber (g) | Vitamin A (%) | Vitamin C (%) | Calcium (%) | Iron (%) |
|---|---|---|---|---|---|---|---|---|---|
| 19 | 15 | 29 | 1220 | na | na | 15 | 2 | 30 | 10 |
| 11 | 43 | 20 | 1000 | na | na | * | * | 6 | 10 |
| 15 | 52 | 22 | 920 | na | na | * | * | 8 | 15 |
| | | | | | | | | | |
| 10 | 27 | 12 | 400 | na | na | 10 | * | 6 | 8 |
| 14 | 36 | 22 | 1180 | na | na | * | * | 10 | 10 |
| | | | | | | | | | |
| 7 | 14 | 23 | 380 | na | na | * | * | 6 | 10 |
| 7 | 14 | 19 | 380 | na | na | * | * | 6 | 8 |
| 11 | 16 | 26 | 690 | na | na | * | * | 6 | 10 |
| | | | | | | | | | |
| 13 | 19 | 34 | 760 | na | na | * | * | 6 | 10 |
| 10 | 37 | 14 | 680 | na | na | * | * | 4 | 10 |
| 7 | 19 | 14 | 710 | na | na | * | * | 4 | 6 |
| 15 | 39 | 16 | 600 | na | na | * | * | 4 | 15 |
| | | | | | | | | | |
| | | | | | | | | | |
| 26 | 31 | 20 | 1030 | na | na | 8 | 10 | 10 | 15 |
| 25 | 28 | 24 | 1010 | na | na | 2 | 8 | 15 | 20 |
| 19 | 31 | 11 | 1500 | na | na | 100 | 30 | 6 | 10 |
| 19 | 44 | 15 | 870 | na | na | 20 | 25 | 50 | 15 |
| 26 | 36 | 13 | 1020 | na | na | 20 | 10 | 4 | 20 |
| 20 | 28 | 20 | 880 | na | na | 6 | * | 10 | 15 |
| | | | | | | | | | |
| 22 | 38 | 7 | 1020 | na | na | 45 | 15 | 4 | 8 |

| FOOD NAME | Serving Size | Calories |
|---|---|---|
| Sweet and Sour Chicken | 11.25 oz | 400 |
| Veal Parmigiana | 11.5 oz | 390 |
| Yankee Pot Roast | 10 oz | 330 |
| *Le Menu LightStyle* | | |
| Cheese Tortellini | 10 oz | 230 |
| Glazed Chicken Breast | 10 oz | 230 |
| Herb Roasted Chicken | 10 oz | 240 |
| Salisbury Steak | 10 oz | 280 |
| Sliced Turkey | 10 oz | 210 |
| Sweet and Sour Chicken | 10 oz | 250 |
| 3-Cheese Stuffed Shells | 10 oz | 280 |
| Turkey Divan | 10 oz | 260 |
| Veal Marsala | 10 oz | 230 |
| *Stouffer's* | | |
| Baked Chicken Breast with Gravy | 10 oz | 300 |
| Barbecue-Style Chicken | 10.5 oz | 390 |
| Cheese Stuffed Shells | 11 oz | 310 |
| Chicken Florentine | 11 oz | 430 |
| Chicken Parmigiana | 11.5 oz | 360 |
| Chicken with Supreme Sauce | 11.38 oz | 360 |
| Fried Chicken | 11.63 oz | 450 |
| Glazed Ham Steak | 10.5 oz | 380 |
| Homestyle Meatloaf | 12.13 oz | 410 |
| Roast Turkey Breast | 10.75 oz | 330 |
| Salisbury Steak with Gravy & Mushrooms | 11.63 oz | 400 |

| Protein (g) | Carbohydrates (g) | Fat (g) | Sodium (mg) | Cholesterol (mg) | Fiber (g) | Vitamin A (%) | Vitamin C (%) | Calcium (%) | Iron (%) |
|---|---|---|---|---|---|---|---|---|---|
| 19 | 41 | 18 | 1020 | na | na | 20 | 6 | 6 | 10 |
| 24 | 36 | 17 | 840 | na | na | 15 | 10 | 20 | 15 |
| 26 | 27 | 13 | 700 | na | na | 120 | 10 | 4 | 20 |
| | | | | | | | | | |
| 10 | 35 | 6 | 460 | 15 | na | 4 | 70 | 10 | 15 |
| 25 | 25 | 3 | 480 | 55 | na | 70 | 8 | 6 | 8 |
| 27 | 18 | 7 | 400 | 70 | na | 8 | 30 | 6 | 8 |
| 18 | 31 | 9 | 400 | 35 | na | 100 | * | 10 | 15 |
| 21 | 21 | 5 | 540 | 30 | na | 70 | 60 | 6 | 6 |
| 18 | 29 | 7 | 530 | 2 | na | 40 | 60 | 2 | 6 |
| 17 | 34 | 8 | 690 | 25 | na | 25 | 50 | 25 | 10 |
| 25 | 23 | 7 | 420 | 60 | na | 15 | 60 | 10 | 8 |
| 22 | 28 | 3 | 700 | 75 | na | 40 | * | 4 | 10 |
| | | | | | | | | | |
| 30 | 20 | 11 | 830 | na | na | 15 | 10 | 2 | 6 |
| 22 | 24 | 23 | 1250 | na | na | 8 | 15 | 15 | 10 |
| 16 | 29 | 14 | 1050 | na | na | 15 | 10 | 35 | 10 |
| 33 | 32 | 18 | 930 | na | na | 120 | 10 | 20 | 10 |
| 31 | 25 | 15 | 1150 | na | na | 15 | 10 | 25 | 10 |
| 33 | 29 | 12 | 990 | na | na | 80 | 60 | 10 | 6 |
| 25 | 35 | 23 | 990 | na | na | 35 | 35 | 10 | 8 |
| 25 | 35 | 15 | 1960 | na | na | 20 | 35 | 20 | 10 |
| 25 | 29 | 22 | 1170 | na | na | 20 | 10 | 4 | 10 |
| 27 | 32 | 10 | 1290 | na | na | 20 | 15 | 6 | 15 |
| 25 | 24 | 23 | 1230 | na | na | 15 | 10 | 15 | 20 |

| FOOD NAME | Serving Size | Calories |
|---|---|---|
| Veal Parmigiana | 11.25 oz | 350 |
| *Swanson Hungry Man* | | |
| Pot Pie, Beef | 16 oz | 610 |
| Pot Pie, Chicken | 16 oz | 630 |
| Pot Pie, Turkey | 16 oz | 650 |
| Salisbury Steak | 16.5 oz | 680 |
| Sliced Beef | 15.25 oz | 450 |
| Turkey | 17 oz | 550 |
| Veal Parmigiana | 18.25 oz | 590 |
| *Swanson's* | | |
| Beans and Franks | 10.5 oz | 440 |
| Beef | 11.25 oz | 310 |
| Beef in Barbecue Sauce | 11 oz | 460 |
| Beef Enchiladas | 13.75 oz | 480 |
| Chicken Nuggets | 8.75 oz | 470 |
| Chopped Sirloin Beef | 10.75 oz | 340 |
| Fish 'n' Chips | 10 oz | 500 |
| Fried Chicken, BBQ Flavored | 10 oz | 540 |
| Fried Chicken, White Meat | 10.25 oz | 550 |
| Fried Chicken, Dark Meat | 9.75 oz | 560 |
| Loin of Pork | 10.75 oz | 280 |
| Macaroni and Beef | 12 oz | 370 |
| Macaroni and Cheese | 12.25 oz | 370 |
| Meatloaf | 10.75 oz | 360 |
| Mexican Style Combination | 14.25 oz | 490 |

| Protein (g) | Carbohydrates (g) | Fat (g) | Sodium (mg) | Cholesterol (mg) | Fiber (g) | Vitamin A (%) | Vitamin C (%) | Calcium (%) | Iron (%) |
|---|---|---|---|---|---|---|---|---|---|
| 27 | 30 | 13 | 1090 | na | na | 10 | 10 | 30 | 15 |
| | | | | | | | | | |
| 24 | 58 | 31 | 1360 | na | na | 45 | 6 | 4 | 25 |
| 22 | 57 | 35 | 1600 | na | na | 60 | * | 6 | 20 |
| 24 | 57 | 36 | 1470 | na | na | 60 | * | 6 | 20 |
| 41 | 37 | 41 | 1730 | na | na | 8 | 10 | 30 | 25 |
| 37 | 49 | 12 | 1060 | na | na | 10 | 10 | 4 | 25 |
| 36 | 61 | 18 | 1810 | na | na | 8 | 15 | 8 | 25 |
| 32 | 57 | 26 | 1840 | na | na | 20 | 25 | 20 | 25 |
| | | | | | | | | | |
| 14 | 53 | 19 | 900 | na | na | 6 | 15 | 15 | 20 |
| 26 | 38 | 6 | 770 | na | na | 6 | 8 | 4 | 25 |
| 30 | 51 | 17 | 860 | na | na | 25 | 8 | 8 | 25 |
| 17 | 55 | 21 | 1350 | na | na | 25 | 6 | 20 | 15 |
| 19 | 47 | 23 | 650 | na | na | 2 | 6 | 2 | 10 |
| 20 | 28 | 16 | 790 | na | na | 100 | 6 | 6 | 15 |
| 20 | 60 | 21 | 960 | na | na | 8 | 4 | 6 | 10 |
| 25 | 61 | 22 | 1160 | na | na | 10 | 4 | 8 | 20 |
| 22 | 60 | 25 | 1460 | na | na | 2 | 4 | 6 | 15 |
| 22 | 55 | 28 | 1130 | na | na | 2 | 6 | 6 | 15 |
| 20 | 27 | 12 | 790 | na | na | 100 | 10 | 4 | 6 |
| 12 | 48 | 15 | 930 | na | na | 8 | 20 | 10 | 10 |
| 13 | 48 | 15 | 1070 | na | na | 70 | 10 | 25 | 15 |
| 15 | 41 | 15 | 960 | na | na | 15 | 15 | 10 | 20 |
| 19 | 62 | 18 | 1760 | na | na | 30 | * | 20 | 15 |

| FOOD NAME | Serving Size | Calories | |
|---|---|---|---|
| *Tyson* | | | |
| Beef Champignon | 10.5 oz | 370 | |
| Chicken à L'Orange | 9.5 oz | 300 | |
| Chicken Francais | 9.5 oz | 280 | |
| Chicken Kiev | 9.25 oz | 450 | |
| Chicken Marsala | 9 oz | 200 | |
| Chicken Parmigiana | 11.25 oz | 380 | |
| Chicken Piccata | 9 oz | 200 | |
| Mesquite Chicken | 9 oz | 320 | |
| Short Ribs | 11 oz | 470 | |
| Sweet & Sour Chicken | 11 oz | 420 | |
| Turkey with Gravy | 9.5 oz | 320 | |
| *Tyson Healthy Portion* | | | |
| BBQ Chicken | 12.5 oz | 470 | |
| Chicken Marinara | 13.75 oz | 330 | |
| Herb Chicken | 13.75 oz | 340 | |
| Honey Mustard Chicken | 13.75 oz | 380 | |
| Italian Style Chicken | 13.75 oz | 320 | |
| Mesquite Chicken | 13.25 oz | 330 | |
| Salsa Chicken | 13.75 oz | 370 | |
| Sesame Chicken | 13.5 oz | 390 | |
| FROZEN ENTREES | | | |
| *Buitoni* | | | |
| Fettucine Alfredo | 10 oz | 440 | |
| Fettucine Carbonara | 10 oz | 440 | |

| Protein (g) | Carbohydrates (g) | Fat (g) | Sodium (mg) | Cholesterol (mg) | Fiber (g) | Vitamin A (%) | Vitamin C (%) | Calcium (%) | Iron (%) |
|---|---|---|---|---|---|---|---|---|---|
| 27 | 31 | 15 | 830 | 51 | na | na | na | na | na |
| 21 | 36 | 8 | 670 | 54 | na | na | na | na | na |
| 19 | 20 | 14 | 1130 | 54 | na | na | na | na | na |
| 18 | 39 | 25 | 950 | 78 | na | na | na | na | na |
| 22 | 19 | 4 | 670 | 52 | na | na | na | na | na |
| 19 | 37 | 17 | 1100 | 26 | na | na | na | na | na |
| 24 | 18 | 4 | 550 | 60 | na | na | na | na | na |
| 23 | 39 | 8 | 660 | 55 | na | na | na | na | na |
| 25 | 38 | 24 | 950 | 70 | na | na | na | na | na |
| 22 | 50 | 15 | 850 | na | na | na | na | na | na |
| 19 | 34 | 12 | 900 | 35 | na | na | na | na | na |
| 44 | 56 | 8 | 600 | 50 | na | na | na | na | na |
| 31 | 37 | 7 | 590 | 45 | na | na | na | na | na |
| 32 | 43 | 4 | 550 | 50 | na | na | na | na | na |
| 31 | 52 | 5 | 520 | 50 | na | na | na | na | na |
| 30 | 38 | 4 | 600 | 50 | na | na | na | na | na |
| 34 | 38 | 5 | 600 | 45 | na | na | na | na | na |
| 27 | 52 | 6 | 470 | 45 | na | na | na | na | na |
| 27 | 58 | 5 | 410 | 45 | na | na | na | na | na |
| na | 36 | 26 | 1119 | na | na | 4 | 6 | 50 | 15 |
| na | 36 | 28 | 1062 | na | na | 6 | 4 | 40 | 20 |

| FOOD NAME | Serving Size | Calories |
|---|---|---|
| Fettucine Primavera | 10 oz | 440 |
| Lasagna, Deep Dish | 11 oz | 390 |
| Lasagna, Deep Dish with Meat Sauce | 10.5 oz | 400 |
| Lasagna Florentine | 9.5 oz | 480 |
| Lasagna with Meat Sauce | 14 oz | 540 |
| *Celentano* | | |
| Lasagna | 16 oz | 708 |
| Ravioli | 13 oz | 852 |
| Stuffed Shells | 8 oz | 330 |
| *Healthy Choice* | | |
| Baked Cheese Ravioli | 9 oz | 250 |
| Baked Potato with Broccoli and Cheese Sauce | 10 oz | 240 |
| Barbecue Beef Ribs | 11 oz | 330 |
| Beef Fajitas | 7 oz | 210 |
| Beef Pepper Steak | 9.5 oz | 250 |
| Cacciatore Chicken | 12.5 oz | 310 |
| Cheese Manicotti | 9.25 oz | 220 |
| Chicken à L'Orange | 9 oz | 240 |
| Chicken and Vegetables | 11.5 oz | 210 |
| Chicken Chow Mein | 8.5 oz | 220 |
| Chicken Enchiladas | 9.5 oz | 280 |
| Chicken Fajitas | 7 oz | 200 |
| Chicken Fettucini | 8.5 oz | 240 |
| Fettucini Alfredo | 8 oz | 240 |
| Fettucini with Turkey and Vegetables | 12.5 oz | 350 |

| Protein (g) | Carbohydrates (g) | Fat (g) | Sodium (mg) | Cholesterol (mg) | Fiber (g) | Vitamin A (%) | Vitamin C (%) | Calcium (%) | Iron (%) |
|---|---|---|---|---|---|---|---|---|---|
| na | 86 | 7 | 1099 | na | na | 10 | 25 | 10 | 15 |
| na | 55 | 10 | 1535 | na | na | 35 | 15 | 25 | 10 |
| na | 45 | 14 | 410 | na | na | 30 | 2 | 10 | 20 |
| na | 36 | 29 | 1100 | na | na | 30 | * | 50 | 10 |
| na | 64 | 18 | 1850 | na | na | 30 | * | 35 | 15 |
|  |  |  |  |  |  |  |  |  |  |
| 34 | 76 | 30 | 1476 | na | na | 72 | * | 4 | 30 |
| 42 | 104 | 30 | 1124 | na | na | 16 | * | 46 | 44 |
| 18 | 41 | 11 | 680 | na | na | na | na | na | na |
|  |  |  |  |  |  |  |  |  |  |
| 14 | 44 | 2 | 420 | 20 | na | 50 | 8 | 25 | 15 |
| 8 | 41 | 5 | 510 | 15 | na | <2 | 25 | 10 | 15 |
| 28 | 40 | 6 | 530 | 70 | na | 6 | 8 | 6 | 10 |
| 19 | 26 | 4 | 250 | 35 | na | 10 | 10 | 10 | 15 |
| 18 | 36 | 4 | 340 | 40 | na | 4 | 45 | 2 | 10 |
| 26 | 47 | 3 | 430 | 35 | na | 10 | 10 | 4 | 15 |
| 15 | 34 | 3 | 310 | 30 | na | 25 | 10 | 15 | 15 |
| 20 | 36 | 2 | 220 | 45 | na | 15 | 45 | 2 | 8 |
| 20 | 31 | 1 | 490 | 35 | na | 15 | 15 | 4 | 15 |
| 18 | 31 | 3 | 440 | 45 | na | 8 | 6 | 2 | 8 |
| 11 | 46 | 6 | 510 | 30 | na | 8 | 35 | 10 | 8 |
| 17 | 25 | 3 | 310 | 35 | na | 15 | 15 | 8 | 15 |
| 22 | 29 | 4 | 370 | 45 | na | <2 | <2 | 8 | 10 |
| 10 | 36 | 7 | 370 | 45 | na | <2 | <2 | 10 | 10 |
| 29 | 45 | 6 | 480 | 60 | na | 15 | <2 | 15 | 15 |

| FOOD NAME | Serving Size | Calories |
|---|---|---|
| Glazed Chicken | 8.5 oz | 220 |
| Lasagna with Meat Sauce | 10 oz | 260 |
| Linguini with Shrimp | 9.5 oz | 230 |
| Macaroni and Cheese | 9 oz | 280 |
| Mandarin Chicken | 11 oz | 260 |
| Rigatoni in Meat Sauce | 9.5 oz | 260 |
| Rigatoni with Chicken | 12.5 oz | 360 |
| Roasted Turkey and Mushrooms in Gravy | 8.5 oz | 200 |
| Salisbury Steak with Mushroom Gravy | 11 oz | 280 |
| Seafood Newburg | 8 oz | 200 |
| Sliced Turkey with Gravy and Dressing | 10 oz | 270 |
| Sole with Lemon Butter Sauce | 8.25 oz | 230 |
| Spaghetti with Meat Sauce | 10 oz | 280 |
| Stuffed Pasta Shells in Tomato Sauce | 12 oz | 330 |
| Teriyaki Pasta with Chicken | 12.6 oz | 350 |
| Zesty Tomato Sauce over Ziti | 12 oz | 350 |
| Zucchini Lasagna | 11.5 oz | 250 |
| *Le Menu* | | |
| Chicken à la King | 8.25 oz | 240 |
| Chicken Dijon | 8 oz | 240 |
| Chicken Enchiladas | 8 oz | 280 |
| Empress Chicken | 8.25 oz | 210 |
| Garden Vegetables Lasagna | 10.5 oz | 260 |
| Glazed Turkey | 8.25 oz | 260 |
| Herb Roasted Chicken | 7.75 oz | 260 |

| Protein (g) | Carbohydrates (g) | Fat (g) | Sodium (mg) | Cholesterol (mg) | Fiber (g) | Vitamin A (%) | Vitamin C (%) | Calcium (%) | Iron (%) |
|---|---|---|---|---|---|---|---|---|---|
| 21 | 27 | 3 | 390 | 45 | na | <2 | <2 | <2 | 6 |
| 18 | 37 | 5 | 420 | 20 | na | 15 | 4 | 10 | 15 |
| 13 | 40 | 2 | 420 | 60 | na | 10 | 20 | 6 | 10 |
| 12 | 45 | 6 | 520 | 20 | na | <2 | <2 | 15 | 10 |
| 23 | 39 | 2 | 400 | 50 | na | 25 | 15 | 2 | 10 |
| 16 | 34 | 6 | 540 | 30 | na | 20 | 4 | 15 | 15 |
| 31 | 50 | 4 | 430 | 60 | na | 6 | 15 | 10 | 10 |
| 18 | 26 | 3 | 380 | 40 | na | 20 | <2 | 2 | 8 |
| 21 | 35 | 6 | 500 | 55 | na | 2 | <2 | 6 | 15 |
| 13 | 30 | 3 | 440 | 55 | na | <2 | 6 | 6 | 6 |
| 27 | 30 | 4 | 530 | 50 | na | 15 | <2 | 6 | 10 |
| 16 | 33 | 4 | 430 | 45 | na | <2 | <2 | 6 | 4 |
| 14 | 42 | 6 | 480 | 20 | na | 25 | 8 | 6 | 20 |
| 24 | 53 | 3 | 470 | 35 | na | 10 | <2 | 40 | 15 |
| 24 | 58 | 3 | 370 | 45 | na | 10 | 10 | 6 | 15 |
| 16 | 59 | 5 | 530 | 30 | na | 6 | <2 | 6 | 20 |
| 14 | 41 | 3 | 400 | 15 | na | 35 | 10 | 25 | 15 |
|  |  |  |  |  |  |  |  |  |  |
| 19 | 29 | 5 | 670 | 30 | na | 2 | * | 8 | 4 |
| 22 | 21 | 7 | 500 | 40 | na | 25 | 10 | 8 | 8 |
| 21 | 32 | 8 | 530 | 35 | na | 2 | 15 | 20 | 10 |
| 16 | 26 | 5 | 690 | 30 | na | 30 | 15 | 2 | 6 |
| 11 | 35 | 8 | 500 | 25 | na | 25 | 80 | 15 | 10 |
| 18 | 34 | 6 | 720 | 35 | na | 2 | 6 | 2 | 6 |
| 22 | 29 | 6 | 500 | 45 | na | 70 | 2 | 2 | 6 |

| FOOD NAME | Serving Size | Calories | |
|---|---|---|---|
| Lasagna with Meat Sauce | 10 oz | 290 | |
| Meat Sauce & Cheese Tortellini | 8 oz | 250 | |
| Spaghetti with Beef Sauce | | | |
|    and Mushrooms | 9 oz | 280 | |
| Swedish Meatballs | 8 oz | 260 | |
| Traditional Turkey | 8 oz | 200 | |
| *Mrs. Paul's* | | | |
| Batter Dipped Fish Fillets | 2 | 330 | |
| Battered Fish Portions | 2 | 300 | |
| Battered Fish Sticks | 4 | 210 | |
| Cod Fillet | 1 | 240 | |
| Crispy Crunchy Breaded Fish Portions | 2 | 230 | |
| Crispy Crunchy Breaded Fish Sticks | 4 | 140 | |
| Crispy Crunchy Fish Fillets | 2 | 220 | |
| Crispy Crunchy Fish Sticks | 4 | 190 | |
| Crunchy Batter Fish Fillets | 2 | 280 | |
| Crunchy Batter Flounder Fillets | 2 | 220 | |
| Crunchy Batter Haddock Fillets | 2 | 190 | |
| Deviled Crab Miniatures | 3.5 oz | 240 | |
| Deviled Crabs | 1 | 180 | |
| Flounder Fillet | 1 | 240 | |
| Fish Cakes | 2 | 190 | |
| Fish Dijon | 8.75 oz | 200 | |
| Fish Florentine | 8 oz | 220 | |
| Fish Mornay | 9 oz | 230 | |

| Protein (g) | Carbohydrates (g) | Fat (g) | Sodium (mg) | Cholesterol (mg) | Fiber (g) | Vitamin A (%) | Vitamin C (%) | Calcium (%) | Iron (%) |
|---|---|---|---|---|---|---|---|---|---|
| 19 | 36 | 8 | 510 | 30 | na | 25 | 30 | 15 | 20 |
| 11 | 34 | 8 | 480 | 15 | na | 10 | 70 | 8 | 15 |
| | | | | | | | | | |
| 12 | 45 | 6 | 450 | 15 | na | 15 | 60 | 4 | 2 |
| 18 | 30 | 8 | 700 | 40 | na | 25 | * | 6 | 15 |
| 19 | 19 | 5 | 610 | 25 | na | 30 | 20 | 4 | 15 |
| | | | | | | | | | |
| 16 | 28 | 17 | 650 | 60 | na | * | * | 2 | 2 |
| 11 | 21 | 19 | 540 | 33 | na | * | * | 2 | 4 |
| 7 | 15 | 12 | 590 | 25 | na | * | * | * | 4 |
| 15 | 22 | 11 | 430 | 50 | na | * | * | 2 | 6 |
| 10 | 14 | 15 | 300 | 25 | na | * | * | 2 | 4 |
| 7 | 14 | 6 | 340 | 20 | na | * | * | 2 | 4 |
| 13 | 23 | 9 | 380 | 22 | na | * | * | 4 | 4 |
| 9 | 18 | 8 | 560 | 25 | na | * | * | 4 | 4 |
| 12 | 26 | 14 | 730 | 22 | na | * | * | 2 | 2 |
| 12 | 23 | 9 | 560 | 40 | na | * | * | 2 | 2 |
| 14 | 22 | 5 | 580 | 25 | na | * | * | * | 4 |
| 9 | 25 | 12 | 540 | 20 | na | * | * | 6 | 6 |
| 8 | 18 | 9 | 480 | 20 | na | * | * | 6 | 6 |
| 16 | 20 | 10 | 450 | 50 | na | 2 | * | 4 | 4 |
| 9 | 24 | 7 | 690 | 20 | na | * | * | 2 | 2 |
| 21 | 17 | 5 | 650 | 60 | na | * | 6 | 20 | 4 |
| 25 | 10 | 8 | 820 | 95 | na | 2 | 8 | 40 | 6 |
| 24 | 12 | 10 | 670 | 80 | na | 2 | 35 | 30 | 4 |

| FOOD NAME | Serving Size | Calories |
|---|---|---|
| Fried Clams | 2.5 oz | 200 |
| Fried Scallops | 3 oz | 160 |
| Haddock Fillet | 1 | 220 |
| Light Fillets in Butter Sauce | 1 | 140 |
| Seafood Lasagna | 9.5 oz | 290 |
| Seafood Rotini | 9 oz | 240 |
| Shrimp and Clams with Linguini | 10 oz | 240 |
| Sole Fillet | 1 | 240 |
| *Stouffer's* | | |
| Beef Chop Suey with Rice | 12 oz | 300 |
| Beef Pie | 10 oz | 500 |
| Beef Short Rib in Gravy | 9 oz | 350 |
| Beef Stroganoff | 9.75 oz | 390 |
| Beef Teriyaki | 9.75 oz | 290 |
| Cashew Chicken | 9.5 oz | 380 |
| Cheese Enchiladas | 10.13 oz | 590 |
| Chicken à la King | 9.5 oz | 290 |
| Chicken Chow Mein | 8 oz | 130 |
| Chicken Divan | 8.5 oz | 320 |
| Chicken Enchiladas | 10 oz | 490 |
| Chicken Pie | 10 oz | 530 |
| Chili con Carne | 8.75 oz | 260 |
| Creamed Chicken | 6.5 oz | 300 |
| Creamed Chipped Beef | 5.5 oz | 230 |
| Escalloped Chicken and Noodles | 10 oz | 420 |

| Protein (g) | Carbohydrates (g) | Fat (g) | Sodium (mg) | Cholesterol (mg) | Fiber (g) | Vitamin A (%) | Vitamin C (%) | Calcium (%) | Iron (%) |
|---|---|---|---|---|---|---|---|---|---|
| 10 | 21 | 9 | 450 | 15 | na | * | * | * | 6 |
| 8 | 18 | 7 | 320 | 10 | na | * | * | 2 | * |
| 17 | 15 | 9 | 350 | 45 | na | * | * | 2 | 2 |
| 20 | 1 | 6 | 520 | 40 | na | * | * | * | * |
| 14 | 39 | 8 | 750 | 57 | na | 2 | 4 | 25 | 8 |
| 12 | 34 | 6 | 570 | 25 | na | * | 2 | 20 | 10 |
| 12 | 36 | 5 | 750 | 40 | na | * | 2 | 4 | 15 |
| 16 | 20 | 10 | 450 | 50 | na | 2 | * | 4 | 4 |
| | | | | | | | | | |
| 16 | 38 | 9 | 1170 | na | na | 2 | 15 | 2 | 8 |
| 20 | 33 | 32 | 1300 | na | na | 70 | 4 | 4 | 15 |
| 30 | 12 | 20 | 900 | na | na | 40 | 6 | 4 | 15 |
| 24 | 28 | 20 | 1090 | na | na | 4 | 2 | 6 | 15 |
| 22 | 33 | 8 | 1450 | na | na | 2 | 15 | 4 | 10 |
| 31 | 29 | 16 | 1140 | na | na | 2 | 2 | 2 | 10 |
| 23 | 34 | 40 | 880 | na | na | 15 | 10 | 60 | 8 |
| 19 | 34 | 9 | 890 | na | na | 2 | 6 | 8 | 4 |
| 13 | 11 | 4 | 1080 | na | na | 8 | 20 | 2 | 4 |
| 24 | 11 | 20 | 780 | na | na | 6 | 30 | 20 | 4 |
| 22 | 34 | 29 | 910 | na | na | 6 | 4 | 30 | 6 |
| 22 | 35 | 33 | 1260 | na | na | 50 | 2 | 10 | 10 |
| 19 | 24 | 10 | 1270 | na | na | 20 | 25 | 8 | 20 |
| 19 | 8 | 21 | 670 | na | na | * | * | 8 | 4 |
| 12 | 9 | 16 | 850 | na | na | * | 2 | 10 | 6 |
| 21 | 27 | 25 | 1230 | na | na | 2 | * | 10 | 8 |

| FOOD NAME | Serving Size | Calories |
|---|---|---|
| Fiesta Lasagna | 10.25 oz | 430 |
| Green Pepper Steak | 10.5 oz | 330 |
| Ham & Asparagus Bake | 9.5 oz | 510 |
| Homestyle Chicken and Noodles | 10 oz | 310 |
| Lasagna | 10.5 oz | 360 |
| Lobster Newburg | 6.5 oz | 380 |
| Macaroni & Beef | 5.75 oz | 170 |
| Macaroni & Cheese | 6 oz | 250 |
| Pasta Shells | 9.25 oz | 330 |
| Salisbury Steak | 9.87 oz | 250 |
| Spaghetti with Meatballs | 12.63 oz | 380 |
| Spaghetti with Meat Sauce | 12.87 oz | 370 |
| Stuffed Green Peppers | 7.75 oz | 200 |
| Swedish Meatballs | 11 oz | 480 |
| Tortellini (Beef) with Marinara Sauce | 10 oz | 360 |
| Tortellini (Cheese) in Alfredo Sauce | 8.87 oz | 600 |
| Tortellini (Cheese) with Tomato Sauce | 9.63 oz | 360 |
| Tortellini (Cheese) with Vinaigrette Dressing | 6.87 oz | 400 |
| Tortilla Grande | 9.63 oz | 530 |
| Tuna Noodle Casserole | 10 oz | 310 |
| Turkey Casserole | 9.75 oz | 360 |
| Turkey Pie | 10 oz | 540 |
| Turkey Tetrazzini | 10 oz | 380 |
| Vegetable Lasagna | 10.5 oz | 420 |

| Protein (g) | Carbohydrates (g) | Fat (g) | Sodium (mg) | Cholesterol (mg) | Fiber (g) | Vitamin A (%) | Vitamin C (%) | Calcium (%) | Iron (%) |
|---|---|---|---|---|---|---|---|---|---|
| 24 | 35 | 22 | 960 | na | na | 10 | 10 | 25 | 10 |
| 21 | 36 | 11 | 1440 | na | na | 4 | 10 | 2 | 10 |
| 18 | 31 | 35 | 900 | na | na | 6 | 60 | 20 | 8 |
| 23 | 21 | 15 | 1090 | na | na | 30 | 2 | 15 | 6 |
| 28 | 33 | 13 | 1020 | na | na | 15 | 10 | 25 | 10 |
| 14 | 9 | 32 | 870 | na | na | 4 | * | 10 | 2 |
| 11 | 15 | 7 | 810 | na | na | 6 | 10 | 4 | 8 |
| 12 | 22 | 13 | 730 | na | na | 2 | * | 25 | 2 |
| 17 | 32 | 15 | 850 | na | na | 6 | 10 | 35 | 6 |
| 21 | 9 | 14 | 1070 | na | na | 30 | 10 | 2 | 15 |
| 20 | 42 | 15 | 1510 | na | na | 20 | 10 | 10 | 15 |
| 18 | 49 | 11 | 1510 | na | na | 15 | 10 | 10 | 15 |
| 11 | 19 | 9 | 940 | na | na | 6 | 10 | 4 | 8 |
| 24 | 37 | 26 | 1510 | na | na | 2 | 2 | 6 | 15 |
| 18 | 45 | 12 | 780 | na | na | 10 | 10 | 10 | 15 |
| 28 | 32 | 40 | 930 | na | na | 4 | 6 | 50 | 8 |
| 18 | 37 | 16 | 860 | na | na | 20 | 10 | 30 | 8 |
| | | | | | | | | | |
| 15 | 24 | 27 | 540 | na | na | 35 | 45 | 25 | 6 |
| 24 | 34 | 33 | 910 | na | na | 20 | 15 | 40 | 15 |
| 17 | 31 | 13 | 1340 | na | na | 2 | * | 15 | 6 |
| 23 | 29 | 17 | 1090 | na | na | 4 | * | 10 | 10 |
| 20 | 35 | 36 | 1300 | na | na | 25 | * | 10 | 10 |
| 22 | 28 | 20 | 1170 | na | na | 2 | * | 10 | 8 |
| 23 | 29 | 24 | 970 | na | na | 50 | 2 | 60 | 6 |

| FOOD NAME | Serving Size | Calories |
|---|---|---|
| Welsh Rarebit | 5 oz | 350 |
| *Stouffer's Lean Cuisine* | | |
| Beef and Bean Enchiladas | 9.25 oz | 280 |
| Beef and Pork Cannelloni | 9.63 oz | 260 |
| Beefsteak Ranchero | 9.25 oz | 270 |
| Breast of Chicken in Herb Cream Sauce | 9.5 oz | 260 |
| Breast of Chicken Marsala | 8.13 oz | 190 |
| Breast of Chicken Parmesan | 10 oz | 260 |
| Cheese Cannelloni | 9.13 oz | 260 |
| Chicken à l'Orange | 8 oz | 260 |
| Chicken and Vegetables with Vermicelli | 11.75 oz | 270 |
| Chicken Cacciatore with Vermicelli | 10.87 oz | 250 |
| Chicken Chow Mein | 11.25 oz | 250 |
| Chicken Enchanadas | 9.87 oz | 270 |
| Chicken Oriental | 9.37 oz | 230 |
| Fiesta Chicken | 8.5 oz | 250 |
| Filet of Fish Divan | 12.37 oz | 260 |
| Filet of Fish Florentine | 9 oz | 230 |
| Filet of Fish Jardiniere | 11.25 oz | 290 |
| Glazed Chicken | 8.5 oz | 270 |
| Lasagna | 10.25 oz | 270 |
| Linguini with Clam Sauce | 9.63 oz | 270 |
| Meatball Stew | 10 oz | 250 |
| Oriental Beef | 8.63 oz | 250 |
| Rigatoni Bake | 9.75 oz | 260 |

| Protein (g) | Carbohydrates (g) | Fat (g) | Sodium (mg) | Cholesterol (mg) | Fiber (g) | Vitamin A (%) | Vitamin C (%) | Calcium (%) | Iron (%) |
|---|---|---|---|---|---|---|---|---|---|
| 13 | 8 | 30 | 680 | na | na | 6 | * | 40 | 2 |
| 15 | 32 | 10 | 890 | 60 | na | 20 | 10 | 15 | 15 |
| 17 | 25 | 10 | 950 | 45 | na | 25 | * | 20 | 8 |
| 16 | 30 | 9 | 950 | 40 | na | 6 | 10 | 4 | 8 |
| 26 | 17 | 10 | 910 | 80 | na | 25 | 4 | 10 | 6 |
| 25 | 11 | 5 | 400 | 80 | na | 25 | 15 | 2 | 6 |
| 27 | 19 | 8 | 870 | 80 | na | 10 | 10 | 15 | 8 |
| 21 | 22 | 10 | 910 | 35 | na | 15 | 10 | 30 | 4 |
| 24 | 30 | 5 | 430 | 55 | na | 6 | 10 | 2 | 4 |
| 20 | 29 | 8 | 980 | 45 | na | 20 | 20 | 10 | 8 |
| 21 | 26 | 7 | 860 | 45 | na | 10 | 15 | 6 | 15 |
| 14 | 36 | 5 | 980 | 35 | na | 2 | 15 | 4 | 4 |
| 17 | 31 | 9 | 850 | 65 | na | 25 | 10 | 15 | 15 |
| 22 | 23 | 6 | 790 | 100 | na | 4 | 25 | 4 | 10 |
| 21 | 29 | 6 | 880 | 45 | na | 15 | 20 | 2 | 6 |
| 31 | 17 | 7 | 750 | 85 | na | 6 | 50 | 20 | 6 |
| 26 | 13 | 8 | 700 | 100 | na | 10 | * | 15 | 6 |
| 31 | 18 | 10 | 840 | 110 | na | 20 | * | 15 | 2 |
| 26 | 23 | 8 | 810 | 55 | na | 2 | 4 | 2 | 4 |
| 25 | 24 | 8 | 970 | 60 | na | 8 | 10 | 20 | 10 |
| 16 | 35 | 7 | 890 | 30 | na | * | * | 2 | 10 |
| 21 | 20 | 10 | 940 | 85 | na | 30 | 6 | 4 | 15 |
| 18 | 28 | 7 | 900 | 45 | na | 15 | * | 2 | 8 |
| 18 | 25 | 10 | 870 | 40 | na | 20 | 10 | 20 | 10 |

| FOOD NAME | Serving Size | Calories | |
|---|---|---|---|
| Salisbury Steak with Italian Style Sauce | 9.5 oz | 280 | |
| Shrimp and Chicken Cantonese | 10.13 oz | 270 | |
| Sliced Turkey Breast in Mushroom Sauce | 8 oz | 240 | |
| Spaghetti with Beef and Mushroom Sauce | 11.5 oz | 280 | |
| Stuffed Cabbage | 10.75 oz | 220 | |
| Szechuan Beef | 9.25 oz | 260 | |
| Tuna Lasagna | 9.75 oz | 270 | |
| Turkey Dijon | 9.5 oz | 270 | |
| Vegetable and Pasta Mornay with Ham | 9.37 oz | 280 | |
| Zucchini Lasagna | 11 oz | 260 | |
| *Stouffer's Right Course* | | | |
| Beef Dijon | 9.5 oz | 290 | |
| Beef Ragout | 10 oz | 300 | |
| Chicken Tenderloins in Barbecue Sauce | 8.75 oz | 270 | |
| Chicken Tenderloins in Peanut Sauce | 9.25 oz | 330 | |
| Chicken Italiano | 9.63 oz | 280 | |
| Fiesta Beef | 8.87 oz | 270 | |
| Homestyle Pot Roast | 9.25 oz | 220 | |
| Sesame Chicken | 10 oz | 320 | |
| Sliced Turkey in a Mild Curry Sauce | 8.75 oz | 320 | |
| Shrimp Primavera | 9.63 oz | 240 | |
| Vegetarian Chili | 9.75 oz | 280 | |
| *Swanson* | | | |
| Chicken Cacciatore | 10.95 oz | 260 | |
| Chicken Nibbles | 4.25 oz | 340 | |

| Protein (g) | Carbohydrates (g) | Fat (g) | Sodium (mg) | Cholesterol (mg) | Fiber (g) | Vitamin A (%) | Vitamin C (%) | Calcium (%) | Iron (%) |
|---|---|---|---|---|---|---|---|---|---|
| 25 | 12 | 15 | 840 | 100 | na | 10 | 10 | 15 | 15 |
| 22 | 25 | 9 | 920 | 100 | na | 10 | 6 | 4 | 6 |
| 23 | 20 | 7 | 790 | 50 | na | 10 | 4 | 2 | 4 |
| 16 | 38 | 7 | 940 | 25 | na | 8 | 10 | 8 | 15 |
| 14 | 19 | 10 | 930 | 55 | na | 15 | 10 | 6 | 10 |
| 20 | 22 | 10 | 680 | 100 | na | 25 | 20 | 4 | 10 |
| 17 | 29 | 10 | 890 | 35 | na | 40 | 6 | 25 | 8 |
| 24 | 22 | 10 | 900 | 60 | na | 50 | 2 | 15 | 6 |
| 15 | 29 | 11 | 970 | 35 | na | 30 | 25 | 15 | 6 |
| 20 | 28 | 7 | 950 | 25 | na | 30 | 10 | 30 | 8 |
| | | | | | | | | | |
| 20 | 31 | 9 | 580 | 580 | na | 25 | 2 | 4 | 15 |
| 19 | 38 | 8 | 550 | 50 | na | 20 | 10 | 4 | 10 |
| 20 | 35 | 6 | 590 | 40 | na | 35 | 45 | 6 | 8 |
| 27 | 32 | 10 | 570 | 50 | na | 6 | 10 | 8 | 10 |
| 24 | 29 | 8 | 560 | 45 | na | 4 | 25 | 10 | 10 |
| 18 | 33 | 7 | 590 | 30 | na | 15 | 10 | 6 | 15 |
| 17 | 22 | 7 | 550 | 35 | na | 50 | 8 | 2 | 8 |
| 25 | 34 | 9 | 590 | 50 | na | 10 | 20 | 4 | 10 |
| 23 | 40 | 8 | 570 | 50 | na | 10 | 10 | 10 | 8 |
| 12 | 32 | 7 | 590 | 50 | na | 30 | 4 | 8 | 10 |
| 9 | 45 | 7 | 590 | 0 | na | 20 | 25 | 8 | 10 |
| | | | | | | | | | |
| 15 | 33 | 8 | 1030 | na | na | 15 | 35 | 8 | 15 |
| 10 | 29 | 20 | 730 | na | na | * | 4 | 2 | 8 |

| FOOD NAME | Serving Size | Calories |
|---|---|---|
| Chicken Pie | 8 oz | 410 |
| Chili con Carne | 8.25 oz | 270 |
| Fish & Fries | 6.5 oz | 340 |
| Fried Chicken | 7 oz | 390 |
| Lasagna | 10.5 oz | 400 |
| Macaroni and Cheese | 10 oz | 390 |
| Pot Pie, Beef | 7 oz | 370 |
| Pot Pie, Chicken | 7 oz | 380 |
| Pot Pie, Macaroni and Cheese | 7 oz | 200 |
| Pot Pie, Turkey | 7 oz | 380 |
| Salisbury Steak | 10 oz | 320 |
| Scalloped Potatoes | 9 oz | 300 |
| Seafood Creole | 9 oz | 240 |
| Sirloin Tips in Burgundy Sauce | 7 oz | 160 |
| Spaghetti with Italian Style Meatballs | 13 oz | 490 |
| Swedish Meatballs | 8.5 oz | 360 |
| Turkey with Dressing | 9 oz | 290 |
| Veal Parmigiana | 10 oz | 330 |
| GARLIC | 1 clove | 4 |
| GELATIN | | |
| D-Zerta Low Calorie, all flavors, average values | ½ cup | 8 |
| Jell-O Brand, all flavors, average values | ½ cup | 80 |
| Jell-O Brand 1-2-3, all flavors, average values | ⅔ cup | 130 |
| GRAPES | 10 | 35 |

| Protein (g) | Carbohydrates (g) | Fat (g) | Sodium (mg) | Cholesterol (mg) | Fiber (g) | Vitamin A (%) | Vitamin C (%) | Calcium (%) | Iron (%) |
|---|---|---|---|---|---|---|---|---|---|
| 15 | 41 | 21 | 1030 | na | na | 30 | 4 | 4 | 10 |
| 20 | 26 | 10 | 740 | na | na | 25 | 6 | 6 | 20 |
| 11 | 37 | 16 | 670 | na | na | * | 4 | 2 | 10 |
| 18 | 33 | 21 | 1100 | na | na | * | 6 | 4 | 10 |
| 26 | 39 | 15 | 1070 | na | na | 15 | 10 | 50 | 15 |
| 17 | 37 | 19 | 1150 | na | na | 2 | 2 | 45 | 10 |
| 12 | 36 | 19 | 730 | na | na | 25 | * | 2 | 15 |
| 11 | 35 | 22 | 760 | na | na | 40 | * | 2 | 10 |
| 7 | 24 | 8 | 740 | na | na | 8 | * | 15 | 6 |
| 11 | 36 | 21 | 720 | na | na | 35 | * | 2 | 10 |
| 21 | 22 | 16 | 980 | na | na | * | * | 4 | 15 |
| 19 | 26 | 13 | 1080 | na | na | 4 | 15 | 35 | 10 |
| 7 | 40 | 6 | 810 | na | na | 15 | 50 | 10 | 8 |
| 12 | 16 | 5 | 550 | na | na | 80 | 45 | 4 | 10 |
| 23 | 60 | 18 | 940 | na | na | 25 | 20 | 10 | 30 |
| 19 | 26 | 20 | 790 | na | na | 6 | * | 8 | 15 |
| 18 | 30 | 11 | 1010 | na | na | * | 4 | 4 | 10 |
| 19 | 33 | 13 | 960 | na | na | 6 | 10 | 8 | 10 |
| 0 | 1 | 0 | 1 | 0 | 0.1 | * | * | * | * |
| | | | | | | | | | |
| 2 | 0 | 0 | 0 | 0 | 0 | * | * | * | * |
| 2 | 19 | 0 | 50-75 | 0 | 0 | * | * | * | * |
| 2 | 27 | 2 | 55 | 0 | 0 | * | * | * | * |
| 0 | 9 | 0 | 1 | 0 | 0.4 | 1 | 3 | 1 | 1 |

| FOOD NAME | Serving Size | Calories | |
|---|---|---|---|
| **GRAPE DRINK** | | | |
| (Kool-Aid Sugar-Sweetened) | 8 fl oz | 80 | |
| (Kool-Aid Sugar Free) | 8 fl oz | 4 | |
| **GRAPE JUICE** | 8 fl oz | 165 | |
| **GRAPEFRUIT** | ½ | 50 | |
| **GRAPEFRUIT JUICE** Unsweetened | 8 fl oz | 100 | |
| **GRAVY** | | | |
| Au jus (Franco-American) | 2 oz | 10 | |
| Beef (Franco-American) | 2 oz | 25 | |
| Chicken (Franco-American) | 2 oz | 45 | |
| Chicken Giblet (Franco-American) | 2 oz | 30 | |
| Cream (Franco-American) | 2 oz | 35 | |
| Mushroom (Franco-American) | 2 oz | 25 | |
| Pork (Franco-American) | 2 oz | 40 | |
| Turkey (Franco-American) | 2 oz | 30 | |
| **GREEN BEANS** | | | |
| *Fresh*, Cooked | 1 cup | 30 | |
| *Frozen* | | | |
| Cut (Birds Eye) | 3 oz | 25 | |
| French Cut (Birds Eye) | 3 oz | 25 | |
| Italian (Birds Eye) | 3 oz | 30 | |
| Petite (Birds Eye) | 2.6 oz | 20 | |
| Whole (Birds Eye) | 4 oz | 30 | |
| (Green Giant) | ½ cup | 14 | |
| Cut (Green Giant) | ½ cup | 16 | |

| Protein (g) | Carbohydrates (g) | Fat (g) | Sodium (mg) | Cholesterol (mg) | Fiber (g) | Vitamin A (%) | Vitamin C (%) | Calcium (%) | Iron (%) |
|---|---|---|---|---|---|---|---|---|---|
| 0 | 20 | 0 | 0 | 0 | 0 | * | 10 | * | * |
| 0 | 0 | 0 | 5 | 0 | 0 | * | 10 | * | * |
| 1 | 42 | 0 | 8 | 0 | 0 | * | * | 3 | 4 |
| 1 | 13 | 0 | 1 | 0 | 0.3 | 11 | 73 | 2 | 3 |
| 1 | 24 | 0 | 3 | 0 | 0 | * | 140 | 2 | 6 |
| | | | | | | | | | |
| 0 | 2 | 0 | 330 | na | na | * | * | * | * |
| 0 | 4 | 1 | 340 | na | na | * | * | * | * |
| 0 | 3 | 4 | 240 | na | na | 4 | * | * | * |
| 1 | 3 | 2 | 310 | na | na | * | * | * | * |
| 0 | 4 | 2 | 220 | na | na | * | * | * | * |
| 0 | 3 | 1 | 290 | na | na | * | * | * | * |
| 0 | 3 | 3 | 330 | na | na | * | * | * | * |
| 0 | 3 | 2 | 290 | na | na | * | * | * | * |
| | | | | | | | | | |
| 2 | 7 | 0 | 5 | 0 | 2.2 | 14 | 25 | 6 | 4 |
| | | | | | | | | | |
| 1 | 6 | 0 | 0 | 0 | 2 | 10 | 15 | 4 | 4 |
| 1 | 6 | 0 | 0 | 0 | 2 | 8 | 15 | 4 | 4 |
| 2 | 7 | 0 | 0 | 0 | 3 | 8 | 25 | 4 | 4 |
| 1 | 5 | 0 | 0 | 0 | 2 | 10 | 15 | 2 | 4 |
| 2 | 7 | 0 | 0 | 0 | 2 | 15 | 20 | 4 | 4 |
| 1 | 4 | 0 | 10 | 0 | 1 | 2 | 4 | 2 | 2 |
| 1 | 4 | 0 | 95 | 0 | 1 | 2 | 6 | 2 | 4 |

| FOOD NAME | Serving Size | Calories | |
|---|---|---|---|
| Cut, in Butter Sauce (Green Giant) | ½ cup | 30 | |
| *Frozen combinations* | | | |
| Broccoli, Green Beans, Pearl Onions | | | |
| and Red Peppers (Birds Eye) | 4 oz | 35 | |
| French Green Beans with Toasted | | | |
| Almonds (Birds Eye) | 3 oz | 50 | |
| **GREENS** | | | |
| Beet, fresh, cooked | 1 cup | 25 | |
| Collard, fresh, cooked | 1 cup | 65 | |
| Dandelion, fresh, cooked | 1 cup | 35 | |
| Mustard, fresh, cooked | 1 cup | 30 | |
| Turnip, fresh, cooked | 1 cup | 30 | |
| **HADDOCK** Breaded and fried | 4 oz | 187 | |
| **HALIBUT** Baked or broiled | 4 oz | 159 | |
| **HAM** | | | |
| Cured, roasted, lean and fat | 4 oz | 276 | |
| Cured, roasted, lean and fat, diced | 1 cup | 341 | |
| Cured, roasted, lean only | 4 oz | 178 | |
| Cured, roasted, lean only, diced | 1 cup | 219 | |
| Roasted, lean and fat | 4 oz | 333 | |
| Roasted, lean and fat, diced | 1 cup | 520 | |
| Roasted, lean only | 4 oz | 249 | |
| Roasted, lean only, diced | 1 cup | 300 | |
| **HAMBURGER MIX** | | | |
| Beef Romanoff (Hamburger Helper) | 1 cup | 350 | |

| Protein (g) | Carbohydrates (g) | Fat (g) | Sodium (mg) | Cholesterol (mg) | Fiber (g) | Vitamin A (%) | Vitamin C (%) | Calcium (%) | Iron (%) |
|---|---|---|---|---|---|---|---|---|---|
| 1 | 4 | 1 | 230 | 5 | 1.5 | 4 | 4 | 2 | 2 |
| 2 | 7 | 0 | 15 | 0 | 3 | 30 | 60 | 6 | 6 |
| 3 | 8 | 2 | 340 | 0 | 2 | 8 | 15 | 4 | 2 |
| 2 | 5 | 0 | 110 | 0 | na | 148 | 37 | 14 | 16 |
| 7 | 10 | 1 | 24 | 0 | na | 296 | 240 | 36 | 8 |
| 2 | 7 | 1 | 46 | 0 | na | 246 | 32 | 15 | 11 |
| 3 | 6 | 1 | 25 | 0 | na | 162 | 112 | 19 | 14 |
| 3 | 5 | 0 | 42 | 0 | 4.4 | 165 | 113 | 25 | 8 |
| 23 | 7 | 7 | 199 | 84 | 0 | * | 5 | 5 | 7 |
| 30 | 0 | 3 | 78 | 46 | 0 | 10 | * | 2 | 4 |
| 25 | 0 | 19 | 1346 | 70 | 0 | * | * | * | 10 |
| 30 | 0 | 24 | 1661 | 86 | 0 | * | * | 2 | 20 |
| 28 | 0 | 6 | 1505 | 62 | 0 | * | * | * | 15 |
| 35 | 0 | 8 | 1858 | 78 | 0 | * | * | 2 | 25 |
| 28 | 0 | 29 | 67 | 105 | 0 | * | * | * | 15 |
| 35 | 0 | 29 | 83 | 131 | 0 | * | * | 2 | 25 |
| 32 | 0 | 13 | 73 | 107 | 7 | * | * | 2 | 20 |
| 40 | 0 | 15 | 90 | 131 | 0 | * | * | 2 | 30 |
| 22 | 31 | 16 | 1070 | na | na | * | * | 6 | 15 |

| FOOD NAME | Serving Size | Calories |
|---|---|---|
| Chili Tomato (Hamburger Helper) | 1 cup | 330 |
| Lasagna (Hamburger Helper) | 1 cup | 340 |
| Tamale Pie (Hamburger Helper) | 1 cup | 380 |
| HERRING Canned, kippered, smoked | 1 fillet | 200 |
| HOLLANDAISE SAUCE Mix (French's) | 3 tbsp | 45 |
| HONEY | 1 tbsp | 60 |
| HONEYDEW MELON | ⅒ | 46 |
| HORSERADISH | | |
| (Kraft) | 1 tbsp | 10 |
| Cream Style (Kraft) | 1 tbsp | 12 |
| Mustard (Kraft) | 1 tbsp | 14 |
| Sauce (Kraft) | 1 tbsp | 50 |
| ICE CREAM | | |
| Butter Almond (Breyers) | ½ cup | 170 |
| Butter Pecan (Breyers) | ½ cup | 180 |
| Butter Pecan (Lady Borden) | ½ cup | 180 |
| Cherry Vanilla (Breyers) | ½ cup | 150 |
| Chocolate (Häagen Dazs) | ½ cup | 270 |
| Chocolate (Baskin-Robbins) | 1 scoop | 270 |
| Coffee (Breyers) | ½ cup | 140 |
| Dutch Chocolate (Borden) | ½ cup | 130 |
| Dutch Chocolate Almond (Borden) | ½ cup | 160 |
| French Vanilla (Lady Borden) | ½ cup | 170 |
| Maple Walnut (Sealtest) | ½ cup | 150 |
| Strawberry (Borden) | ½ cup | 130 |

| Protein (g) | Carbohydrates (g) | Fat (g) | Sodium (mg) | Cholesterol (mg) | Fiber (g) | Vitamin A (%) | Vitamin C (%) | Calcium (%) | Iron (%) |
|---|---|---|---|---|---|---|---|---|---|
| 20 | 31 | 14 | 1410 | na | na | 8 | * | 2 | 20 |
| 21 | 33 | 14 | 1050 | na | na | 10 | * | 2 | 15 |
| 19 | 39 | 16 | 940 | na | na | 6 | * | 4 | 15 |
| 16 | 0 | 6 | 1000 | 93 | 0 | * | * | 2 | 4 |
| Tr | 2 | 4 | 290 | 75 | 0 | * | * | 2 | * |
| 0 | 16 | 0 | 1 | 0 | 0 | * | * | * | * |
| <1 | 8 | Tr | 13 | 0 | 0.8 | 1 | 57 | 2 | 3 |
| | | | | | | | | | |
| 0 | 1 | 0 | 140 | 0 | 0.2 | * | 2 | * | * |
| 0 | 1 | 1 | 85 | 0 | na | * | * | * | * |
| 1 | 1 | 1 | 135 | 0 | na | * | * | * | * |
| 0 | 2 | 5 | 105 | 5 | na | * | * | * | * |
| | | | | | | | | | |
| 4 | 15 | 10 | 125 | 25 | na | na | na | na | na |
| 3 | 15 | 11 | 125 | 25 | na | na | na | na | na |
| na | 16 | 12 | na | na | na | 8 | * | 8 | * |
| 3 | 17 | 7 | 45 | 20 | na | na | na | na | na |
| 5 | 24 | 17 | 50 | na | 0 | na | na | na | na |
| 5 | 32 | 14 | 160 | 37 | 0 | 8 | * | 8 | * |
| 3 | 15 | 8 | 50 | 30 | 0 | na | na | na | na |
| 2 | 16 | 6 | 65 | na | 0 | 4 | * | 8 | * |
| na | 18 | 9 | na | na | 0 | 6 | * | 10 | * |
| na | 20 | 9 | na | na | 0 | 6 | * | 10 | * |
| 3 | 16 | 9 | 50 | 20 | 0 | na | na | na | na |
| 2 | 18 | 6 | 55 | na | 0 | 4 | * | 6 | * |

| FOOD NAME | Serving Size | Calories |
|---|---|---|
| Strawberry (Häagen Dazs) | ½ cup | 250 |
| Vanilla (Borden) | ½ cup | 130 |
| Vanilla (Breyers) | ½ cup | 150 |
| Vanilla (Frusen Glädjé) | ½ cup | 230 |
| Vanilla (Häagen Dazs) | ½ cup | 260 |
| Vanilla (Sealtest) | ½ cup | 140 |
| Vanilla Fudge (Sealtest) | ½ cup | 140 |
| Vanilla Swiss Almond (Frusen Glädjé) | ½ cup | 270 |
| Vanilla Swiss Almond (Häagen Dazs) | ½ cup | 290 |
| **ICE CREAM BAR** | | |
| Chip Candy Crunch (Good Humor) | 1 | 255 |
| Chocolate Eclair (Good Humor) | 1 | 180 |
| Chocolate Fudge Cake (Good Humor) | 1 | 214 |
| Dark Chocolate Coating (Häagen Dazs) | 1 | 390 |
| Toasted Almond (Good Humor) | 1 | 190 |
| Toasted Caramel (Good Humor) | 1 | 170 |
| Vanilla (Good Humor) | 1 | 198 |
| Vanilla (Häagen Dazs) | 1 | 390 |
| **ICE CREAM SANDWICH** | | |
| Vanilla (Good Humor) | 1 | 191 |
| Vanilla (Klondike) | 1 | 230 |
| **ICE MILK** | | |
| Hard | ½ cup | 92 |
| Soft | ½ cup | 112 |

| Protein (g) | Carbohydrates (g) | Fat (g) | Sodium (mg) | Cholesterol (mg) | Fiber (g) | Vitamin A (%) | Vitamin C (%) | Calcium (%) | Iron (%) |
|---|---|---|---|---|---|---|---|---|---|
| 4 | 23 | 15 | 40 | na | 0 | na | na | na | na |
| 2 | 15 | 7 | 55 | na | 0 | 6 | * | 8 | * |
| 3 | 15 | 8 | 50 | 30 | 0 | na | na | na | na |
| 5 | 16 | 17 | 70 | 90 | 0 | na | na | na | na |
| 5 | 23 | 17 | 55 | na | 0 | na | na | na | na |
| 2 | 16 | 7 | 50 | 20 | 0 | na | na | na | na |
| 3 | 19 | 7 | 55 | 15 | 0 | na | na | na | na |
| 6 | 18 | 19 | 65 | 85 | 0 | na | na | na | na |
| 5 | 24 | 19 | 55 | na | 0 | na | na | na | na |
| | | | | | | | | | |
| 2 | 21 | 18 | 40 | na | na | 4 | * | 6 | * |
| 2 | 23 | 10 | 54 | na | na | 2 | * | 4 | * |
| 2 | 18 | 15 | 50 | na | na | 4 | * | 6 | * |
| | | | | | | | | | |
| 5 | 32 | 27 | 60 | na | na | na | na | na | na |
| 2 | 24 | 12 | 34 | na | na | 2 | * | 4 | * |
| na | 21 | 9 | 55 | na | na | 4 | * | 6 | * |
| 2 | 17 | 14 | 44 | na | na | 4 | * | 6 | * |
| 5 | 32 | 27 | 65 | na | 0 | na | na | na | na |
| | | | | | | | | | |
| 4 | 31 | 6 | 155 | na | na | na | na | na | na |
| 5 | 33 | 9 | 220 | na | na | na | na | na | na |
| | | | | | | | | | |
| 3 | 15 | 3 | 52 | 9 | 0 | 3 | 1 | 10 | * |
| 4 | 19 | 2 | 81 | 7 | 0 | 4 | 2 | 13 | 1 |

## FOOD NAME

| FOOD NAME | Serving Size | Calories | |
|---|---|---|---|
| **ICE CREAM SUBSTITUTE** | | | |
| Tofutti (Lite-Lite, all flavors) | ½ cup | 90 | |
| **JALAPEÑO PEPPERS** Mexican Hot (Vlasic) | 1 oz | 8 | |
| **JELLIES, JAMS AND PRESERVES** | | | |
| Grape Jelly (Kraft Reduced Calorie) | 1 tsp | 6 | |
| Jam, all varieties (Kraft) | 1 tsp | 17 | |
| Jams, all flavors (Smucker's) | 1 tsp | 18 | |
| Jams, all flavors (Welch's) | 1 tsp | 18 | |
| Jelly, all varieties (Kraft) | 1 tsp | 17 | |
| Jelly, all flavors (Polaner's) | 1 tsp | 18 | |
| Jelly, all flavors (Smucker's) | 1 tsp | 18 | |
| Jelly, all flavors (Welch's) | 1 tsp | 18 | |
| Preserves, all varieties (Kraft) | 1 tsp | 17 | |
| Preserves, all flavors (Smucker's) | 1 tsp | 18 | |
| Preserves, all flavors (Welch's) | 1 tsp | 18 | |
| Strawberry Preserves | | | |
| (Kraft Reduced Calorie) | 1 tsp | 6 | |
| **KALE** Fresh, boiled, drained | 1 cup | 45 | |
| **KETCHUP** | 1 tbsp | 15 | |
| **KIDNEY BEANS** | | | |
| *Fresh* | | | |
| Red, dry, cooked, drained | 1 cup | 220 | |
| *Canned* | | | |
| Dark Red (Green Giant) | ½ cup | 90 | |
| Dark Red, 50% less salt (Green Giant) | ½ cup | 90 | |

| Protein (g) | Carbohydrates (g) | Fat (g) | Sodium (mg) | Cholesterol (mg) | Fiber (g) | Vitamin A (%) | Vitamin C (%) | Calcium (%) | Iron (%) |
|---|---|---|---|---|---|---|---|---|---|
| 2 | 20 | <1 | 80 | 0 | na | na | na | na | na |
| 0 | 2 | 0 | 380 | 0 | na | 2 | * | * | 2 |
| | | | | | | | | | |
| 0 | 2 | 0 | 5 | 0 | na | * | * | * | * |
| 0 | 4 | 0 | 0 | 0 | na | * | * | * | * |
| 0 | 4 | 0 | 0 | 0 | na | * | * | * | * |
| 0 | 4 | 0 | <3 | 0 | na | na | na | na | na |
| 0 | 4 | 0 | 0 | 0 | na | * | * | * | * |
| 0 | 5 | 0 | na | 0 | 0 | na | na | na | na |
| 0 | 4 | 0 | 0 | 0 | na | * | * | * | * |
| 0 | 4 | 0 | <3 | 0 | 0 | na | na | na | na |
| 0 | 4 | 0 | 0 | 0 | na | * | * | * | * |
| 0 | 4 | 0 | 0 | 0 | na | * | * | * | * |
| 0 | 4 | 0 | <3 | 0 | na | na | na | na | na |
| | | | | | | | | | |
| 0 | 2 | 0 | 5 | 0 | na | * | * | * | * |
| 2 | 7 | 1 | 47 | 0 | 1 | 183 | 170 | 20 | 10 |
| 0 | 4 | 0 | 156 | 0 | 0 | 4 | 3 | * | 1 |
| | | | | | | | | | |
| | | | | | | | | | |
| na | 40 | 1 | 6 | 0 | 10 | * | * | 6 | 25 |
| | | | | | | | | | |
| 7 | 20 | <1 | 330 | 0 | 5 | * | * | 6 | 10 |
| 7 | 20 | <1 | 165 | 0 | 5 | * | * | 6 | 10 |

| FOOD NAME | Serving Size | Calories |
|---|---|---|
| Light Red (Green Giant) | ½ cup | 90 |
| Light Red, 50% less salt (Green Giant) | ½ cup | 90 |
| Light Red (Van Camp's) | 1 cup | 184 |
| Red (Hunt's) | 4 oz | 120 |
| Red (Progresso) | 8 oz | 190 |
| KIELBASA | | |
| Eckrich Polska | 1 oz | 95 |
| Eckrich Lean Supreme Polska | 1 oz | 72 |
| Eckrich Skinless | 1 link | 180 |
| Hillshire Farm Polska Flavorsea | 2 oz | 190 |
| Hormel | 3 oz | 220 |
| KNOCKWURST | | |
| Hebrew National | 1 | 263 |
| Hillshire Farm | 1 | 180 |
| KUMQUAT | 1 med | 12 |
| LAMB | | |
| Chop, cooked, lean and fat | 2.2 oz | 220 |
| Chop, cooked, lean only | 1.7 oz | 135 |
| Chop, loin, broiled, lean and fat | 2.8 oz | 235 |
| Chop, loin, broiled, lean only | 2.3 oz | 140 |
| Leg, roasted, lean and fat | 3 oz | 205 |
| Leg, roasted, lean only | 2.6 oz | 140 |
| Rib, roasted, lean and fat | 3 oz | 315 |
| Rib, roasted, lean only | 2 oz | 130 |
| LEMON | 1 | 20 |

| Protein (g) | Carbohydrates (g) | Fat (g) | Sodium (mg) | Cholesterol (mg) | Fiber (g) | Vitamin A (%) | Vitamin C (%) | Calcium (%) | Iron (%) |
|---|---|---|---|---|---|---|---|---|---|
| 7 | 20 | <1 | 330 | 0 | 5 | * | * | 6 | 10 |
| 7 | 20 | <1 | 165 | 0 | 5 | * | * | 6 | 10 |
| 12 | 33 | <1 | 688 | 0 | 2.2 | na | na | na | na |
| 7 | 21 | 0 | 400 | 0 | na | * | * | 4 | 18 |
| 12 | 34 | 1 | 1080 | 0 | na | na | na | na | na |
| | | | | | | | | | |
| 4 | 1 | 9 | 260 | na | 0 | * | 8 | * | 2 |
| 4 | 1 | 6 | 224 | na | 0 | na | na | na | na |
| 7 | 2 | 16 | 420 | na | 0 | * | 20 | 2 | 4 |
| 8 | 2 | 17 | 540 | na | 0 | na | na | na | na |
| 12 | 1 | 19 | 904 | na | 0 | na | na | na | na |
| | | | | | | | | | |
| 10 | <1 | 25 | 877 | na | 0 | na | na | na | na |
| 7 | 1 | 16 | 460 | na | 0 | na | na | na | na |
| Tr | 3 | 0 | 1 | 0 | 0.7 | 2 | 10 | 2 | * |
| | | | | | | | | | |
| 20 | 0 | 15 | 46 | 77 | 0 | * | * | * | 8 |
| 17 | 0 | 7 | 36 | 59 | 0 | * | * | * | 7 |
| 22 | 0 | 16 | 62 | 78 | 0 | * | * | * | 8 |
| 19 | 0 | 6 | 54 | 60 | 0 | * | * | * | 7 |
| 22 | 0 | 13 | 57 | 78 | 0 | * | * | * | 9 |
| 20 | 0 | 6 | 50 | 65 | 0 | * | * | * | 8 |
| 18 | 0 | 26 | 60 | 77 | 0 | * | * | * | 8 |
| 15 | 0 | 7 | 46 | 50 | 0 | * | * | * | 6 |
| 1 | 6 | 0 | 1 | 0 | 0 | * | 65 | 2 | 2 |

| FOOD NAME | Serving Size | Calories |
|---|---|---|
| **LEMONADE** | | |
| Crystal Light Sugar Free Drink Mix | 8 fl oz | 4 |
| Kool-Aid Sugar-Sweetened Soft Drink Mix | 8 fl oz | 80 |
| Kool-Aid Sugar Free Soft Drink Mix | 8 fl oz | 4 |
| Sunkist Frozen | 8 fl oz | 92 |
| Veryfine | 8 fl oz | 120 |
| Pink Country Time Sugar-Sweet | | |
| Drink Mix | 8 fl oz | 80 |
| Pink Kool-Aid Unsweetened | | |
| Soft Drink Mix | 8 fl oz | 2 |
| Punch Country Time Sugar- | | |
| Sweet Drink Mix | 8 fl oz | 80 |
| **LENTILS** Dry, cooked | 1 cup | 230 |
| **LETTUCE** | | |
| Bibb or Boston | 1 leaf | 2 |
| Iceburg | ½ head | 35 |
| Looseleaf, Shredded | 1 cup | 10 |
| **LIMA BEANS** | | |
| Dry, cooked | 1 cup | 260 |
| *Frozen* | | |
| Baby (Birds Eye) | 3.3 oz | 130 |
| Baby (Green Giant) | ½ cup | 80 |
| Baby (Seabrook) | 3.3 oz | 130 |
| Baby in Butter (Seabrook) | 3.3 oz | 140 |
| In Butter Sauce (Green Giant) | ½ cup | 100 |

| Protein (g) | Carbohydrates (g) | Fat (g) | Sodium (mg) | Cholesterol (mg) | Fiber (g) | Vitamin A (%) | Vitamin C (%) | Calcium (%) | Iron (%) |
|---|---|---|---|---|---|---|---|---|---|
| 0 | 0 | 0 | 0 | 0 | 0 | * | 10 | * | * |
| 0 | 20 | 0 | 25 | 0 | 0 | * | 10 | * | * |
| 0 | 0 | 0 | 0 | 0 | 0 | * | 10 | * | * |
| Tr | 24 | 0 | 1 | 0 | 0 | na | na | na | na |
| Tr | 30 | 0 | 24 | 0 | 0 | na | na | na | na |
| 0 | 20 | 0 | 20 | 0 | 0 | * | 10 | * | * |
| 0 | 0 | 0 | 0 | 0 | 0 | * | 10 | * | * |
| 0 | 20 | 0 | 15 | 0 | 0 | * | 10 | * | * |
| 18 | 40 | Tr | 2 | 0 | 4 | * | * | 4 | 25 |
| Tr | Tr | Tr | 1 | 0 | 0.5 | 2 | 2 | * | 2 |
| <3 | 6 | <1 | 24 | 0 | 2.7 | 16 | 30 | 4 | 8 |
| <1 | 2 | Tr | 6 | 0 | 0.4 | 20 | 15 | 4 | 4 |
| 12 | 49 | 1 | 4 | 0 | 7.2 | * | * | 6 | 35 |
| 7 | 24 | 0 | 115 | 0 | na | 4 | 30 | 4 | 10 |
| 6 | 18 | 0 | 170 | 0 | 4 | * | 4 | 2 | 8 |
| 7 | 24 | 0 | 125 | 0 | 2 | na | na | na | na |
| 7 | 26 | 1 | 213 | 0 | 2 | na | na | na | na |
| 6 | 17 | 3 | 390 | 5 | 4.5 | 2 | 6 | * | 10 |

| FOOD NAME | Serving Size | Calories |
|---|---|---|
| Fordhook (Birds Eye) | 3.3 oz | 100 |
| LIME | 1 | 20 |
| LIVER | | |
| Beef, fried | 3 oz | 200 |
| Calf, fried | 3 oz | 220 |
| LIVER CHEESE  (Oscar Mayer) | 1 slice | 115 |
| LIVERWURST SPREAD | | |
| Canned (Hormel) | ½ can | 35 |
| Canned (Underwood) | ½ can | 220 |
| LOBSTER  Northern, boiled or steamed | 3 oz | 80 |
| LOGANBERRIES  Raw | 1 cup | 90 |
| LUNCHEON LOAF | | |
| Oscar Mayer | 1 slice | 75 |
| Oscar Mayer Old Fashioned | 1 slice | 65 |
| Oscar Mayer Olive | 1 slice | 60 |
| Oscar Mayer Pickle and Pimento | 1 slice | 65 |
| Oscar Mayer Picnic | 1 slice | 60 |
| MACADAMIA NUTS | 1 oz | 200 |
| MACARONI | | |
| Cooked, elbow, shell, twist | 1 cup | 155 |
| Dry, elbow, shell, twist | 2 oz | 210 |
| MACARONI & CHEESE | | |
| Kraft | ¾ cup | 290 |
| Kraft Deluxe | ¾ cup | 260 |
| Kraft Dinomac | ¾ cup | 310 |

| Protein (g) | Carbohydrates (g) | Fat (g) | Sodium (mg) | Cholesterol (mg) | Fiber (g) | Vitamin A (%) | Vitamin C (%) | Calcium (%) | Iron (%) |
|---|---|---|---|---|---|---|---|---|---|
| 6 | 19 | 0 | 100 | 0 | na | 4 | 30 | 2 | 8 |
| <1 | 7 | 1 | 1 | 0 | 0.3 | * | 33 | 3 | 2 |
| | | | | | | | | | |
| 24 | 5 | 9 | 156 | 410 | 0 | 910 | 40 | * | 40 |
| 25 | <5 | 6 | 100 | 280 | 0 | 560 | 50 | 2 | 70 |
| 6 | Tr | 10 | 420 | 80 | 0 | na | na | na | na |
| | | | | | | | | | |
| 2 | 0 | 3 | na | na | 0 | na | * | * | na |
| 8 | 4 | 16 | 470 | na | 0 | 80 | * | * | 25 |
| 17 | 1 | 2 | 179 | 60 | 0 | * | * | 6 | 4 |
| 1 | 22 | 1 | 1 | 0 | 4.3 | 6 | 60 | 4 | 10 |
| | | | | | | | | | |
| 4 | 2 | 6 | 345 | 20 | 0 | na | na | na | na |
| 4 | 2 | 5 | 325 | 15 | 0 | na | na | na | na |
| 3 | 3 | 4 | 380 | 10 | 0 | na | na | na | na |
| 3 | 4 | 4 | 370 | 15 | 0 | na | na | na | na |
| 4 | 1 | 4 | 335 | 15 | 0 | na | na | na | na |
| 2 | 4 | 21 | 1 | 0 | 1.5 | * | * | 6 | * |
| | | | | | | | | | |
| 5 | 32 | 1 | 2 | 0 | 1 | * | * | * | 7 |
| 7 | 41 | 1 | 4 | 0 | 1.4 | * | * | * | 10 |
| | | | | | | | | | |
| 9 | 34 | 13 | 530 | 5 | na | 10 | * | 8 | 10 |
| 11 | 36 | 8 | 590 | 20 | na | * | * | 10 | 10 |
| 9 | 36 | 14 | 560 | 10 | na | 8 | * | 10 | 10 |

| FOOD NAME | Serving Size | Calories |
|---|---|---|
| Kraft Family Size | ¾ cup | 290 |
| Kraft Spirals | ¾ cup | 340 |
| Kraft Teddy Bears | ¾ cup | 310 |
| Kraft Wild Wheels | ¾ cup | 310 |
| MACKEREL | | |
| Atlantic, fresh, broiled | | |
| with butter | 3 oz | 200 |
| Canned | 4 oz | 200 |
| MANGO Fresh | 1 cup | 108 |
| MARGARINE | | |
| Chiffon Soft Margarine Cup | 1 tbsp | 90 |
| Chiffon Soft Stick | 1 tbsp | 100 |
| Chiffon Soft Unsalted | 1 tbsp | 90 |
| Chiffon Whipped | 1 tbsp | 70 |
| Kraft Touch of Butter Bowl, 40% fat | 1 tbsp | 50 |
| Kraft Touch of Butter Stick, 70% fat | 1 tbsp | 90 |
| Miracle Brand Whipped Cup | 1 tbsp | 60 |
| Miracle Brand Whipped Stick | 1 tbsp | 70 |
| Parkay | 1 tbsp | 100 |
| Parkay Soft | 1 tbsp | 100 |
| Parkay Soft Reduced Calorie | 1 tbsp | 50 |
| Parkay Spread, 50% vegetable oil | 1 tbsp | 60 |
| Prkay Squeeze Spread | 1 tbsp | 90 |
| Parkay Whipped Cup | 1 tbsp | 70 |
| Parkay Whipped Stick | 1 tbsp | 70 |

| Protein (g) | Carbohydrates (g) | Fat (g) | Sodium (mg) | Cholesterol (mg) | Fiber (g) | Vitamin A (%) | Vitamin C (%) | Calcium (%) | Iron (%) |
|---|---|---|---|---|---|---|---|---|---|
| 9 | 34 | 13 | 490 | 5 | na | 10 | * | 8 | 10 |
| 9 | 36 | 18 | 600 | 10 | na | 10 | * | 10 | 10 |
| 9 | 36 | 14 | 560 | 10 | na | 8 | * | 10 | 10 |
| 9 | 36 | 14 | 560 | 10 | na | 8 | * | 10 | 10 |
| | | | | | | | | | |
| | | | | | | | | | |
| 20 | 0 | 14 | 70 | 62 | 0 | 8 | * | * | 6 |
| 24 | 0 | 11 | 430 | 90 | 0 | 1 | na | 30 | 14 |
| <1 | 28 | Tr | 4 | 0 | 1.8 | 158 | 97 | 2 | 4 |
| | | | | | | | | | |
| 0 | 0 | 10 | 95 | 0 | 0 | 6 | * | * | * |
| 0 | 0 | 11 | 105 | 0 | 0 | 8 | * | * | * |
| 0 | 0 | 10 | 0 | 0 | 0 | 6 | * | * | * |
| 0 | 0 | 8 | 80 | 0 | 0 | 4 | * | * | * |
| 0 | 0 | 6 | 110 | 0 | 0 | 10 | * | * | * |
| 0 | 0 | 10 | 110 | 0 | 0 | 10 | * | * | * |
| 0 | 0 | 7 | 70 | 0 | 0 | 6 | * | * | * |
| 0 | 0 | 7 | 65 | 0 | 0 | 6 | * | * | * |
| 0 | 0 | 11 | 105 | 0 | 0 | 10 | * | * | * |
| 0 | 0 | 11 | 105 | 0 | 0 | 10 | * | * | * |
| 0 | 0 | 6 | 110 | 0 | 0 | 10 | * | * | * |
| 0 | 0 | 7 | 110 | 0 | 0 | 10 | * | * | * |
| 0 | 0 | 10 | 110 | 0 | 0 | 10 | * | * | * |
| 0 | 0 | 7 | 70 | 0 | 0 | 6 | * | * | * |
| 0 | 0 | 7 | 65 | 0 | 0 | 6 | * | * | * |

| FOOD NAME | Serving Size | Calories |
|---|---|---|
| **MARSHMALLOWS** | | |
| Funmallows | 1 | 30 |
| Funmallows Miniature | 10 | 18 |
| Kraft Creme | 1 oz | 90 |
| Kraft Jet-Puffed | 1 | 25 |
| Kraft Miniature | 10 | 18 |
| **MAYONNAISE** | | |
| Hellman's | 1 tbsp | 100 |
| Hellman's Cholesterol Free | 1 tbsp | 50 |
| Hellman's Light | 1 tbsp | 50 |
| Kraft | 1 tbsp | 100 |
| Kraft Free Nonfat | 1 tbsp | 12 |
| Kraft Light | 1 tbsp | 50 |
| **MAYONNAISE, IMITATION** | | |
| Miracle Whip | 1 tbsp | 70 |
| Miracle Whip Free Nonfat | 1 tbsp | 20 |
| Miracle Whip Light | 1 tbsp | 45 |
| **MILK** | | |
| Whole | 1 cup | 150 |
| Lowfat 2% | 1 cup | 125 |
| Lowfat 1% | 1 cup | 105 |
| Skim | 1 cup | 85 |
| Buttermilk | 1 cup | 100 |
| Evaporated Whole | 1 cup | 340 |
| Evaporated Lowfat | 1 cup | 220 |

| Protein (g) | Carbohydrates (g) | Fat (g) | Sodium (mg) | Cholesterol (mg) | Fiber (g) | Vitamin A (%) | Vitamin C (%) | Calcium (%) | Iron (%) |
|---|---|---|---|---|---|---|---|---|---|
| 0 | 7 | 0 | 15 | 0 | 0 | * | * | * | * |
| 0 | 5 | 0 | 5 | 0 | 0 | * | * | * | * |
| 0 | 23 | 0 | 20 | 0 | 0 | * | * | * | * |
| 0 | 6 | 0 | 5 | 0 | 0 | * | * | * | * |
| 0 | 5 | 0 | 5 | 0 | 0 | * | * | * | * |
| 0 | 0 | 11 | 80 | 5 | 0 | * | * | * | * |
| 0 | 1 | 5 | 80 | 0 | 0 | * | * | * | * |
| 0 | 1 | 5 | 115 | 5 | 0 | * | * | * | * |
| 0 | 0 | 12 | 70 | 5 | 0 | * | * | * | * |
| 0 | 3 | 0 | 190 | 0 | 0 | * | * | * | * |
| 0 | 1 | 5 | 110 | 0 | 0 | * | * | * | * |
| 0 | 2 | 7 | 85 | 5 | 0 | * | * | * | * |
| 0 | 5 | 0 | 210 | 0 | 0 | * | * | * | * |
| 0 | 2 | 4 | 125 | 0 | 0 | * | * | * | * |
| 8 | 11 | 8 | 122 | 30 | 0 | 6 | 3 | 29 | 1 |
| 9 | 12 | 5 | 150 | 15 | 0 | 10 | 3 | 31 | 1 |
| 9 | 12 | 2 | 122 | 10 | 0 | 10 | 3 | 31 | 1 |
| 8 | 12 | 0 | 127 | <1 | 0 | 10 | 3 | 30 | 1 |
| 8 | 12 | 2 | 257 | 15 | 0 | 2 | 3 | 29 | 1 |
| 17 | 25 | 19 | 266 | na | 0 | 12 | 8 | 66 | 3 |
| 18 | 24 | 6 | 276 | na | 0 | 20 | * | 60 | * |

| FOOD NAME | Serving Size | Calories |
|---|---|---|
| Nonfat Dry Powder | 1 cup | 245 |
| Malted (Kraft Instant Natural | 3 tsp | 90 |
| Malted (Kraft Instant Chocolate) | 3 tsp | 90 |
| MOLASSES | 1 tbsp | 65 |
| MOUSSE, CHOCOLATE (Pillsbury, from mix) | 1/16 | 260 |
| MUFFIN | | |
| Apple Spice (Healthy Choice) | 1 | 190 |
| Banana Nut (Healthy Choice) | 1 | 180 |
| Blueberry (Healthy Choice) | 1 | 190 |
| Blueberry (Pepperidge Farm) | 1 | 170 |
| Bran'nola | 1 | 160 |
| Corn | 1 | 125 |
| English (Pepperidge Farm Cinnamon Apple) | 1 | 140 |
| English (Pepperidge Farm Cinnamon Chip) | 1 | 160 |
| English (Pepperidge Farm Cinnamon Raisin) | 1 | 150 |
| English (Pepperidge Farm Plain) | 1 | 140 |
| English (Pepperidge Farm Sourdough) | 1 | 135 |
| English (Thomas') | 1 | 130 |
| Extra Crisp (Arnold) | 1 | 150 |
| Oatbran with Apple (Pepperidge Farm Cholesterol Free) | 1 | 190 |
| Plain | 1 | 120 |
| Raisin (Arnold) | 1 | 170 |
| Raisin Bran (Pepperidge Farm Cholesterol Free) | 1 | 170 |

| Protein (g) | Carbohydrates (g) | Fat (g) | Sodium (mg) | Cholesterol (mg) | Fiber (g) | Vitamin A (%) | Vitamin C (%) | Calcium (%) | Iron (%) |
|---|---|---|---|---|---|---|---|---|---|
| 24 | 35 | 0 | 373 | 12 | 0 | 32 | 7 | 84 | 1 |
| 3 | 16 | 2 | 100 | na | na | * | 2 | 6 | * |
| 1 | 18 | 1 | 45 | na | na | * | * | * | 2 |
| 0 | 15 | 0 | 30 | 0 | 0 | * | * | 2 | 4 |
| 3 | 37 | 12 | 310 | 40 | na | * | * | 2 | 6 |
| | | | | | | | | | |
| 3 | 40 | 4 | 90 | 0 | na | <2 | 8 | 10 | 10 |
| 3 | 32 | 5 | 80 | 0 | na | <2 | <2 | 10 | 10 |
| 3 | 39 | 4 | 110 | 0 | na | <2 | 6 | 10 | 8 |
| 2 | 27 | 7 | 250 | 25 | na | * | 2 | 2 | 2 |
| 6 | 30 | 1 | 260 | na | na | * | * | 6 | 10 |
| 3 | 19 | 4 | 192 | na | na | 2 | * | 4 | 4 |
| 4 | 27 | 1 | 210 | 0 | na | * | * | 4 | 8 |
| 4 | 28 | 3 | 180 | 0 | na | * | * | 2 | 8 |
| 5 | 29 | 2 | 200 | 0 | na | * | * | 2 | 8 |
| 5 | 27 | 1 | 220 | 0 | na | * | * | 2 | 8 |
| 4 | 27 | 1 | 260 | 0 | na | * | * | 2 | 10 |
| 4 | 26 | 1 | 215 | na | na | * | * | 4 | 7 |
| 5 | 30 | 1 | 310 | na | na | * | * | 2 | 10 |
| | | | | | | | | | |
| 3 | 29 | 7 | 200 | 0 | na | * | * | 4 | 6 |
| 3 | 17 | 4 | 176 | na | na | 1 | * | 4 | 3 |
| 6 | 35 | 1 | 350 | na | na | * | * | 6 | 10 |
| | | | | | | | | | |
| 4 | 30 | 6 | 280 | 0 | na | * | * | 2 | 2 |

| FOOD NAME | Serving Size | Calories | |
|---|---|---|---|
| Stone Ground Wheat (Pepperidge Farm) | 1 | 130 | |
| **MUSHROOMS** | | | |
| Fresh, sliced | 1 cup | 20 | |
| Canned (B In B, Pieces & Stems, Whole, Broiled in Butter) | ¼ cup | 12 | |
| Canned (B In B, Sliced with Garlic) | ¼ can | 12 | |
| Canned (Green Giant Pieces & Stems, Sliced, Whole) | ¼ cup | 12 | |
| Canned (Green Giant Whole Straw Mushrooms) | ¼ cup | 12 | |
| **MUSSELS** Cooked | 3 oz | 150 | |
| **MUSTARD** | | | |
| Bold 'n Spicy (French's) | 1 tbsp | 16 | |
| Brown (Heinz) | 1 tbsp | 24 | |
| Horseradish (French's) | 1 tbsp | 16 | |
| Horseradish (Kraft) | 1 tbsp | 14 | |
| Medford (French's) | 1 tbsp | 16 | |
| Prepared Yellow (French's) | 1 tbsp | 10 | |
| Pure Prepared (Kraft) | 1 tbsp | 11 | |
| With Onion (French's) | 1 tbsp | 25 | |
| **MUSTARD GREENS** Fresh, cooked | 1 cup | 30 | |
| **NAVY BEANS** Cooked, drained | 1 cup | 220 | |
| **NECTARINE** | 1 | 67 | |
| **NOODLES** | | | |
| Egg, Dry (Buitoni) | 2 oz | 220 | |

| Protein (g) | Carbohydrates (g) | Fat (g) | Sodium (mg) | Cholesterol (mg) | Fiber (g) | Vitamin A (%) | Vitamin C (%) | Calcium (%) | Iron (%) |
|---|---|---|---|---|---|---|---|---|---|
| 5 | 25 | 2 | 340 | na | na | na | na | na | na |
| 2 | 3 | 0 | 7 | 0 | 1 | * | 3 | * | 3 |
| 1 | 2 | 0 | 240 | 0 | 1 | * | * | * | 2 |
| 1 | 2 | 0 | 200 | 0 | 1 | * | * | * | * |
| 1 | 2 | 0 | 220 | 0 | 1 | * | * | * | * |
| 1 | 2 | 0 | 290 | 0 | 1 | * | * | * | * |
| 20 | 6 | 4 | 315 | 48 | 0 | * | * | 28 | 30 |
| 1 | 1 | 1 | 145 | 0 | 0 | * | * | * | * |
| na | <2 | 1 | 174 | 0 | 0 | * | * | * | * |
| 1 | 1 | 1 | 265 | 0 | na | * | * | * | * |
| 1 | 1 | 1 | 135 | 0 | na | * | * | * | * |
| 1 | 1 | 1 | 240 | 0 | 0 | * | * | * | * |
| 1 | 1 | 1 | 180 | 0 | 0 | * | * | * | * |
| 1 | 1 | 1 | 160 | 0 | 0 | * | * | * | * |
| 1 | 5 | 1 | 190 | 0 | 0 | * | * | * | * |
| 3 | 6 | 1 | 25 | 0 | na | 162 | 112 | 19 | 14 |
| 24 | 41 | 1 | 13 | 0 | 6.9 | * | * | 10 | 30 |
| 1 | 16 | <1 | Tr | Tr | 2.2 | 45 | 30 | * | 4 |
| 8 | 40 | 3 | na | na | na | * | * | 2 | 10 |

| FOOD NAME | Serving Size | Calories |
|---|---|---|
| Egg, Dry (Creamette) | 2 oz | 221 |
| Egg, Dry (Mueller's) | 2 oz | 220 |
| Egg, Dry (Pennsylvania Dutch) | 2 oz | 220 |
| NOODLE DISHES, Mix | | |
| Kraft Egg Noodle and Cheese | ¾ cup | 340 |
| Kraft Egg Noodle with Chicken | ¾ cup | 240 |
| Lipton Noodles and Sauce Alfredo | ½ cup | 220 |
| Lipton Noodles and Sauce Beef Flavor | ½ cup | 180 |
| Lipton Noodles and Sauce Butter Flavor | ½ cup | 200 |
| Lipton Noodles and Sauce Butter and Herb Flavor | ½ cup | 190 |
| Lipton Noodles and Sauce Cheese Flavor | ½ cup | 190 |
| Lipton Noodles and Sauce Chicken Flavor | ½ cup | 180 |
| Lipton Noodles and Sauce Sour Cream and Chives | ½ cup | 200 |
| Lipton Noodles and Sauce Stroganoff | ½ cup | 200 |
| OATS AND OATMEAL *(see also Cereal, Hot)* | 1 cup | 130 |
| Instant (Quaker Apple Cinnamon) | 1 pkt | 140 |
| Instant (Quaker Cinnamon Spice) | 1 pkt | 164 |
| Instant (Quaker Raisin and Cinnamon) | 1 pkt | 129 |
| Old-fashioned (Quaker) | ⅔ cup | 110 |
| OCEAN PERCH Atlantic, fried | 3 oz | 190 |
| OIL | | |
| Almond | 1 tbsp | 120 |
| Avocado | 1 tbsp | 124 |

| Protein (g) | Carbohydrates (g) | Fat (g) | Sodium (mg) | Cholesterol (mg) | Fiber (g) | Vitamin A (%) | Vitamin C (%) | Calcium (%) | Iron (%) |
|---|---|---|---|---|---|---|---|---|---|
| 8 | 40 | <3 | 3 | 70 | 0.8 | * | * | 2 | 10 |
| 8 | 40 | 3 | 10 | 55 | na | na | na | na | na |
| 8 | 40 | 3 | 15 | na | na | * | * | * | 10 |
| | | | | | | | | | |
| 10 | 37 | 17 | 670 | 50 | na | 15 | * | 10 | 10 |
| 8 | 32 | 9 | 1050 | 45 | na | * | * | 2 | 10 |
| 7 | 24 | 10 | 580 | na | na | 8 | * | 10 | 6 |
| 5 | 23 | 7 | 700 | na | na | 4 | * | * | 4 |
| 6 | 23 | 10 | 510 | na | na | 4 | * | * | 4 |
| | | | | | | | | | |
| 5 | 23 | 9 | 520 | na | na | 4 | * | * | 4 |
| 5 | 25 | 8 | 530 | na | na | 4 | * | 4 | 4 |
| 5 | 23 | 8 | 450 | na | na | 4 | * | * | 4 |
| | | | | | | | | | |
| 5 | 24 | 9 | 500 | na | na | 4 | * | * | 4 |
| 7 | 23 | 9 | 410 | na | na | 4 | * | 4 | 8 |
| 5 | 23 | 2 | 1 | 0 | 5 | * | * | 2 | 8 |
| 4 | 26 | 2 | 260 | 0 | 3 | 20 | * | 10 | 25 |
| 5 | 35 | 2 | 322 | 0 | 3.1 | na | na | na | na |
| 4 | 27 | 2 | 110 | 0 | 2.7 | na | na | na | na |
| 5 | 18 | 2 | 9 | 0 | 2.7 | * | * | * | 4 |
| 20 | 6 | 12 | 130 | 61 | 0 | * | * | 2 | 6 |
| | | | | | | | | | |
| 0 | 0 | 14 | 0 | 0 | 0 | * | * | * | * |
| 0 | 0 | 14 | 0 | 0 | 0 | * | * | * | * |

| FOOD NAME | Serving Size | Calories | |
|---|---|---|---|
| Cocoa Butter | 1 tbsp | 120 | |
| Coconut | 1 tbsp | 120 | |
| Cod Liver | 1 tbsp | 120 | |
| Corn | 1 tbsp | 120 | |
| Cottonseed | 1 tbsp | 120 | |
| Hazelnut | 1 tbsp | 120 | |
| Olive | 1 tbsp | 120 | |
| Palm | 1 tbsp | 120 | |
| Peanut | 1 tbsp | 120 | |
| Poppyseed | 1 tbsp | 120 | |
| Safflower | 1 tbsp | 120 | |
| Sesame | 1 tbsp | 120 | |
| Soybean | 1 tbsp | 120 | |
| Sunflower | 1 tbsp | 120 | |
| Vegetable | 1 tbsp | 120 | |
| Walnut | 1 tbsp | 120 | |
| OKRA | | | |
| Fresh, cooked | 10 pods | 30 | |
| Frozen (Birds Eye Cut) | 3.3 oz | 25 | |
| Frozen (Birds Eye Whole) | 3.3 oz | 30 | |
| OLIVES | | | |
| Green | 4 | 20 | |
| Ripe | 4 | 20 | |
| ONIONS | | | |
| Chopped | 1 cup | 65 | |

| Protein (g) | Carbohydrates (g) | Fat (g) | Sodium (mg) | Cholesterol (mg) | Fiber (g) | Vitamin A (%) | Vitamin C (%) | Calcium (%) | Iron (%) |
|---|---|---|---|---|---|---|---|---|---|
| 0 | 0 | 14 | 0 | 0 | 0 | * | * | * | * |
| 0 | 0 | 14 | 0 | 0 | 0 | * | * | * | * |
| 0 | 0 | 14 | 0 | 80 | 0 | na | na | na | na |
| 0 | 0 | 14 | 0 | 0 | 0 | * | * | * | * |
| 0 | 0 | 14 | 0 | 0 | 0 | * | * | * | * |
| 0 | 0 | 14 | 0 | 0 | 0 | * | * | * | * |
| 0 | 0 | 14 | 0 | 0 | 0 | * | * | * | * |
| 0 | 0 | 14 | 0 | 0 | 0 | * | * | * | * |
| 0 | 0 | 14 | 0 | 0 | 0 | * | * | * | * |
| 0 | 0 | 14 | 0 | 0 | 0 | * | * | * | * |
| 0 | 0 | 14 | 0 | 0 | 0 | * | * | * | * |
| 0 | 0 | 14 | 0 | 0 | 0 | * | * | * | * |
| 0 | 0 | 14 | 0 | 0 | 0 | * | * | * | * |
| 0 | 0 | 14 | 0 | 0 | 0 | * | * | * | * |
| 0 | 0 | 14 | 0 | 0 | 0 | * | * | * | * |
| 0 | 0 | 14 | 0 | 0 | 0 | * | * | * | * |
| 2 | 6 | 0 | 2 | 0 | 2 | 10 | 35 | 10 | 3 |
| 2 | 6 | 0 | 5 | 0 | na | 10 | 15 | 8 | 2 |
| 2 | 7 | 0 | 5 | 0 | na | 8 | 25 | 8 | 2 |
| 0 | Tr | 2 | 360 | 0 | 0.4 | * | * | * | 2 |
| 0 | Tr | 2 | 82 | 0 | 0.4 | * | * | 2 | 2 |
| 3 | 15 | 0 | 17 | 0 | 2.6 | * | 28 | 5 | 5 |

| FOOD NAME | Serving Size | Calories | |
|---|---|---|---|
| Green | 6 | 15 | |
| ONION RINGS Frozen (Mrs. Paul's Crispy) | 2.2 oz | 190 | |
| ORANGE | 1 | 65 | |
| Chopped | 1 cup | 90 | |
| ORANGE JUICE | | | |
| Fresh | 6 fl oz | 83 | |
| Boxed (Minute Maid) | 6 fl oz | 85 | |
| Frozen (Minute Maid) | 6 fl oz | 90 | |
| ORANGE JUICE DRINK | | | |
| Kool-Aid Sugar-Sweetened Soft Drink Mix | 8 fl oz | 80 | |
| Kool-Aid Koolers | 8.5 fl oz | 110 | |
| Tang Fruit Box | 8.5 oz | 130 | |
| OYSTERS | | | |
| Eastern, Raw | 12 med | 150 | |
| Pacific, Raw | 6 med | 220 | |
| PANCAKES | | | |
| *Mix* | | | |
| Buttermilk (Aunt Jemima) | 3 4" | 300 | |
| Buttermilk (Hungry Jack) | 3 | 200 | |
| Buttermilk Complete (Hungry Jack) | 3 | 180 | |
| Buckwheat (Aunt Jemima) | 3 4" | 200 | |
| Complete (Aunt Jemima) | 3 | 240 | |
| Extra Lights (Hungry Jack) | 3 | 200 | |
| Regular (Aunt Jemima) | 3 4" | 220 | |
| Whole Wheat (Aunt Jemima) | 3 | 250 | |

| Protein (g) | Carbohydrates (g) | Fat (g) | Sodium (mg) | Cholesterol (mg) | Fiber (g) | Vitamin A (%) | Vitamin C (%) | Calcium (%) | Iron (%) |
|---|---|---|---|---|---|---|---|---|---|
| 0 | 3 | 0 | 2 | 0 | 1.2 | * | 13 | 1 | 1 |
| 2 | 19 | 12 | 230 | na | na | * | * | 2 | 2 |
| 1 | 16 | 0 | 1 | 0 | 0.6 | 5 | 110 | 5 | 3 |
| 2 | 22 | 0 | 2 | 0 | 0.8 | 7 | 150 | 7 | 4 |
| | | | | | | | | | |
| 1 | 19 | Tr | 2 | 0 | 0.2 | 9 | 150 | 1 | 1 |
| 1 | 20 | Tr | 1 | 0 | 0.2 | 6 | 90 | 2 | * |
| 1 | 21 | Tr | 1 | 0 | 0.2 | 8 | 150 | 2 | * |
| | | | | | | | | | |
| 0 | 20 | 0 | 15 | 0 | na | * | 10 | * | * |
| 0 | 30 | 0 | 10 | 0 | na | * | 10 | * | 10 |
| 0 | 31 | 0 | 10 | 0 | na | * | 100 | * | * |
| | | | | | | | | | |
| 12 | 7 | 3 | 160 | 188 | 0 | 14 | * | 20 | 65 |
| 30 | 16 | 6 | 300 | na | 0 | 15 | * | 20 | 100 |
| | | | | | | | | | |
| 10 | 40 | 11 | 990 | 1 | 1.3 | 6 | * | 30 | 10 |
| 6 | 28 | 7 | 570 | 55 | 0.5 | * | * | 6 | 4 |
| 5 | 38 | 1 | 720 | 5 | 1 | * | * | 15 | 6 |
| 7 | 25 | 8 | 520 | na | 5 | 4 | * | 15 | 6 |
| 6 | 47 | 3 | 870 | 16 | 2.1 | * | * | 10 | 8 |
| 6 | 28 | 7 | 495 | 0 | 0.5 | 4 | * | 15 | 4 |
| 7 | 26 | 8 | 550 | 19 | 1.8 | 4 | * | 15 | 6 |
| 10 | 32 | 9 | 725 | 0 | 3.6 | 4 | * | 20 | 10 |

| FOOD NAME | Serving Size | Calories | |
|---|---|---|---|
| Wild Blueberry (Hungry Jack) | 3 | 320 | |
| *Frozen* | | | |
| With Bacon (Swanson) | 4.5 oz | 400 | |
| And Sausages (Swanson) | 6 oz | 460 | |
| Silver Dollar Pancakes and Sausage (Swanson) | 3.75 oz | 310 | |
| Whole Wheat Pancakes with | | | |
| Lite Links (Swanson) | 5.5 oz | 350 | |
| *Microwave* | | | |
| Blueberry (Hungry Jack) | 3 | 230 | |
| Buttermilk (Aunt Jemima) | 3.5 oz | 210 | |
| Buttermilk (Hungry Jack) | 3 | 260 | |
| Harvest Wheat (Hungry Jack) | 3 | 230 | |
| Oat Bran (Hungry Jack) | 3 | 230 | |
| Original (Aunt Jemima) | 3.5 oz | 211 | |
| Original (Hungry Jack) | 3 | 240 | |
| Original (Pillsbury) | 3 | 240 | |
| PANCAKE SYRUP | | | |
| Aunt Jemima Lite | 1 fl oz | 54 | |
| Aunt Jemima Original | 1 fl oz | 109 | |
| Golden Griddle | 1 tbsp | 50 | |
| Hungry Jack Lite | 2 tbsp | 50 | |
| Hungry Jack Regular | 2 tbsp | 100 | |
| Karo | 1 tbsp | 60 | |
| Mrs. Butterworth's | 3 tbsp | 165 | |
| PAPAYA Fresh, cubed | 1 cup | 55 | |

| Protein (g) | Carbohydrates (g) | Fat (g) | Sodium (mg) | Cholesterol (mg) | Fiber (g) | Vitamin A (%) | Vitamin C (%) | Calcium (%) | Iron (%) |
|---|---|---|---|---|---|---|---|---|---|
| 6 | 41 | 14 | 820 | 45 | na | 4 | 2 | 10 | 10 |
| 11 | 43 | 20 | 1000 | na | na | * | * | 6 | 10 |
| 15 | 52 | 22 | 920 | na | na | * | * | 8 | 15 |
| 10 | 37 | 14 | 680 | na | na | * | * | 4 | 10 |
| 15 | 39 | 16 | 600 | na | na | * | * | 4 | 15 |
| 5 | 47 | 4 | 550 | 10 | 1 | * | 2 | 8 | 10 |
| 6 | 41 | 3 | 860 | 20 | 1.8 | na | na | na | na |
| 5 | 51 | 4 | 590 | 10 | 1 | * | * | 8 | 10 |
| 6 | 46 | 4 | 560 | 10 | 3 | * | * | 8 | 10 |
| 6 | 45 | 4 | 580 | 10 | 3 | * | * | 8 | 10 |
| 6 | 40 | <4 | 801 | na | 1.8 | na | na | na | na |
| 5 | 49 | 4 | 570 | 10 | 2 | * | * | 8 | 10 |
| 6 | 47 | 4 | 550 | na | na | na | na | na | na |
| 0 | 13 | Tr | 92 | 0 | 0.3 | na | na | na | na |
| 0 | 27 | 0 | 32 | 0 | 0 | na | na | na | na |
| 0 | 13 | 0 | 20 | 0 | na | * | * | * | * |
| 0 | 14 | 0 | 105 | 0 | 0 | * | * | * | * |
| 0 | 26 | 0 | 25 | 0 | 0 | * | * | * | * |
| 0 | 15 | 0 | 35 | 0 | na | * | * | * | * |
| 0 | 40 | <1 | na | 0 | na | * | * | * | * |
| 1 | 14 | 0 | 3 | 0 | 1.2 | 49 | 130 | 3 | 2 |

| FOOD NAME | Serving Size | Calories |
|---|---|---|
| PARSLEY Fresh, chopped | 1 tbsp | 2 |
| PARSNIPS Boiled, drained | 1 cup | 100 |
| PASTA | | |
| Cooked | 1 cup | 200 |
| Dry | 2 oz | 211 |
| *Canned* | | |
| Beef RavioliO's in Meat Sauce | 7½ oz | 250 |
| CircusO's in Tomato and Cheese Sauce | 7⅜ oz | 170 |
| CircusO's with Meatballs in Tomato Sauce | 7⅜ oz | 210 |
| Macaroni and Cheese (Franco-American) | 7⅜ oz | 170 |
| Spaghetti in Tomato Sauce with Cheese | | |
| (Franco-American) | 7⅜ oz | 180 |
| Spaghetti with Meatballs in Tomato Sauce | | |
| (Franco-American) | 7⅜ oz | 220 |
| SpaghettiO's in Tomato & Cheese Sauce | 7½ oz | 170 |
| SpaghettiO's with Meatballs | 7⅜ oz | 220 |
| SpaghettiO's with Sliced Franks | 7⅜ oz | 220 |
| SportyO's in Tomato & Cheese Sauce | 7½ oz | 170 |
| SportyO's with Meatballs in | | |
| Tomato Sauce | 7⅜ oz | 210 |
| TeddyO's in Tomato & Cheese Sauce | 7½ oz | 170 |
| TeddyO's with Meatballs | 7⅜ oz | 210 |
| *Frozen* | | |
| Bavarian Style Recipe Green Beans and | | |
| Spaetzle (Birds Eye) | 3.3 oz | 100 |

| Protein (g) | Carbohydrates (g) | Fat (g) | Sodium (mg) | Cholesterol (mg) | Fiber (g) | Vitamin A (%) | Vitamin C (%) | Calcium (%) | Iron (%) |
|---|---|---|---|---|---|---|---|---|---|
| Tr | Tr | Tr | 2 | 0 | Tr | 6 | 10 | * | * |
| 2 | 23 | 1 | 12 | 0 | 4.2 | * | 25 | 6 | 4 |
| | | | | | | | | | |
| 7 | 40 | 0 | 1 | 0 | 3.1 | * | * | * | 7 |
| 7 | 43 | 1 | 4 | 0 | 1.4 | * | * | * | 10 |
| | | | | | | | | | |
| 10 | 35 | 8 | 920 | na | na | 10 | 10 | 2 | 10 |
| 5 | 33 | 2 | 860 | na | na | 10 | * | 2 | 6 |
| 9 | 25 | 8 | 950 | na | na | 10 | 6 | 2 | 10 |
| 6 | 24 | 6 | 870 | na | na | 10 | * | 8 | 6 |
| | | | | | | | | | |
| 5 | 36 | 2 | 840 | na | na | 8 | * | 2 | 8 |
| | | | | | | | | | |
| 10 | 28 | 8 | 870 | na | na | 8 | * | 2 | 10 |
| 5 | 33 | 2 | 860 | na | na | 10 | * | 2 | 6 |
| 9 | 25 | 9 | 950 | na | na | 8 | * | 2 | 10 |
| 8 | 26 | 9 | 1000 | na | na | 8 | * | 2 | 8 |
| 5 | 33 | 2 | 860 | na | na | 10 | * | 2 | 6 |
| | | | | | | | | | |
| 9 | 25 | 8 | 950 | na | na | 10 | 6 | 2 | 10 |
| 5 | 33 | 2 | 900 | na | na | 10 | * | 4 | 8 |
| 9 | 25 | 8 | 950 | na | na | 10 | 6 | 2 | 10 |
| | | | | | | | | | |
| | | | | | | | | | |
| 2 | 11 | 5 | 350 | 10 | 2 | 10 | 6 | 4 | 4 |

| FOOD NAME | Serving Size | Calories |
|---|---|---|
| Broccoli, Carrots & Rotini in Cheese Flavored Sauce (Green Giant) | 1 pkg | 100 |
| Cheese Tortellini in Tomato Sauce (Birds Eye) | 5.5 oz | 210 |
| Chow Mein Vegetables in Oriental Sauce (Birds Eye) | 4.6 oz | 80 |
| Fettucine Primavera (Green Giant) | 1 pkg | 230 |
| Pasta and Vegetables in Creamy Stroganoff Sauce (Birds Eye) | 4.6 oz | 120 |
| Pasta and Vegetables with White Cheese Sauce (Birds Eye) | 4.6 oz | 150 |
| Pasta Accents Vegetables, Creamy Cheddar (Green Giant) | ½ cup | 90 |
| Pasta Accents Vegetables, Garden Herb Seasoning (Green Giant) | ½ cup | 80 |
| Pasta Accents Vegetables, Garlic Seasoning (Green Giant) | ½ cup | 100 |
| Pasta Accents Vegetables, Primavera (Green Giant) | ½ cup | 110 |
| Pasta Dijon (Green Giant) | 1 pkg | 260 |
| Pasta Florentine (Green Giant) | 1 pkg | 230 |
| Pasta Parmesan with Sweet Peas (Green Giant) | 1 pkg | 160 |
| Rotini Cheddar (Green Giant) | 1 pkg | 230 |
| Tortellini Provençale (Green Giant) | 1 pkg | 260 |
| *Mix* | | |
| Bits of Bacon Shells and Cheese (Velveeta) | ½ cup | 240 |

| Protein (g) | Carbohydrates (g) | Fat (g) | Sodium (mg) | Cholesterol (mg) | Fiber (g) | Vitamin A (%) | Vitamin C (%) | Calcium (%) | Iron (%) |
|---|---|---|---|---|---|---|---|---|---|
| 5 | 17 | 2 | 440 | 5 | 3 | 170 | 10 | 6 | 6 |
| 11 | 31 | 5 | 500 | 30 | 0 | 20 | 20 | 10 | 10 |
| 3 | 14 | 2 | 570 | 0 | 1 | 10 | 20 | 4 | 4 |
| 13 | 26 | 8 | 610 | 25 | 6 | 15 | 20 | 15 | 10 |
| 5 | 15 | 5 | 700 | 30 | 0 | 6 | 4 | 4 | 4 |
| 7 | 19 | 6 | 440 | 15 | 1 | 80 | 15 | 8 | 4 |
| 4 | 14 | 3 | 280 | 5 | 2 | 30 | 4 | 6 | 2 |
| 3 | 12 | 3 | 290 | 5 | 3 | 10 | 6 | 2 | 2 |
| 3 | 14 | 4 | 260 | 5 | 2 | 20 | 2 | 2 | 2 |
| 5 | 15 | 4 | 190 | 5 | 2.5 | 4 | 8 | 6 | 4 |
| 7 | 21 | 17 | 630 | 55 | 4 | 25 | 50 | 8 | 8 |
| 14 | 27 | 9 | 840 | 25 | 4 | 190 | 10 | 30 | 10 |
| 9 | 21 | 5 | 420 | 10 | 2.5 | 4 | 2 | 15 | 8 |
| 9 | 32 | 10 | 570 | 20 | 4.5 | 100 | 50 | 15 | 6 |
| 10 | 44 | 6 | 840 | 20 | 3 | 150 | 2 | 20 | 15 |
| 10 | 27 | 8 | 630 | 25 | na | 6 | * | 15 | 8 |

| FOOD NAME | Serving Size | Calories |
|---|---|---|
| Garden Primavera Pasta Salad (Kraft) | ½ cup | 170 |
| Homestyle Pasta Salad (Kraft) | ½ cup | 240 |
| Light Italian Pasta Salad (Kraft) | ½ cup | 130 |
| Light Rancher's Choice Pasta Salad (Kraft) | ½ cup | 170 |
| Pasta & Cheese Cheddar Broccoli (Kraft) | ½ cup | 180 |
| Pasta & Cheese Chicken (Kraft) | ½ cup | 170 |
| Pasta & Cheese Fettucine Alfredo (Kraft) | ½ cup | 180 |
| Pasta & Cheese Parmesan (Kraft) | ½ cup | 180 |
| Pasta & Cheese Sour Cream with Chives (Kraft) | ½ cup | 180 |
| Pasta & Cheese 3-Cheese with Vegetables (Kraft) | ½ cup | 180 |
| Pasta Salad & Dressing Broccoli & Vegetables (Kraft) | ½ cup | 210 |
| Rancher's Choice Pasta Salad and Dressing with Bacon (Kraft) | ½ cup | 250 |
| Shells and Cheese (Velveeta) | ½ cup | 210 |
| Touch of Mexican Shells and Cheese (Velveeta) | ½ cup | 210 |
| PASTA SAUCE | | |
| Enrico's All Natural | 4 oz | 60 |
| Enrico's All Natural No Salt | 4 oz | 60 |
| French's Italian, from mix | ½ cup | 80 |
| French's Thick, from mix | ½ cup | 97 |
| Hunt's No Salt Added | 4 oz | 80 |
| Hunt's Traditional | 4 oz | 70 |
| Prego Marinara | 4 oz | 100 |

| Protein (g) | Carbohydrates (g) | Fat (g) | Sodium (mg) | Cholesterol (mg) | Fiber (g) | Vitamin A (%) | Vitamin C (%) | Calcium (%) | Iron (%) |
|---|---|---|---|---|---|---|---|---|---|
| 5 | 21 | 7 | 450 | 0 | na | 4 | 2 | 6 | 4 |
| 4 | 21 | 16 | 300 | 10 | na | 2 | * | * | 8 |
| 5 | 20 | 3 | 420 | 0 | na | 4 | 2 | 6 | 8 |
| 5 | 23 | 7 | 350 | 0 | na | 2 | * | 2 | 8 |
| 6 | 19 | 8 | 620 | 30 | na | 6 | * | 10 | 6 |
| 5 | 21 | 7 | 550 | 25 | na | 4 | * | 6 | 4 |
| 7 | 19 | 9 | 590 | 30 | na | 4 | * | 10 | 4 |
| 6 | 19 | 8 | 630 | 30 | na | 4 | * | 10 | 6 |
| 5 | 22 | 8 | 360 | 25 | na | 4 | * | 4 | 4 |
| 6 | 19 | 8 | 630 | 25 | na | 6 | * | 10 | 6 |
| 4 | 15 | 16 | 290 | 10 | na | 8 | 4 | 2 | 6 |
| 5 | 21 | 16 | 350 | 10 | na | 2 | * | * | 8 |
| 10 | 25 | 8 | 570 | 20 | na | 6 | * | 15 | 8 |
| 10 | 27 | 8 | 630 | 20 | na | 6 | * | 15 | 8 |
| 2 | 9 | 1 | 345 | 0 | na | na | na | na | na |
| 2 | 9 | 1 | 30 | 0 | na | na | na | na | na |
| 2 | 12 | 3 | 720 | na | 0 | 28 | 24 | 2 | 6 |
| 2 | 14 | 4 | 831 | na | 0 | 29 | 29 | 1 | 6 |
| 2 | 13 | 2 | 30 | na | na | 30 | 35 | 2 | 10 |
| 2 | 12 | 2 | 530 | 0 | na | na | na | na | na |
| 2 | 10 | 6 | 620 | na | na | 15 | 30 | 2 | 4 |

| FOOD NAME | Serving Size | Calories |
|---|---|---|
| Prego Meat Flavored | 4 oz | 140 |
| Prego Mushroom | 4 oz | 130 |
| Prego No Salt Added | 4 oz | 110 |
| Prego Onion and Garlic | 4 oz | 110 |
| Prego Regular | 4 oz | 130 |
| Prego Three Cheese | 4 oz | 100 |
| Prego Tomato & Basil | 4 oz | 100 |
| Prego Extra Chunky Garden Combination | 4 oz | 80 |
| Prego Extra Chunky Mushroom and Green Pepper | 4 oz | 100 |
| Prego Extra Chunky Mushroom and Onion | 4 oz | 100 |
| Prego Extra Chunky Mushroom and Tomato | 4 oz | 110 |
| Prego Extra Chunky Mushroom with Extra Spice | 4 oz | 100 |
| Prego Extra Chunky Sausage & Green Pepper | 4 oz | 160 |
| Prego Extra Chunky Tomato and Onion | 4 oz | 110 |
| Ragu | 4 oz | 80 |
| Ragu Chunky Garden Style | 4 oz | 70 |
| Ragu Fresh Italian | 4 oz | 90 |
| Ragu Homestyle | 4 oz | 50 |
| Ragu Thick & Hearty | 4 oz | 100 |
| PASTRAMI (Oscar Mayer 98% Fat Free) | 1 sl | 15 |
| PATÉ (Underwood) | ½ can | 220 |
| PEACHES | | |
| Fresh | 1 | 39 |

| Protein (g) | Carbohydrates (g) | Fat (g) | Sodium (mg) | Cholesterol (mg) | Fiber (g) | Vitamin A (%) | Vitamin C (%) | Calcium (%) | Iron (%) |
|---|---|---|---|---|---|---|---|---|---|
| 2 | 20 | 6 | 660 | na | na | 20 | 25 | 4 | 6 |
| 2 | 20 | 5 | 630 | na | na | 20 | 25 | 4 | 4 |
| 2 | 11 | 6 | 25 | na | na | 30 | 30 | 4 | 6 |
| 1 | 16 | 4 | 510 | na | na | 20 | 8 | 2 | 6 |
| 2 | 20 | 5 | 630 | na | na | 20 | 30 | 4 | 6 |
| 3 | 17 | 2 | 410 | na | na | 15 | 35 | 4 | 8 |
| 2 | 18 | 2 | 370 | na | na | 20 | 35 | 4 | 6 |
| 2 | 14 | 2 | 420 | na | na | 20 | 40 | 4 | 6 |
| | | | | | | | | | |
| 2 | 14 | 4 | 410 | na | na | 15 | 20 | 2 | 6 |
| 2 | 13 | 4 | 490 | na | na | 10 | 20 | 2 | 6 |
| 1 | 14 | 5 | 500 | na | na | 10 | 20 | 2 | 6 |
| | | | | | | | | | |
| 2 | 17 | 3 | 450 | na | na | 15 | 35 | 4 | 6 |
| 3 | 19 | 8 | 500 | na | na | 20 | 30 | 4 | 6 |
| 2 | 14 | 5 | 490 | na | na | 10 | 20 | 2 | 6 |
| 2 | 9 | 4 | 740 | 0 | na | 15 | 10 | 2 | 4 |
| 2 | 10 | 3 | 440 | 0 | na | na | na | na | na |
| 2 | 13 | 3 | 490 | 0 | na | na | na | na | na |
| 2 | 6 | 2 | 390 | 0 | na | na | na | na | na |
| 2 | 15 | 3 | 460 | 0 | na | na | na | na | na |
| 3 | <1 | <1 | 215 | 5 | 0 | * | 10 | * | 4 |
| 12 | 3 | 19 | 570 | na | 0 | 80 | * | * | 25 |
| | | | | | | | | | |
| <1 | 10 | Tr | Tr | 0 | 1.4 | 25 | 10 | * | 2 |

| FOOD NAME | Serving Size | Calories |
|---|---|---|
| Sliced | 1 cup | 70 |
| *Canned* | | |
| In heavy syrup, cling (Del Monte) | ½ cup | 80 |
| In heavy syrup, cling (Del Monte Lite) | ½ cup | 50 |
| Freestone (Del Monte) | ½ cup | 90 |
| Freestone (Del Monte Lite) | ½ cup | 60 |
| Spiced, with pits, cling (Del Monte) | 3.5 oz | 80 |
| *Dried* | 1 cup | 400 |
| Del Monte | 2 oz | 140 |
| PEACH JUICE (Dole) | 6 fl oz | 90 |
| PEACH NECTAR (Libby's) | 6 fl oz | 100 |
| PEANUTS | ½ cup | 428 |
| Salted | ½ cup | 420 |
| PEANUT BUTTER | | |
| Bama Creamy | 2 tbsp | 200 |
| Bama Chunky | 2 tbsp | 200 |
| Jif Creamy, Low Sugar, Low Salt | 2 tbsp | 180 |
| Peter Pan Creamy, No Sugar Added, Salt Free | 2 tbsp | 190 |
| Peter Pan Extra Crunchy | 2 tbsp | 190 |
| Skippy Cream | 2 tbsp | 190 |
| Skippy Super Chunk | 2 tbsp | 190 |
| Smucker's Goober Grape | 2 tbsp | 180 |
| Smucker's Natural | 2 tbsp | 200 |
| Smucker's Natural Chunky | 2 tbsp | 200 |

| Protein (g) | Carbohydrates (g) | Fat (g) | Sodium (mg) | Cholesterol (mg) | Fiber (g) | Vitamin A (%) | Vitamin C (%) | Calcium (%) | Iron (%) |
|---|---|---|---|---|---|---|---|---|---|
| 1 | 17 | Tr | 2 | 0 | 2.8 | 45 | 20 | 2 | 4 |
| | | | | | | | | | |
| 0 | 22 | 0 | 9 | 0 | na | 6 | 4 | * | * |
| 0 | 13 | 0 | 9 | 0 | na | 6 | 4 | * | * |
| 0 | 23 | 0 | 9 | 0 | na | 2 | 2 | * | * |
| 0 | 13 | 0 | 9 | 0 | na | 2 | 2 | * | * |
| 0 | 20 | 0 | 9 | 0 | na | 6 | 25 | * | * |
| 6 | 100 | 1 | 12 | 0 | 13.2 | 125 | 50 | 8 | 60 |
| 2 | 35 | 0 | 9 | 0 | na | 25 | * | * | 10 |
| 0 | 24 | 0 | 10 | 0 | na | na | na | na | na |
| 0 | 24 | 0 | 5 | 0 | na | na | na | na | na |
| 17 | 16 | 36 | 4 | 4 | 5.8 | * | * | 5 | 8 |
| 17 | 14 | 36 | 300 | 0 | 5.8 | * | * | 5 | 8 |
| | | | | | | | | | |
| 7 | 6 | 17 | 140 | 0 | 0.6 | * | * | * | 2 |
| 7 | 6 | 17 | 115 | 0 | na | * | * | 2 | 2 |
| 9 | 5 | 16 | 65 | 0 | na | * | * | * | 2 |
| | | | | | | | | | |
| 9 | 5 | 17 | 0 | 0 | na | * | * | 2 | 4 |
| 9 | 5 | 16 | 122 | 0 | na | * | * | 2 | 4 |
| 9 | 4 | 17 | 150 | 0 | 0.6 | * | * | * | 2 |
| 9 | 4 | 17 | 130 | 0 | 0.6 | * | * | * | 2 |
| 6 | 18 | 10 | 120 | 0 | na | * | * | * | 2 |
| 8 | 6 | 16 | 125 | 0 | na | na | na | na | na |
| 8 | 6 | 16 | 125 | 0 | na | na | na | na | na |

| FOOD NAME | Serving Size | Calories | |
|---|---|---|---|
| PEAR | | | |
| Fresh | 1 | 100 | |
| Sliced | 1 cup | 100 | |
| *Canned* | | | |
| Bartlett (Del Monte) | ½ cup | 80 | |
| Bartlett (Del Monte Lite) | ½ cup | 50 | |
| *Dried* | 1 cup | 480 | |
| PEAR NECTAR | 6 fl oz | 112 | |
| PEAS | | | |
| *Fresh* | | | |
| Cooked | 1 cup | 110 | |
| *Canned* | | | |
| Green Giant 50% Less Sal | ½ cup | 50 | |
| Green Giant, With Tiny Pearl Onions | ½ cup | 50 | |
| Green Giant Very Young Small Early | ½ cup | 50 | |
| Green Giant Very Young Small Sweet | ½ cup | 50 | |
| Green Giant Very Young Tender Sweet | ½ cup | 50 | |
| *Frozen* | | | |
| Birds Eye | 3.3 oz | 80 | |
| Birds Eye Tender Tiny | 3.3 oz | 60 | |
| Green Giant | ½ cup | 50 | |
| Green Giant, With Butter Sauce | ½ cup | 80 | |
| Le Sueur Baby Early | ½ cup | 60 | |
| Le Sueur Baby Early, With Butter Sauce | ½ cup | 80 | |
| Sugar Snap | ½ cup | 30 | |

| Protein (g) | Carbohydrates (g) | Fat (g) | Sodium (mg) | Cholesterol (mg) | Fiber (g) | Vitamin A (%) | Vitamin C (%) | Calcium (%) | Iron (%) |
|---|---|---|---|---|---|---|---|---|---|
| 1 | 25 | <1 | 0 | 0 | 4 | * | 10 | 2 | 2 |
| <1 | 25 | <1 | 0 | 0 | 4 | * | 10 | 2 | 2 |
| | | | | | | | | | |
| 0 | 22 | 0 | 9 | 0 | na | * | 2 | * | * |
| 0 | 14 | 0 | 9 | 0 | na | * | 2 | * | * |
| na | 120 | 3 | 13 | 0 | na | 2 | 20 | 6 | 15 |
| Tr | 30 | Tr | 7 | 0 | 1.2 | na | na | na | na |
| | | | | | | | | | |
| 8 | 25 | Tr | 4 | 0 | 6 | 15 | 60 | 4 | 15 |
| | | | | | | | | | |
| 4 | 11 | 0 | 195 | 0 | 3 | 6 | 10 | * | 4 |
| 4 | 11 | 0 | 510 | 0 | 4 | 6 | 10 | 2 | 6 |
| 3 | 12 | 0 | 390 | 0 | 3 | 6 | 10 | 2 | 6 |
| 4 | 12 | 0 | 390 | 0 | 4 | 6 | 15 | 2 | 8 |
| 4 | 11 | 0 | 390 | 0 | 4 | 6 | 10 | 2 | 6 |
| | | | | | | | | | |
| 5 | 13 | 0 | 130 | 0 | 4 | 15 | 30 | 2 | 8 |
| 4 | 11 | 0 | 120 | 0 | 4 | 15 | 30 | * | 6 |
| 4 | 12 | 0 | 135 | 0 | 3 | 6 | 10 | 2 | 6 |
| 5 | 14 | 2 | 410 | 5 | 4 | 10 | 15 | 2 | 8 |
| 4 | 12 | 1 | 140 | 0 | 3 | 10 | 25 | 2 | 6 |
| 5 | 14 | 2 | 440 | 5 | 3 | 10 | 15 | 2 | 6 |
| 2 | 8 | 0 | 100 | 0 | 2 | 4 | 10 | 2 | 2 |

| FOOD NAME | Serving Size | Calories |
|---|---|---|
| *Frozen combinations* | | |
| Birds Eye, with Cream Sauce | 5 oz | 180 |
| Birds Eye, with Pearl Onions | 3.3 oz | 70 |
| Birds Eye, with Pearl Onions in Cheese Sauce | 5 oz | 140 |
| Birds Eye, with Potatoes in Cream Sauce | 5 oz | 190 |
| Le Sueur Baby Early with Mushrooms | ½ cup | 60 |
| PECANS Halves | 1 cup | 720 |
| PEPPERS | | |
| *Fresh* | | |
| Sweet Green or Red | 1 | 20 |
| Sweet Green or Red, cooked, drained | 1 cup | 25 |
| *Bottled* | | |
| Hot Banana Pepper Rings (Vlasic) | 1 oz | 4 |
| Hot Cherry Peppers (Vlasic) | 1 oz | 10 |
| Mexican Hot Jalapeño Peppers (Vlasic) | 1 oz | 8 |
| Mexican Tiny Hot Peppers (Vlasic) | 1 oz | 6 |
| Mild Cherry Peppers (Vlasic) | 1 oz | 8 |
| Mild Greek Pepperoncini Salad (Vlasic) | 1 oz | 4 |
| PEPPERONI | | |
| (Eckrich Sliced) | 2 oz | 270 |
| (Hormel Chunk) | 2 oz | 280 |
| PERCH Fried | 1 fillet | 195 |
| PICKLE AND PIMIENTO LOAF (Oscar Mayer) | 1 slice | 60 |
| PICKLES | | |
| Bread & Butter (Vlasic Chips) | 1 oz | 30 |

| Protein (g) | Carbohydrates (g) | Fat (g) | Sodium (mg) | Cholesterol (mg) | Fiber (g) | Vitamin A (%) | Vitamin C (%) | Calcium (%) | Iron (%) |
|---|---|---|---|---|---|---|---|---|---|
| 5 | 16 | 11 | 480 | 0 | 3 | 15 | 10 | 6 | 6 |
| 5 | 13 | 0 | 440 | 0 | 3 | 15 | 30 | * | 4 |
| 6 | 17 | 5 | 470 | 5 | 3 | 40 | 25 | 10 | 6 |
| 4 | 17 | 12 | 490 | 0 | 2 | 15 | 10 | 4 | 4 |
| 4 | 11 | 0 | 95 | 0 | 4 | 8 | 20 | 2 | 6 |
| 8 | 20 | 73 | 1 | 0 | 7 | 2 | 4 | 8 | 15 |
| | | | | | | | | | |
| <1 | 5 | Tr | 1 | 0 | 1.2 | 6 | 160 | * | 4 |
| <1 | 5 | Tr | 2 | 0 | 0.6 | 10 | 220 | 2 | 4 |
| | | | | | | | | | |
| 0 | 1 | 0 | 465 | 0 | na | * | 15 | * | 2 |
| 0 | 2 | 0 | 425 | 0 | na | 2 | 25 | * | * |
| 0 | 2 | 0 | 380 | 0 | na | 2 | * | * | 2 |
| 0 | 2 | 0 | 430 | 0 | na | * | 2 | * | * |
| 0 | 2 | 0 | 410 | 0 | na | 2 | 10 | * | 2 |
| 0 | 1 | 0 | 450 | 0 | na | * | * | * | 2 |
| | | | | | | | | | |
| 12 | 2 | 24 | 1000 | 46 | 0 | * | * | 2 | 6 |
| 12 | 0 | 24 | 846 | na | 0 | na | na | na | na |
| 16 | 6 | 11 | 128 | 7 | 0 | * | * | 3 | 6 |
| 4 | 1 | 4 | 335 | 15 | na | na | na | na | na |
| | | | | | | | | | |
| 0 | 7 | 0 | 160 | 0 | na | * | * | * | * |

| FOOD NAME | Serving Size | Calories |
|---|---|---|
| Bread & Butter (Vlasic Chunks) | 1 oz | 25 |
| Bread & Butter (Vlasic Stix) | 1 oz | 18 |
| Half-the-Salt (Vlasic Hamburger Dill Chips) | 1 oz | 2 |
| Half-the-Salt (Vlasic Kosher Crunchy Dills) | 1 oz | 4 |
| Half-the-Salt (Vlasic Kosher Dill Spears) | 1 oz | 4 |
| Half-the-Salt (Vlasic Sweet Butter Chips) | 1 oz | 30 |
| Hot & Spicy (Vlasic Cauliflower) | 1 oz | 4 |
| Hot & Spicy (Vlasic Garden Mix) | 1 oz | 4 |
| Kosher (Vlasic Baby Dills) | 1 oz | 4 |
| Kosher (Vlasic Crunchy Dills) | 1 oz | 4 |
| Kosher (Vlasic Dill Gherkins) | 1 oz | 4 |
| Kosher (Vlasic Dill Spears) | 1 oz | 4 |
| Kosher (Vlasic Snack Chunks) | 1 oz | 4 |
| No Garlic (Vlasic Dill Spears) | 1 oz | 4 |
| Original (Vlasic Crunchy Dills) | 1 oz | 4 |
| Original (Vlasic Dills) | 1 oz | 2 |
| Original (Vlasic Polish Snack Chunks) | 1 oz | 4 |
| Original (Vlasic Zesty Dill Snack Chunks) | 1 oz | 4 |
| Original (Vlasic Zesty Dill Spears) | 1 oz | 4 |
| Refrigerated (Vlasic Deli Bread & Butter) | 1 oz | 25 |
| Refrigerated (Vlasic Deli Dill Halves) | 1 oz | 4 |
| PIE | | |
| Apple (Banquet frozen) | ⅙ | 250 |
| Apple (Mrs. Smith's frozen) | ⅛ | 210 |
| Banana Cream (Banquet frozen) | ⅙ | 180 |

| Protein (g) | Carbohydrates (g) | Fat (g) | Sodium (mg) | Cholesterol (mg) | Fiber (g) | Vitamin A (%) | Vitamin C (%) | Calcium (%) | Iron (%) |
|---|---|---|---|---|---|---|---|---|---|
| 0 | 6 | 0 | 120 | 0 | na | * | * | * | * |
| 0 | 5 | 0 | 110 | 0 | na | * | * | * | * |
| 0 | 1 | 0 | 175 | 0 | na | * | * | * | * |
| 0 | 1 | 0 | 125 | 0 | na | * | * | * | * |
| 0 | 1 | 0 | 120 | 0 | na | * | * | * | * |
| 0 | 7 | 0 | 80 | 0 | na | * | * | * | * |
| 0 | 1 | 0 | 435 | 0 | na | * | * | * | 2 |
| 0 | 1 | 0 | 380 | 0 | na | 2 | 6 | * | 2 |
| 0 | 1 | 0 | 210 | 0 | na | * | * | * | 2 |
| 0 | 1 | 0 | 210 | 0 | na | * | * | * | 2 |
| 0 | 1 | 0 | 210 | 0 | na | * | * | * | 2 |
| 0 | 1 | 0 | 175 | 0 | na | * | * | * | * |
| 0 | 1 | 0 | 220 | 0 | na | * | * | * | * |
| 0 | 1 | 0 | 210 | 0 | na | * | * | * | 2 |
| 0 | 1 | 0 | 250 | 0 | na | * | * | * | * |
| 0 | 1 | 0 | 375 | 0 | na | * | * | * | * |
| 0 | 1 | 0 | 300 | 0 | na | * | 2 | * | * |
| 0 | 1 | 0 | 290 | 0 | na | * | * | * | * |
| 0 | 1 | 0 | 230 | 0 | na | * | * | * | * |
| 0 | 6 | 0 | 120 | 0 | na | * | * | * | * |
| 0 | 1 | 0 | 290 | 0 | na | * | * | * | * |
|  |  |  |  |  |  |  |  |  |  |
| 2 | 37 | 11 | 290 | 0 | na | 1 | 4 | 1 | 6 |
| 2 | 29 | 9 | 250 | 0 | na | 4 | * | * | 4 |
| 2 | 21 | 10 | 150 | 0 | na | * | * | 2 | 5 |

Pie

| FOOD NAME | Serving Size | Calories |
|---|---|---|
| Banana Cream (Mrs. Smith's frozen) | ⅛ | 240 |
| Banana Cream (Pet-Ritz frozen) | ⅙ | 180 |
| Blackberry (Banquet frozen) | ⅙ | 270 |
| Blueberry (Mrs. Smith's frozen) | ⅛ | 220 |
| Boston Cream (Betty Crocker mix) | ⅛ | 260 |
| Boston Cream (Mrs. Smith's frozen) | ⅛ | 260 |
| Cherry (Banquet frozen) | ⅙ | 250 |
| Cherry (Mrs. Smith's frozen) | ⅛ | 220 |
| Cherry Lattice (Mrs. Smith's frozen) | ⅛ | 350 |
| Chocolate Cream (Mrs. Smith's frozen) | ⅛ | 270 |
| Chocolate Cream (Mrs. Smith's frozen) | ⅙ | 190 |
| Coconut Cream (Banquet frozen) | ⅙ | 190 |
| Coconut Cream (Mrs. Smith's frozen) | ⅛ | 270 |
| Coconut Cream (Pet-Ritz frozen) | ⅙ | 190 |
| Coconut Custard (Mrs. Smith's frozen) | ⅛ | 330 |
| Egg Custard (Mrs. Smith's frozen) | ⅛ | 300 |
| Lemon Cream (Banquet frozen) | ⅙ | 170 |
| Lemon Cream (Mrs. Smith's frozen) | ⅛ | 245 |
| Lemon Cream (Pet-Ritz frozen) | ⅙ | 190 |
| Lemon Meringue (Mrs. Smith's frozen) | ⅛ | 210 |
| Mincemeat (Banquet frozen) | ⅙ | 260 |
| Neapolitan Cream (Pet-Ritz frozen) | ⅙ | 180 |
| Peach (Banquet frozen) | ⅙ | 245 |
| Peach (Mrs. Smith's frozen) | ⅛ | 365 |
| Pecan (Mrs. Smith's frozen) | ⅛ | 510 |

| Protein (g) | Carbohydrates (g) | Fat (g) | Sodium (mg) | Cholesterol (mg) | Fiber (g) | Vitamin A (%) | Vitamin C (%) | Calcium (%) | Iron (%) |
|---|---|---|---|---|---|---|---|---|---|
| 2 | 31 | 12 | 180 | 0 | na | * | * | 4 | 2 |
| 2 | 22 | 9 | 155 | 0 | na | * | * | 2 | 5 |
| 3 | 40 | 11 | 350 | 0 | na | * | 15 | * | 4 |
| 2 | 32 | 9 | 240 | 0 | na | 4 | * | * | 2 |
| 2 | 48 | 6 | 405 | na | na | 2 | * | 15 | 2 |
| 2 | 44 | 8 | 225 | na | na | 2 | * | 2 | 2 |
| 3 | 36 | 11 | 260 | 0 | na | 2 | * | 2 | 4 |
| 2 | 32 | 9 | 200 | 0 | na | 2 | * | 2 | 4 |
| 3 | 59 | 11 | 490 | 0 | na | 10 | * | * | 2 |
| 2 | 35 | 13 | 235 | na | na | 2 | * | 2 | 2 |
| 1 | 27 | 8 | 145 | na | 0 | 2 | * | 2 | 2 |
| 2 | 22 | 11 | 120 | na | na | * | * | 2 | 2 |
| 2 | 33 | 14 | 220 | na | na | * | * | 2 | 2 |
| 2 | 27 | 8 | 145 | na | na | na | na | na | na |
| 9 | 40 | 15 | 550 | na | na | 2 | * | 10 | 6 |
| 10 | 45 | 9 | 490 | na | na | * | * | 15 | 4 |
| 2 | 23 | 9 | 120 | na | na | 2 | * | * | 2 |
| 2 | 32 | 12 | 185 | na | na | 2 | * | * | 2 |
| 2 | 26 | 9 | 150 | na | na | na | na | na | na |
| 2 | 38 | 5 | 130 | na | na | 4 | * | * | 2 |
| 3 | 38 | 11 | 370 | na | na | na | na | na | na |
| 1 | 17 | 10 | 185 | na | na | na | na | na | na |
| 3 | 35 | 11 | 280 | na | na | 2 | * | * | 4 |
| 3 | 53 | 16 | 435 | na | na | 2 | * | * | 4 |
| 2 | 70 | 23 | 510 | na | na | 6 | * | * | 4 |

| FOOD NAME | Serving Size | Calories |
|---|---|---|
| Pumpkin (Banquet frozen) | ⅙ | 200 |
| Pumpkin Custard (Mrs. Smith's frozen) | ⅛ | 310 |
| Strawberry Cream (Banquet frozen) | ⅙ | 170 |
| Strawberry Cream (Pet-Ritz frozen) | ⅙ | 170 |
| **PIE CRUST** | | |
| Mix (Pillsbury) | ⅛ | 200 |
| Shell (Mrs. Smith's frozen) | ⅛ | 90 |
| Shell (Pet-Ritz frozen) | ⅙ | 110 |
| **PIE FILLING** | | |
| Apple (Comstock) | 3.5 oz | 120 |
| Banana Cream (Jell-O) | ½ cup | 170 |
| Butter Pecan (Jell-O) | ½ cup | 170 |
| Butterscotch (Royal) | ½ cup | 186 |
| Chocolate (Royal) | ½ cup | 190 |
| Chocolate (D-Zerta) | ½ cup | 70 |
| Chocolate Fudge (Jell-O) | ½ cup | 180 |
| Coconut (Royal) | ½ cup | 170 |
| Custard & Flan (Royal) | ½ cup | 150 |
| French Vanilla (Jell-O) | ½ cup | 170 |
| Lemon (Jell-O) | ½ cup | 180 |
| Milk Chocolate (Jell-O) | ½ cup | 170 |
| Mincemeat (Musselman's) | 4 oz | 190 |
| Peach (Comstock) | 3.5 oz | 110 |
| Pineapple Cream (Jell-O) | ½ cup | 170 |
| Pistachio (Jell-O) | ½ cup | 180 |

| Protein (g) | Carbohydrates (g) | Fat (g) | Sodium (mg) | Cholesterol (mg) | Fiber (g) | Vitamin A (%) | Vitamin C (%) | Calcium (%) | Iron (%) |
|---|---|---|---|---|---|---|---|---|---|
| 3 | 29 | 8 | 350 | na | na | 30 | * | 8 | 4 |
| 3 | 46 | 11 | 495 | na | na | 30 | * | 8 | 4 |
| 2 | 22 | 9 | 120 | na | na | na | na | na | na |
| 2 | 20 | 9 | 145 | na | na | na | na | na | na |
| 3 | 20 | 13 | 300 | 0 | na | * | * | * | 4 |
| 1 | 10 | 5 | 125 | 0 | na | * | * | * | 4 |
| 1 | 11 | 7 | 110 | na | na | * | * | * | 4 |
| 0 | 30 | 0 | 15 | 0 | 0.4 | na | na | na | na |
| 4 | 30 | 4 | 385 | 15 | 0 | 2 | * | 15 | * |
| 4 | 29 | 5 | 385 | 15 | 0 | 2 | * | 15 | * |
| 4 | 29 | 5 | 245 | na | 0 | 4 | 2 | 15 | * |
| 4 | 35 | 4 | 365 | na | 0 | 4 | 2 | 15 | 4 |
| 5 | 11 | 0 | 80 | na | 0 | 4 | 2 | 15 | * |
| 5 | 32 | 5 | 430 | 15 | 0 | 2 | * | 15 | 2 |
| 4 | 30 | 4 | 320 | na | 0 | 4 | 2 | 15 | 2 |
| 4 | 22 | 5 | 130 | na | 0 | 4 | 2 | 15 | * |
| 4 | 30 | 4 | 200 | 15 | 0 | 2 | * | 15 | * |
| 5 | 31 | 4 | 385 | 15 | 0 | 2 | * | 15 | * |
| 5 | 29 | 4 | 180 | 15 | 0 | 2 | * | 15 | * |
| 0 | 48 | 1 | 145 | na | na | na | na | na | na |
| 0 | 26 | 0 | 20 | 0 | 0.2 | na | na | na | na |
| 4 | 30 | 4 | 335 | na | 0 | 2 | * | 15 | * |
| 6 | 30 | 5 | 425 | 15 | 0 | 2 | * | 15 | * |

| FOOD NAME | Serving Size | Calories |
|---|---|---|
| Pumpkin (Comstock) | 3.5 oz | 100 |
| Tapioca, Chocolate (Jell-O) | ½ cup | 170 |
| Tapioca, Vanilla (Jell-O) | ½ cup | 160 |
| Vanilla (D-Zerta) | ½ cup | 70 |
| Vanilla (Jell-O) | ½ cup | 160 |
| PIKE Northern, broiled | 4 oz | 128 |
| PIMENTOS (Dromedary) | 1 oz | 10 |
| PINEAPPLE | | |
| *Fresh* | | |
| Diced | 1 cup | 80 |
| *Canned* | | |
| In heavy syrup (Del Monte) | ½ cup | 90 |
| In juice (Del Monte Chunks or Slices) | ½ cup | 70 |
| In juice (Del Monte Spears) | 2 | 50 |
| Unsweetened (Del Monte) | 6 fl oz | 100 |
| PINTO BEANS Boiled | ½ cup | 117 |
| PISTACHIO NUTS | 1 oz | 164 |
| PIZZA, FROZEN | | |
| *Jeno's* | | |
| Canadian Bacon | ½ | 240 |
| Cheese | ½ | 240 |
| Combination | ½ | 280 |
| Hamburger | ½ | 280 |
| Pepperoni | ½ | 280 |
| Sausage | ½ | 280 |

| Protein (g) | Carbohydrates (g) | Fat (g) | Sodium (mg) | Cholesterol (mg) | Fiber (g) | Vitamin A (%) | Vitamin C (%) | Calcium (%) | Iron (%) |
|---|---|---|---|---|---|---|---|---|---|
| 0 | 24 | 0 | 180 | 0 | na | na | na | na | na |
| 6 | 28 | 5 | 170 | 0 | na | 2 | * | 15 | 2 |
| 5 | 27 | 4 | 170 | 15 | 0 | 2 | * | 15 | * |
| 6 | 12 | 0 | 105 | na | 0 | 4 | 2 | 15 | * |
| 5 | 27 | 4 | 200 | 15 | 0 | 2 | * | 15 | * |
| 28 | 0 | 1 | 56 | 57 | 0 | 4 | 16 | 8 | * |
| 0 | 2 | 0 | 5 | 0 | na | 10 | 15 | * | 8 |
| | | | | | | | | | |
| <1 | 22 | <1 | 2 | 0 | 1.8 | 2 | 45 | 2 | 4 |
| | | | | | | | | | |
| 0 | 23 | 0 | 9 | 0 | na | * | 6 | * | * |
| 0 | 18 | 0 | 9 | 0 | na | * | 6 | * | * |
| 0 | 14 | 0 | 10 | 0 | na | 2 | 4 | 2 | 2 |
| 0 | 25 | 0 | 9 | 0 | na | * | 100 | 2 | 4 |
| 7 | 22 | Tr | 1 | 0 | 3.7 | * | * | 6 | 8 |
| 6 | 7 | 13 | 2 | 0 | 3.1 | 4 | * | 24 | 45 |
| | | | | | | | | | |
| 10 | 28 | 10 | 680 | 5 | 1 | 8 | 4 | 15 | 10 |
| 11 | 28 | 10 | 500 | 10 | 1 | 6 | 4 | 20 | 10 |
| 10 | 27 | 15 | 680 | 15 | 1 | 8 | 4 | 15 | 10 |
| 11 | 28 | 14 | 640 | 15 | 1 | 6 | 4 | 15 | 10 |
| 10 | 28 | 15 | 710 | 15 | 1 | 8 | 4 | 15 | 10 |
| 10 | 27 | 15 | 640 | 10 | 1 | 8 | 4 | 15 | 10 |

# FOOD NAME

| FOOD NAME | Serving Size | Calories |
|---|---|---|
| Sausage & Pepperoni Pizza Pocket | 1 | 360 |
| Pepperoni Pizza Pocket | 1 | 370 |
| Sausage Pizza Pocket | 1 | 360 |
| Supreme Pizza Pocket | 1 | 370 |
| Cheese Pizza Roll | 3 oz | 200 |
| Combination Pizza Roll | 3 oz | 220 |
| Hamburger Pizza Roll | 3 oz | 220 |
| Pepperoni Pizza Roll | 3 oz | 220 |
| Sausage Pizza Roll | 3 oz | 210 |
| *Oven Lovin'* | | |
| Cheese Microwave | ½ | 250 |
| Combination Microwave | ½ | 310 |
| Pepperoni Microwave | ½ | 300 |
| Sausage Microwave | ½ | 290 |
| Supreme Microwave | ½ | 310 |
| Cheese Microwave French Bread | 1 | 350 |
| Combination Microwave French Bread | 1 | 420 |
| Pepperoni Microwave French Bread | 1 | 410 |
| Sausage Microwave French Bread | 1 | 400 |
| *Pappalo's* | | |
| 9" Pepperoni | ½ | 390 |
| 9" Sausage | ½ | 380 |
| 9" Sausage & Pepperoni | ½ | 390 |
| 9" Supreme | ½ | 400 |
| 9" Three Cheese | ½ | 350 |

| Protein (g) | Carbohydrates (g) | Fat (g) | Sodium (mg) | Cholesterol (mg) | Fiber (g) | Vitamin A (%) | Vitamin C (%) | Calcium (%) | Iron (%) |
|---|---|---|---|---|---|---|---|---|---|
| 12 | 35 | 20 | 710 | 20 | na | 8 | 8 | 15 | 10 |
| 12 | 35 | 20 | 790 | 25 | na | 8 | 10 | 15 | 10 |
| 11 | 35 | 19 | 660 | 15 | na | 8 | 8 | 15 | 10 |
| 12 | 36 | 19 | 720 | 20 | na | 10 | 100 | 15 | 15 |
| 9 | 30 | 5 | 370 | 20 | 1.4 | 2 | * | 15 | 4 |
| 10 | 26 | 9 | 230 | 15 | 1.9 | * | * | 6 | 4 |
| 10 | 28 | 8 | 310 | 20 | 2 | * | * | 8 | 4 |
| 9 | 26 | 9 | 350 | 20 | 1.8 | * | * | 6 | 4 |
| 9 | 26 | 7 | 340 | 15 | 1.6 | * | * | 6 | 4 |
| | | | | | | | | | |
| 11 | 24 | 12 | 430 | 10 | na | 8 | 6 | 25 | 10 |
| 13 | 26 | 18 | 580 | 20 | na | 8 | 6 | 25 | 10 |
| 13 | 25 | 17 | 620 | 25 | na | 8 | 6 | 25 | 10 |
| 12 | 26 | 16 | 510 | 15 | na | 8 | 6 | 20 | 10 |
| 13 | 27 | 18 | 570 | 20 | na | 10 | 100 | 25 | 10 |
| 17 | 40 | 14 | 700 | 15 | na | 10 | 8 | 35 | 10 |
| 18 | 41 | 21 | 910 | 30 | na | 10 | 10 | 30 | 10 |
| 18 | 40 | 21 | 980 | 35 | na | 10 | 8 | 30 | 10 |
| 18 | 41 | 20 | 830 | 25 | na | 10 | 8 | 30 | 10 |
| | | | | | | | | | |
| 23 | 47 | 14 | 870 | 45 | 4 | 10 | 2 | 50 | 25 |
| 22 | 47 | 13 | 680 | 40 | 4 | 8 | 2 | 50 | 20 |
| 23 | 45 | 15 | 650 | 45 | 4 | 8 | 2 | 40 | 20 |
| 25 | 46 | 16 | 700 | 45 | 4 | 8 | 2 | 45 | 20 |
| 21 | 47 | 11 | 640 | 30 | 4 | 15 | 2 | 60 | 20 |

| FOOD NAME | Serving Size | Calories | |
|---|---|---|---|
| 12" Pepperoni | ¼ | 350 | |
| 12" Sausage | ¼ | 350 | |
| 12" Sausage & Pepperoni | ¼ | 360 | |
| 12" Supreme | ¼ | 350 | |
| 12" Three Cheese | ¼ | 310 | |
| Pepperoni Pan | ⅕ | 350 | |
| Sausage Pan | ⅕ | 350 | |
| Sausage & Pepperoni Pan | ⅕ | 360 | |
| Supreme Pan | ⅕ | 340 | |
| Three Cheese Pan | ⅕ | 310 | |
| *Stouffer's* | | | |
| Cheese | ½ | 320 | |
| Deluxe | ½ | 370 | |
| Extra Cheese | ½ | 370 | |
| Pepperoni | ½ | 350 | |
| Sausage | ½ | 360 | |
| Sausage & Pepperoni | ½ | 380 | |
| *Stouffer's French Bread* | | | |
| Canadian Style Bacon | ½ | 360 | |
| Cheese | ½ | 340 | |
| Deluxe | ½ | 430 | |
| Hamburger | ½ | 410 | |
| Pepperoni | ½ | 410 | |
| Pepperoni & Mushroom | ½ | 430 | |
| Sausage | ½ | 420 | |

| Protein (g) | Carbohydrates (g) | Fat (g) | Sodium (mg) | Cholesterol (mg) | Fiber (g) | Vitamin A (%) | Vitamin C (%) | Calcium (%) | Iron (%) |
|---|---|---|---|---|---|---|---|---|---|
| 22 | 40 | 11 | 700 | 45 | 4 | 15 | 8 | 30 | 25 |
| 22 | 39 | 12 | 600 | 40 | 4 | 15 | 8 | 30 | 25 |
| 23 | 40 | 12 | 730 | 45 | 4 | 15 | 8 | 30 | 25 |
| 22 | 38 | 12 | 640 | 45 | 4 | 15 | 110 | 25 | 25 |
| 20 | 41 | 7 | 440 | 30 | 4 | 4 | 2 | 35 | 6 |
| 22 | 40 | 11 | 720 | 50 | 3 | 15 | 6 | 30 | 30 |
| 22 | 39 | 11 | 530 | 40 | 3 | 10 | 6 | 30 | 25 |
| 22 | 40 | 12 | 630 | 45 | 3 | 10 | 6 | 30 | 25 |
| 22 | 37 | 12 | 610 | 45 | 3 | 15 | 80 | 30 | 25 |
| 20 | 39 | 8 | 490 | 30 | 3 | 4 | 2 | 30 | 6 |
| | | | | | | | | | |
| 14 | 32 | 15 | 640 | na | na | 5 | 5 | 25 | 10 |
| 16 | 33 | 19 | 590 | na | na | 5 | 5 | 20 | 10 |
| 17 | 33 | 19 | 720 | na | na | 5 | 5 | 30 | 10 |
| 15 | 34 | 18 | 820 | na | na | 10 | 5 | 20 | 10 |
| 16 | 32 | 18 | 830 | na | na | 5 | 5 | 20 | 10 |
| 16 | 33 | 21 | 860 | na | na | 5 | 5 | 15 | 10 |
| | | | | | | | | | |
| 18 | 41 | 14 | 960 | na | na | 8 | 10 | 20 | 10 |
| 15 | 41 | 13 | 840 | na | na | 8 | 10 | 20 | 15 |
| 18 | 41 | 21 | 1130 | na | na | 10 | 10 | 20 | 15 |
| 19 | 40 | 19 | 1010 | na | na | 6 | 10 | 20 | 15 |
| 17 | 41 | 20 | 1120 | na | na | 10 | 10 | 20 | 15 |
| 18 | 40 | 22 | 1340 | na | na | 10 | 10 | 20 | 20 |
| 18 | 41 | 20 | 1110 | na | na | 8 | 10 | 20 | 15 |

| FOOD NAME | Serving Size | Calories | |
|---|---|---|---|
| Sausage & Mushroom | ½ | 410 | |
| Sausage & Pepperoni | ½ | 450 | |
| Vegetable Deluxe | ½ | 420 | |
| *Stouffer's Lean Cuisine French Bread* | | | |
| Cheese | 1 | 310 | |
| Deluxe | 1 | 350 | |
| Extra Cheese | 1 | 350 | |
| Pepperoni | 1 | 340 | |
| Sausage | 1 | 350 | |
| PIZZA CROISSANT | | | |
| Cheese (Pepperidge Farm) | 1 | 430 | |
| Deluxe (Pepperidge Farm) | 1 | 430 | |
| Pepperoni (Pepperidge Farm) | 1 | 420 | |
| PLANTAIN | 1 | 313 | |
| PLUMS | | | |
| Fresh | 1 | 30 | |
| Canned in syrup | 1 cup | 215 | |
| POMPANO Broiled | 4 oz | 239 | |
| POPCORN | | | |
| Popped with oil and salt | 1 cup | 40 | |
| Popped plain | 1 cup | 25 | |
| Microwave (Jiffy Pop) | 4 cups | 140 | |
| Microwave (Orville Redenbacher Gourmet) | 4 cups | 90 | |
| Microwave (Pillsbury) | 2 cups | 120 | |
| Microwave (Planters Natural) | 3 cups | 140 | |

| Protein (g) | Carbohydrates (g) | Fat (g) | Sodium (mg) | Cholesterol (mg) | Fiber (g) | Vitamin A (%) | Vitamin C (%) | Calcium (%) | Iron (%) |
|---|---|---|---|---|---|---|---|---|---|
| 17 | 42 | 19 | 1050 | na | na | 8 | 10 | 20 | 15 |
| 20 | 40 | 23 | 1350 | na | na | 10 | 10 | 20 | 20 |
| 18 | 41 | 20 | 830 | na | na | 25 | 2 | 35 | 15 |
| | | | | | | | | | |
| 16 | 40 | 10 | 750 | 15 | na | 6 | 10 | 25 | 15 |
| 20 | 40 | 12 | 990 | 35 | na | 8 | 10 | 25 | 20 |
| 21 | 39 | 12 | 850 | 20 | na | 4 | 25 | 50 | 20 |
| 18 | 40 | 12 | 970 | 30 | na | 6 | 10 | 25 | 20 |
| 23 | 40 | 11 | 960 | 45 | na | 4 | 10 | 25 | 25 |
| | | | | | | | | | |
| 15 | 41 | 23 | 640 | na | na | 6 | 4 | 35 | 10 |
| 16 | 43 | 23 | 790 | na | na | 4 | 2 | 30 | 15 |
| 14 | 43 | 22 | 690 | na | na | 6 | 6 | 25 | 10 |
| 2 | 57 | 1 | 13 | 0 | 0.9 | * | 62 | 2 | 10 |
| | | | | | | | | | |
| 0 | 8 | 0 | 1 | 0 | 0.4 | 3 | 7 | 1 | 2 |
| 1 | 56 | 0 | 10 | 0 | 0.8 | 63 | 8 | 2 | 13 |
| 26 | 0 | 14 | 86 | 73 | 0 | na | na | na | na |
| | | | | | | | | | |
| 1 | 6 | Tr | na | 0 | na | * | * | * | 2 |
| 1 | 5 | 0 | 1 | 0 | na | * | * | * | 2 |
| 3 | 17 | 7 | 270 | 0 | 3 | na | na | na | na |
| 2 | 18 | 1 | Tr | 0 | na | * | * | * | 4 |
| 2 | 11 | 8 | 348 | na | na | * | * | * | 2 |
| 2 | 14 | 9 | 560 | 0 | na | na | na | na | na |

| FOOD NAME | Serving Size | Calories |
|---|---|---|
| Microwave (Totino's) | 4 cups | 260 |
| **PORK CHOP** | | |
| Loin, lean and fat | 4 oz | 452 |
| Loin, lean only | 4 oz | 300 |
| **PORK ROAST** | | |
| Lean and fat | 4 oz | 413 |
| Lean only | 4 oz | 292 |
| **PORK SHOULDER** | | |
| Roasted, lean and fat | 4 oz | 370 |
| Roasted, lean only | 4 oz | 277 |
| **POTATO** | | |
| Baked | 1 | 145 |
| Boiled | 1 | 105 |
| Mashed with milk | 1 cup | 135 |
| *Canned* | | |
| Del Monte | ½ cup | 45 |
| *Frozen* | | |
| Birds Eye Tiny Taters | 3.2 oz | 200 |
| Birds Eye Whole peeled | 3.2 oz | 60 |
| Ore-Ida Crispy Crowns | 3 oz | 150 |
| Ore-Ida Golden Patties | 2.5 oz | 130 |
| Ore-Ida Cottage Fries | 3 oz | 140 |
| Ore-Ida Golden Crinkles | 3 oz | 12 |
| Ore-Ida Golden Fries | 3 oz | 130 |
| Ore-Ida Tater Tots | 3 oz | 160 |

| Protein (g) | Carbohydrates (g) | Fat (g) | Sodium (mg) | Cholesterol (mg) | Fiber (g) | Vitamin A (%) | Vitamin C (%) | Calcium (%) | Iron (%) |
|---|---|---|---|---|---|---|---|---|---|
| 3 | 28 | 15 | 405 | 0 | na | * | 6 | * | 6 |
| | | | | | | | | | |
| 28 | 0 | 37 | 68 | 116 | 0 | * | * | * | 22 |
| 34 | 0 | 18 | 82 | 108 | 0 | * | * | * | 24 |
| | | | | | | | | | |
| 28 | 0 | 32 | 68 | 110 | 0 | * | * | * | 20 |
| 33 | 0 | 17 | 78 | 109 | 0 | * | * | 2 | 24 |
| | | | | | | | | | |
| 25 | 0 | 29 | 77 | 109 | 0 | * | * | * | 20 |
| 29 | 0 | 17 | 86 | 110 | 0 | * | * | * | 20 |
| | | | | | | | | | |
| 4 | 33 | 0 | 5 | 0 | 1.3 | * | 52 | 1 | 6 |
| 3 | 23 | 0 | 4 | 0 | 2.1 | * | 37 | * | 4 |
| 4 | 27 | 2 | 632 | 4 | 0.6 | 1 | 35 | 5 | 44 |
| | | | | | | | | | |
| 1 | 10 | 0 | 355 | 0 | na | * | 25 | 2 | 2 |
| | | | | | | | | | |
| 1 | 22 | 12 | 280 | na | na | * | 6 | * | 2 |
| 1 | 13 | 0 | 6 | 0 | na | * | 8 | * | * |
| 1 | 18 | 8 | 370 | na | na | * | 4 | * | 2 |
| 1 | 17 | 10 | 340 | na | na | * | 4 | * | 4 |
| 1 | 21 | 6 | 40 | na | na | * | 8 | * | 2 |
| 2 | 20 | 5 | 40 | na | na | * | 6 | * | 2 |
| 2 | 21 | 5 | 40 | na | na | * | 6 | * | 2 |
| 1 | 21 | 8 | 550 | na | na | * | 4 | * | 2 |

| FOOD NAME | Serving Size | Calories | |
|---|---|---|---|
| Ore-Ida Tater Tots, Bacon Flavor | 3 oz | 160 | |
| Ore-Ida Tater Tots, Onion Flavor | 3 oz | 160 | |
| Ore-Ida Hashbrowns | 6 oz | 130 | |
| Ore-Ida Home Style | 3 oz | 110 | |
| Ore-Ida Home Style Potato Planks | 3 oz | 110 | |
| Ore-Ida Potato Thins | 3 oz | 130 | |
| Ore-Ida Shoestring | 3 oz | 160 | |
| Ore-Ida Whole peeled | 3 oz | 80 | |
| *Microwave* | | | |
| Green Giant Au Gratin | ½ cup | 120 | |
| *Mix* | | | |
| Betty Crocker Au Gratin | ½ cup | 150 | |
| Betty Crocker Chicken 'n Herb | ½ cup | 120 | |
| Betty Crocker Creamed Oven | ½ cup | 170 | |
| Betty Crocker Creamed Saucepan | ½ cup | 180 | |
| Betty Crocker Hash Browns | ½ cup | 150 | |
| Betty Crocker Hickory Smoke Cheese | ½ cup | 150 | |
| Betty Crocker Julienne | ½ cup | 130 | |
| Betty Crocker Potato Buds | ½ cup | 130 | |
| Hungry Jack Flakes | ½ cup | 130 | |
| Idaho Mashed Potatoes, Granules | ½ cup | 120 | |
| Idaho Spuds Mashed Potatoes | ½ cup | 130 | |
| Kraft Cheese Au Gratin | ½ cup | 130 | |
| Kraft Cheese Broccoli Au Gratin | ½ cup | 150 | |
| Kraft Cheese Scalloped | ½ cup | 140 | |

| Protein (g) | Carbohydrates (g) | Fat (g) | Sodium (mg) | Cholesterol (mg) | Fiber (g) | Vitamin A (%) | Vitamin C (%) | Calcium (%) | Iron (%) |
|---|---|---|---|---|---|---|---|---|---|
| 2 | 21 | 7 | 720 | na | na | 8 | 4 | * | 2 |
| 1 | 21 | 8 | 600 | na | na | * | 4 | * | 2 |
| 2 | 29 | 0 | 50 | na | na | * | 14 | * | 4 |
| 1 | 17 | 4 | 40 | na | na | * | 8 | * | 2 |
| 1 | 18 | 5 | 30 | na | na | * | 8 | * | 2 |
| 1 | 18 | 6 | 40 | na | na | * | 8 | * | 2 |
| 1 | 24 | 7 | 40 | na | na | * | 4 | * | 2 |
| 1 | 17 | 0 | 40 | 0 | na | * | 10 | * | 2 |
| 3 | 17 | 5 | 430 | 5 | 1.5 | 6 | * | 4 | 2 |
| 2 | 21 | 6 | 605 | na | na | 4 | 2 | 8 | 2 |
| 2 | 19 | 4 | 585 | na | na | 2 | * | 2 | 2 |
| 3 | 22 | 8 | 415 | na | na | 4 | * | 6 | 2 |
| 4 | 23 | 8 | 425 | na | na | 6 | 8 | 8 | 2 |
| 2 | 22 | 6 | 460 | na | na | 4 | * | * | 2 |
| 2 | 21 | 6 | 650 | na | na | 4 | * | 8 | 2 |
| 2 | 17 | 6 | 570 | na | na | 4 | * | 6 | * |
| 2 | 15 | 6 | 355 | na | na | 4 | 2 | 2 | * |
| 2 | 17 | 6 | 85 | 0 | 1 | 6 | 8 | 2 | * |
| 2 | 16 | 5 | 85 | 0 | 1 | 4 | * | 4 | * |
| 3 | 16 | 6 | 105 | 0 | 1 | 6 | * | 4 | * |
| 4 | 19 | 5 | 570 | 40 | na | 2 | * | 10 | * |
| 5 | 20 | 5 | 530 | 40 | na | 2 | * | 10 | 2 |
| 4 | 20 | 5 | 500 | 25 | na | 2 | * | 10 | * |

| FOOD NAME | Serving Size | Calories |
|---|---|---|
| Kraft Cheese Scalloped with Ham | ½ cup | 150 |
| Kraft Cheese Sour Cream with Chives | ½ cup | 150 |
| Kraft Cheese 2-Cheese | ½ cup | 130 |
| Pillsbury Au Gratin | ½ cup | 140 |
| Pillsbury Cheddar & Bacon | ½ cup | 140 |
| Pillsbury Cheesy Scalloped | ½ cup | 150 |
| Pillsbury Creamy White Sauce Scalloped | ½ cup | 150 |
| Pillsbury Sour Cream & Chives | ½ cup | 150 |
| Pillsbury Potato Pancakes | 3-3" | 90 |
| POTATO CHIPS | | |
| Bachman | 1 oz | 160 |
| Bachman Kettle Cooked | 1 oz | 140 |
| Buckeye Ketchup & French Fry Flavor | 1 oz | 160 |
| Cape Cod | 1 oz | 150 |
| Cape Cod No Salt | 1 oz | 150 |
| Eagle Extra Crunchy | 1 oz | 150 |
| Lay's | 1 oz | 150 |
| Lay's Unsalted | 1 oz | 150 |
| Pringle's | 1 oz | 170 |
| Pringle's Light | 1 oz | 150 |
| Ruffles | 1 oz | 150 |
| Ruffles Light | 1 oz | 130 |
| Wise | 1 oz | 160 |
| Wise New York Deli | 1 oz | 160 |
| Wise No Salt | 1 oz | 150 |

| Protein (g) | Carbohydrates (g) | Fat (g) | Sodium (mg) | Cholesterol (mg) | Fiber (g) | Vitamin A (%) | Vitamin C (%) | Calcium (%) | Iron (%) |
|---|---|---|---|---|---|---|---|---|---|
| 5 | 20 | 5 | 510 | 15 | na | 2 | * | 10 | * |
| 5 | 20 | 5 | 610 | 10 | na | 2 | * | 10 | * |
| 4 | 19 | 4 | 540 | 10 | na | 2 | * | 10 | * |
| 3 | 20 | 6 | 520 | 15 | 1 | 4 | 2 | 6 | 2 |
| 3 | 19 | 6 | 480 | 15 | 1 | 2 | 2 | 6 | * |
| 3 | 2 | 6 | 540 | 15 | 1 | 4 | 2 | 6 | 2 |
| 3 | 20 | 6 | 470 | 15 | 1 | 2 | 2 | 4 | 2 |
| 3 | 20 | 6 | 500 | 15 | 1 | 4 | 2 | 6 | 2 |
| 3 | 16 | 2 | 420 | 55 | 1 | * | * | 10 | 4 |
| | | | | | | | | | |
| 2 | 14 | 10 | 270 | 0 | na | * | 10 | * | 2 |
| 2 | 16 | 8 | 115 | 0 | na | * | 10 | *. | 2 |
| 2 | 14 | 11 | 230 | na | na | * | 10 | * | 2 |
| 2 | 16 | 8 | 120 | 0 | na | * | 10 | * | 2 |
| 2 | 16 | 8 | 0 | 0 | na | * | 10 | * | 2 |
| 2 | 16 | 8 | 180 | 0 | na | * | 10 | * | 2 |
| 1 | 15 | 10 | 200 | 0 | na | * | 10 | * | 2 |
| 2 | 15 | 10 | 10 | 0 | na | * | 10 | * | 2 |
| 2 | 12 | 13 | 170 | 0 | na | * | 10 | * | 2 |
| 2 | 17 | 8 | 120 | 0 | na | * | 10 | * | 2 |
| 1 | 15 | 10 | 190 | 0 | na | * | 10 | * | 2 |
| 1 | 19 | 6 | 190 | 0 | na | * | 10 | * | 2 |
| 2 | 14 | 11 | 240 | 0 | na | * | 10 | * | 2 |
| 2 | 14 | 11 | 120 | 0 | na | * | 10 | * | 2 |
| 2 | 14 | 10 | 20 | 0 | na | * | 10 | * | * |

| FOOD NAME | Serving Size | Calories |
|-----------|--------------|----------|
| **PRESERVES** | | |
| All flavors (Bama) | 2 tsp | 30 |
| All flavors (Kraft) | 2 tsp | 34 |
| All flavors (Polaner) | 2 tsp | 35 |
| All flavors (Smucker's) | 2 tsp | 36 |
| All flavors (Welch's) | 2 tsp | 35 |
| **PRETZELS** | | |
| Bachman Nutzels | 1 oz | 110 |
| Bachman Petite | 1 oz | 110 |
| Bachman Rings | 1 oz | 110 |
| Bachman Rods | 1 oz | 110 |
| Bachman Thins | 1 oz | 110 |
| Bachman Twists | 1 oz | 110 |
| Mr. Salty | 1 oz | 110 |
| Mr. Salty Dutch | 1 oz | 110 |
| Mr. Salty Little Shapes | 1 oz | 110 |
| Mr. Salty Sticks | 1 oz | 110 |
| Pepperidge Farm Snack Sticks | 1 oz | 120 |
| Rokeach Baldies | 1 oz | 110 |
| Rokeach No Salt Dutch | 1 oz | 110 |
| Rokeach Party | 1 oz | 110 |
| Quinlan Beer | 1 oz | 110 |
| Quinlan Logs | 1 oz | 103 |
| Quinlan Sticks | 1 oz | 105 |
| Quinlan Thins | 1 oz | 104 |

| Protein (g) | Carbohydrates (g) | Fat (g) | Sodium (mg) | Cholesterol (mg) | Fiber (g) | Vitamin A (%) | Vitamin C (%) | Calcium (%) | Iron (%) |
|---|---|---|---|---|---|---|---|---|---|
| 0 | 8 | 0 | 5 | 0 | na | * | * | * | * |
| 0 | 8 | 0 | 0 | 0 | na | * | * | * | * |
| 0 | 9 | 0 | na | 0 | na | * | * | * | * |
| 0 | 8 | 0 | 0 | 0 | na | * | * | * | * |
| 0 | 9 | 0 | 0 | 0 | na | * | * | * | * |
|  |  |  |  |  |  |  |  |  |  |
| 3 | 21 | 2 | 470 | 0 | na | * | * | * | na |
| 3 | 21 | 2 | 410 | 0 | na | * | * | * | na |
| 3 | 21 | 2 | 410 | 0 | na | * | * | * | * |
| 3 | 21 | 2 | 240 | 0 | na | * | * | * | na |
| 3 | 21 | 2 | 410 | 0 | na | * | * | * | na |
| 3 | 21 | 2 | 410 | 0 | na | * | * | * | na |
| 2 | 22 | 2 | 500 | 0 | na | * | * | * | 4 |
| 3 | 22 | 1 | 440 | 0 | na | * | * | * | 2 |
| 3 | 21 | 1 | 450 | 0 | na | * | * | * | 2 |
| 3 | 22 | 1 | 620 | 0 | na | * | * | * | 6 |
| 3 | 20 | 3 | 430 | 0 | na | * | * | * | * |
| 3 | 20 | 0 | 30 | 0 | na | * | * | * | * |
| 3 | 20 | 0 | 30 | 0 | na | * | * | * | * |
| 3 | 23 | 1 | na | 0 | na | * | * | * | * |
| <3 | 22 | 1 | 446 | 0 | 0.1 | * | * | * | na |
| 3 | 22 | 1 | 480 | 0 | 0.3 | * | * | * | na |
| 3 | 22 | <1 | 538 | 0 | 0.3 | * | * | * | na |
| 3 | 22 | <1 | 765 | 0 | 0.1 | * | * | * | na |

| FOOD NAME | Serving Size | Calories |
|---|---|---|
| Quinlan Ultra Thins | 1 oz | 106 |
| **PRUNES** | | |
| Canned, stewed (Rokeach) | ½ cup | 90 |
| Dried | 5 | 110 |
| **PRUNE JUICE** | | |
| Del Monte | 6 fl oz | 120 |
| Mott's Super | 6 fl oz | 120 |
| **PUDDING** | | |
| D-Zerta Butterscotch | ½ cup | 70 |
| D-Zerta Chocolate | ½ cup | 60 |
| D-Zerta Vanilla | ½ cup | 70 |
| Del Monte Banana Cup | 5 oz | 180 |
| Del Monte Butterscotch Cup | 5 oz | 180 |
| Del Monte Chocolate Cup | 5 oz | 190 |
| Del Monte Chocolate Fudge Cup | 5 oz | 220 |
| Del Monte Tapioca Cup | 5 oz | 180 |
| Del Monte Vanilla Cup | 5 oz | 180 |
| Hunt's Snack Pack Banana | 5 oz | 210 |
| Hunt's Snack Pack Butterscotch | 5 oz | 210 |
| Hunt's Snack Pack Chocolate | 5 oz | 210 |
| Hunt's Snack Pack Chocolate Fudge | 5 oz | 200 |
| Hunt's Snack Pack Chocolate Marshmallow | 5 oz | 200 |
| Hunt's Snack Pack German Chocolate | 5 oz | 220 |
| Hunt's Snack Pack Lemon | 5 oz | 180 |
| Hunt's Snack Pack Rice | 5 oz | 220 |

| Protein (g) | Carbohydrates (g) | Fat (g) | Sodium (mg) | Cholesterol (mg) | Fiber (g) | Vitamin A (%) | Vitamin C (%) | Calcium (%) | Iron (%) |
|---|---|---|---|---|---|---|---|---|---|
| 3 | 23 | <1 | 618 | 0 | 0.1 | * | * | * | na |
| 0 | 25 | 0 | <5 | 0 | 0.8 | 8 | 2 | 2 | 8 |
| 1 | 29 | 0 | 2 | 0 | na | 14 | 2 | 2 | 9 |
| 1 | 33 | 0 | <10 | 0 | na | * | 10 | * | 8 |
| 1 | 30 | 0 | 8 | 0 | na | * | 70 | 2 | 10 |
| 4 | 12 | 0 | 65 | 0 | 0 | 4 | 2 | 15 | * |
| 5 | 11 | 0 | 70 | 0 | 0 | 4 | 2 | 15 | * |
| 4 | 12 | 0 | 65 | 0 | 0 | 4 | 2 | 15 | * |
| 3 | 30 | 5 | 285 | na | 0 | * | * | 10 | * |
| 3 | 31 | 5 | 285 | na | 0 | * | * | 10 | * |
| 4 | 31 | 6 | 280 | na | 0 | * | * | 10 | 2 |
| 2 | 35 | 9 | 155 | na | 0 | * | * | 10 | * |
| 3 | 30 | 4 | 250 | na | 0 | * | * | 10 | * |
| 3 | 32 | 5 | 285 | na | 0 | * | * | 10 | * |
| 2 | 26 | 11 | 215 | na | 0 | * | * | 4 | * |
| 2 | 30 | 9 | 235 | na | 0 | * | * | 4 | * |
| 2 | 30 | 9 | 160 | na | 0 | * | * | 4 | 2 |
| 2 | 28 | 10 | 165 | na | 0 | * | * | 2 | 2 |
| 2 | 30 | 9 | 155 | na | 0 | * | * | * | 2 |
| 2 | 35 | 9 | 155 | na | 0 | * | * | * | 2 |
| 0 | 36 | 4 | 80 | na | 0 | * | * | * | * |
| 3 | 27 | 12 | 230 | na | 0 | * | * | 6 | * |

| FOOD NAME | Serving Size | Calories |
|---|---|---|
| Hunt's Snack Pack Tapioca | 5 oz | 140 |
| Hunt's Snack Pack Vanilla | 5 oz | 210 |
| Jell-O Butterscotch | ½ cup | 170 |
| Jell-O Chocolate | ½ cup | 160 |
| Jell-O Chocolate Fudge | ½ cup | 160 |
| Jell-O Flan | ½ cup | 150 |
| Jell-O French Vanilla | ½ cup | 170 |
| Jell-O Milk Chocolate | ½ cup | 160 |
| Jell-O Vanilla | ½ cup | 160 |
| Jell-O Sugar Free Chocolate | ½ cup | 90 |
| Jell-O Sugar Free Vanilla | ½ cup | 80 |
| Jell-O Instant Banana Cream | ½ cup | 160 |
| Jell-O Instant Butter Pecan | ½ cup | 170 |
| Jell-O Instant Butterscotch | ½ cup | 160 |
| Jell-O Instant Chocolate | ½ cup | 180 |
| Jell-O Instant Chocolate Fudge | ½ cup | 180 |
| Jell-O Instant Coconut Cream | ½ cup | 180 |
| Jell-O Instant French Vanilla | ½ cup | 160 |
| Jell-O Instant Lemon | ½ cup | 170 |
| Jell-O Instant Milk Chocolate | ½ cup | 180 |
| Jell-O Instant Pistachio | ½ cup | 170 |
| Jell-O Instant Vanilla | ½ cup | 170 |
| Jell-O Instant Sugar Free Banana | ½ cup | 80 |
| Jell-O Instant Sugar Free Butterscotch | ½ cup | 90 |
| Jell-O Instant Sugar Free Chocolate | ½ cup | 90 |

| Protein (g) | Carbohydrates (g) | Fat (g) | Sodium (mg) | Cholesterol (mg) | Fiber (g) | Vitamin A (%) | Vitamin C (%) | Calcium (%) | Iron (%) |
|---|---|---|---|---|---|---|---|---|---|
| 3 | 27 | 6 | 170 | na | 0 | * | * | 6 | * |
| 2 | 31 | 9 | 195 | na | 0 | * | * | 4 | * |
| 4 | 30 | 4 | 190 | 15 | 0 | 2 | * | 15 | * |
| 5 | 28 | 4 | 170 | 15 | 0 | 2 | * | 15 | * |
| 5 | 28 | 4 | 170 | 15 | 0 | 2 | * | 15 | * |
| 4 | 26 | 4 | 65 | 15 | 0 | 2 | * | 15 | * |
| 4 | 30 | 4 | 190 | 15 | 0 | 2 | * | 15 | * |
| 4 | 28 | 4 | 170 | 15 | 0 | 2 | * | 15 | * |
| 4 | 26 | 4 | 200 | 15 | 0 | 2 | * | 15 | * |
| 5 | 13 | 3 | 160 | 10 | 0 | 4 | * | 15 | 2 |
| 4 | 11 | 2 | 200 | 10 | 0 | 4 | * | 15 | * |
| 4 | 28 | 4 | 410 | 15 | 0 | 2 | * | 15 | * |
| 4 | 28 | 5 | 410 | 15 | 0 | 2 | * | 15 | * |
| 4 | 28 | 4 | 450 | 15 | 0 | 2 | * | 15 | * |
| 4 | 31 | 4 | 480 | 15 | 0 | 2 | * | 15 | 2 |
| 5 | 31 | 5 | 440 | 15 | 0 | 2 | * | 15 | * |
| 4 | 27 | 6 | 320 | 15 | 0 | 2 | * | 15 | * |
| 4 | 28 | 4 | 400 | 15 | 0 | 2 | * | 15 | * |
| 4 | 29 | 4 | 360 | 15 | 0 | 2 | * | 15 | * |
| 5 | 31 | 5 | 470 | 15 | 0 | 2 | * | 15 | 2 |
| 4 | 28 | 5 | 410 | 15 | 0 | 2 | * | 15 | * |
| 4 | 29 | 4 | 410 | 15 | 0 | 2 | * | 15 | * |
| 4 | 11 | 2 | 390 | 10 | 0 | 4 | * | 15 | * |
| 4 | 12 | 2 | 390 | 10 | 0 | 4 | * | 15 | * |
| 4 | 13 | 3 | 380 | 10 | 0 | 4 | * | 15 | 4 |

| FOOD NAME | Serving Size | Calories |
|---|---|---|
| Jell-O Instant Sugar Free Chocolate Fudge | ½ cup | 100 |
| Jell-O Instant Sugar Free Pistachio | ½ cup | 90 |
| Jell-O Instant Sugar Free Vanilla | ½ cup | 90 |
| Jell-O Microwave Banana Cream | ½ cup | 150 |
| Jell-O Microwave Butterscotch | ½ cup | 170 |
| Jell-O Microwave Chocolate | ½ cup | 170 |
| Jell-O Microwave Milk Chocolate | ½ cup | 160 |
| Jell-O Microwave Vanilla | ½ cup | 160 |
| Jell-O Butterscotch/Chocolate/Vanilla Swirl Snack | 4 oz | 180 |
| Jell-O Chocolate Snack | 4 oz | 170 |
| Jell-O Chocolate Fudge Snack | 4 oz | 170 |
| Jell-O Chocolate/Caramel Swirl Snack | 4 oz | 170 |
| Jell-O Chocolate Fudge/Milk Chocolate Swirl Snack | 4 oz | 170 |
| Jell-O Chocolate/Vanilla Swirl Snack | 4 oz | 170 |
| Jell-O Milk Chocolate Snack | 4 oz | 170 |
| Jell-O Tapioca Snack | 4 oz | 170 |
| Jell-O Vanilla/Chocolate Swirl Snack | 4 oz | 180 |
| Jell-O Vanilla Snack | 4 oz | 180 |
| Jell-O Large Chocolate Snack | 5.5 oz | 230 |
| Jell-O Large Vanilla Snack | 5.5 oz | 250 |
| Jell-O Large Chocolate/Vanilla Swirl Snack | 5.5 oz | 240 |
| Jell-O Light Chocolate Snack | 4 oz | 100 |
| Jell-O Light Chocolate Fudge Snack | 4 oz | 100 |

| Protein (g) | Carbohydrates (g) | Fat (g) | Sodium (mg) | Cholesterol (mg) | Fiber (g) | Vitamin A (%) | Vitamin C (%) | Calcium (%) | Iron (%) |
|---|---|---|---|---|---|---|---|---|---|
| 5 | 14 | 3 | 330 | 10 | 0 | 4 | * | 15 | 4 |
| 4 | 12 | 3 | 390 | 10 | 0 | 4 | * | 15 | * |
| 4 | 12 | 2 | 390 | 10 | 0 | 4 | * | 15 | * |
| 4 | 25 | 4 | 220 | 15 | 0 | 2 | * | 15 | * |
| 4 | 28 | 4 | 180 | 15 | 0 | 2 | * | 15 | * |
| 5 | 28 | 5 | 190 | 15 | 0 | 2 | * | 15 | 2 |
| 4 | 27 | 5 | 190 | 15 | 0 | 2 | * | 15 | 2 |
| 4 | 26 | 4 | 180 | 15 | 0 | 2 | * | 15 | * |
| 3 | 28 | 6 | 140 | 0 | 0 | 2 | * | 10 | * |
| 3 | 28 | 6 | 130 | 0 | 0 | 2 | * | 10 | * |
| 3 | 28 | 6 | 130 | 0 | 0 | 2 | * | 10 | * |
| 3 | 28 | 6 | 130 | 0 | 0 | 2 | * | 10 | * |
| 3 | 28 | 6 | 135 | 0 | 0 | 2 | * | 10 | * |
| 3 | 28 | 6 | 135 | 0 | 0 | 22 | * | 10 | * |
| 4 | 29 | 6 | 135 | 0 | 0 | 2 | * | 10 | * |
| 3 | 27 | 4 | 140 | 0 | 0 | 2 | * | 10 | * |
| 3 | 28 | 6 | 140 | 0 | 0 | 2 | * | 10 | * |
| 3 | 28 | 7 | 140 | 0 | 0 | 2 | * | 10 | * |
| 4 | 38 | 8 | 170 | 0 | 0 | 4 | * | 10 | 4 |
| 4 | 38 | 9 | 190 | 0 | 0 | 4 | * | 15 | * |
| 4 | 39 | 8 | 180 | 0 | 0 | 2 | 10 | 15 | 2 |
| 3 | 21 | 2 | 125 | 5 | 0 | 2 | * | 8 | 2 |
| 3 | 22 | 1 | 125 | 5 | 0 | 2 | * | 8 | 2 |

| FOOD NAME | Serving Size | Calories |
|-----------|--------------|----------|
| Jell-O Light Chocolate Vanilla Combo Snack | 4 oz | 100 |
| Jell-O Light Vanilla Snack | 4 oz | 100 |
| **PUFF PASTRY** | | |
| Apple Dumpling (Pepperidge Farm) | 3 oz | 260 |
| Apple Fruit Square (Pepperidge Farm) | 1 | 220 |
| Apple Turnover (Pepperidge Farm) | 1 | 300 |
| Blueberry Turnover (Pepperidge Farm) | 1 | 310 |
| Broccoli with Cheese Pastry (Pepperidge Farm) | 1 | 230 |
| Cherry Turnover (Pepperidge Farm) | 1 | 310 |
| Flaky Apple Turnover (Pillsbury) | 1 | 170 |
| Flaky Cherry Turnover (Pillsbury) | 1 | 170 |
| Mini Puff Pastry Shell (Pepperidge Farm) | 1 | 50 |
| Puff Pastry Shell (Pepperidge Farm) | 1 | 210 |
| Peach Turnover (Pepperidge Farm) | 1 | 310 |
| Puff Pastry Dough Sheet (Pepperidge Farm) | ¼ sheet | 260 |
| Raspberry Turnover (Pepperidge Farm) | 1 | 310 |
| **PUMPKIN** | | |
| Cooked, drained, mashed | ½ cup | 24 |
| Canned (Del Monte) | ½ cup | 35 |
| **PUMPKIN SEEDS** | 1 cup | 90 |
| **PUNCH** | | |
| Crystal Light Sugar Free Fruit | 8 fl oz | 4 |
| Hawaiian Red | 6 fl oz | 90 |
| Hawaiian Red Lite | 6 fl oz | 60 |
| Hawaiian Tropical | 6 fl oz | 90 |

| Protein (g) | Carbohydrates (g) | Fat (g) | Sodium (mg) | Cholesterol (mg) | Fiber (g) | Vitamin A (%) | Vitamin C (%) | Calcium (%) | Iron (%) |
|---|---|---|---|---|---|---|---|---|---|
| 3 | 21 | 2 | 125 | 5 | 0 | 4 | * | 8 | * |
| 3 | 20 | 2 | 130 | 5 | 0 | 4 | * | 10 | * |
| | | | | | | | | | |
| 2 | 33 | 13 | 230 | na | na | * | 2 | * | 4 |
| 2 | 27 | 12 | 170 | na | na | * | 2 | * | 4 |
| 3 | 34 | 17 | 210 | na | na | * | 4 | * | 4 |
| 3 | 32 | 19 | 230 | na | na | * | 10 | * | 4 |
| 5 | 18 | 16 | 380 | na | na | 8 | 20 | 6 | 8 |
| 3 | 32 | 19 | 280 | na | na | * | * | * | 4 |
| 2 | 23 | 8 | 330 | 0 | na | * | * | * | 4 |
| 2 | 23 | 8 | 330 | 0 | na | * | 6 | * | 4 |
| 1 | 4 | 4 | 40 | na | na | * | * | * | * |
| 3 | 16 | 15 | 180 | na | na | * | * | * | 2 |
| 3 | 34 | 18 | 260 | na | na | 6 | 60 | * | 2 |
| 4 | 22 | 17 | 290 | na | na | * | * | * | 4 |
| 4 | 36 | 17 | 260 | na | na | * | 20 | * | 4 |
| | | | | | | | | | |
| 1 | 6 | Tr | 2 | 0 | 4 | 600 | 8 | 2 | 4 |
| 0 | 9 | 0 | <10 | 0 | 4 | 600 | 8 | 2 | 4 |
| 0 | 22 | 0 | 10 | 0 | na | * | 50 | * | * |
| | | | | | | | | | |
| 0 | 0 | 0 | 0 | 0 | 0 | * | 10 | * | * |
| 0 | 22 | 0 | 20 | 0 | 0 | na | na | na | na |
| 0 | 15 | 0 | 30 | 0 | na | na | na | na | na |
| 0 | 22 | 0 | 30 | 0 | na | na | na | na | na |

| FOOD NAME | Serving Size | Calories |
|---|---|---|
| Hi-C | 6 fl oz | 96 |
| Kool-Aid Tropical | 8 fl oz | 80 |
| Kool-Aid Sugar Free Mountain Berry | 8 fl oz | 4 |
| Kool-Aid Sugar Free Surfin' Berry | 8 fl oz | 4 |
| Kool-Aid Sugar Free Tropical | 8 fl oz | 4 |
| Kool-Aid Koolers Mountain Berry | 8.5 fl oz | 140 |
| Kool-Aid Koolers Rainbow | 8.5 fl oz | 130 |
| Kool-Aid Koolers Tropical | 8.5 fl oz | 130 |
| Mott's | 9.5 fl oz | 160 |
| Wyler's Tropical | 8 fl oz | 90 |
| Wyler's Tropical Sugar Free | 8 fl oz | 4 |
| QUAIL | 1 | 125 |
| RADISHES | 10 med | 10 |
| RAISINS | 1 cup | 420 |
| Del Monte Golden | 3 oz | 260 |
| Del Monte Natural | 3 oz | 250 |
| Dole | ½ cup | 260 |
| Sun-Maid | ½ cup | 290 |
| RASPBERRIES | | |
| Black | 1 cup | 100 |
| Red | 1 cup | 70 |
| Red frozen (Birds Eye) | 5 oz | 100 |
| RASPBERRY DRINK | | |
| Dole | 6 fl oz | 87 |
| Kool-Aid | 8 fl oz | 80 |

| Protein (g) | Carbohydrates (g) | Fat (g) | Sodium (mg) | Cholesterol (mg) | Fiber (g) | Vitamin A (%) | Vitamin C (%) | Calcium (%) | Iron (%) |
|---|---|---|---|---|---|---|---|---|---|
| Tr | 24 | Tr | 17 | 0 | na | * | 100 | * | * |
| 0 | 21 | 0 | 0 | 0 | na | * | 10 | * | * |
| 0 | 0 | 0 | 35 | 0 | na | * | 10 | * | * |
| 0 | 0 | 0 | 25 | 0 | na | * | 10 | * | * |
| 0 | 0 | 0 | 10 | 0 | na | * | 10 | * | * |
| 0 | 37 | 0 | 10 | 0 | na | * | 10 | * | * |
| 0 | 36 | 0 | 10 | 0 | na | * | 10 | * | * |
| 0 | 35 | 0 | 10 | 0 | na | * | 10 | * | * |
| 0 | 40 | 0 | 4 | 0 | na | na | na | na | na |
| 0 | 22 | 0 | na | na | na | * | 15 | * | * |
| 0 | 1 | 0 | 30 | na | na | * | 15 | * | * |
| 20 | 0 | 4 | 47 | na | 0 | na | na | na | na |
| 0 | 2 | Tr | <10 | 0 | 0.2 | * | 20 | 2 | 2 |
| 4 | 112 | 0 | 2 | 0 | 2 | 14 | 2 | 2 | 9 |
| <3 | 58 | 0 | 9 | 0 | 4 | 4 | * | 4 | 8 |
| 3 | 68 | 0 | 15 | 0 | 4 | * | * | 4 | 10 |
| 3 | 63 | 0 | 25 | 0 | 4 | na | na | na | na |
| 3 | 69 | 0 | <15 | 0 | 4 | na | na | na | na |
| | | | | | | | | | |
| 1 | 21 | 2 | 1 | 0 | na | * | 40 | 4 | 6 |
| 1 | 17 | <1 | 1 | 0 | 5.8 | 4 | 50 | 2 | 6 |
| 0 | 26 | 0 | 0 | na | na | * | 10 | * | * |
| | | | | | | | | | |
| Tr | 24 | Tr | 15 | 0 | na | na | na | na | na |
| 0 | 20 | 0 | 25 | 0 | na | * | 10 | * | * |

| FOOD NAME | Serving Size | Calories |
|---|---|---|
| Kool-Aid Unsweetened | 8 fl oz | 2 |
| RASPBERRY JUICE | | |
| Smucker's | 8 fl oz | 120 |
| Welch's | 10 fl oz | 160 |
| RAVIOLI | | |
| Beef (Franco-American) | 7.5 oz | 280 |
| Beef (Franco-American | | |
| Ravioli0's) | 7.5 oz | 250 |
| Beef (Hormel Micro-Cup) | 7.5 oz | 247 |
| Cheese (Buitoni) | 7.5 oz | 190 |
| Cheese (Chef Boyardee) | 7.5 oz | 200 |
| Chicken (Chef Boyardee) | 7.5 oz | 180 |
| In Meat Sauce (Buitoni) | 7.5 oz | 180 |
| RED BEANS | | |
| *Canned* | | |
| B&M, baked-style | 4 oz | 112 |
| Green Giant | ½ cup | 90 |
| Hunt's | 4 oz | 91 |
| RED SNAPPER Broiled | 4 oz | 145 |
| REFRIED BEANS | | |
| Del Monte | ½ cup | 130 |
| Del Monte Spicy | ½ cup | 130 |
| Gebhardt | 4 oz | 130 |
| Little Pancho | ½ cup | 80 |
| Old El Paso | ¼ cup | 50 |

| Protein (g) | Carbohydrates (g) | Fat (g) | Sodium (mg) | Cholesterol (mg) | Fiber (g) | Vitamin A (%) | Vitamin C (%) | Calcium (%) | Iron (%) |
|---|---|---|---|---|---|---|---|---|---|
| 0 | 0 | 0 | 25 | 0 | na | * | 10 | * | * |
| | | | | | | | | | |
| 0 | 30 | 0 | 10 | 0 | na | na | na | na | na |
| 0 | 40 | 0 | 10 | 0 | 0 | na | na | na | na |
| | | | | | | | | | |
| 9 | 35 | 11 | 810 | na | na | 30 | 4 | 2 | 10 |
| | | | | | | | | | |
| 9 | 35 | 8 | 920 | na | na | 30 | 2 | 2 | 10 |
| 8 | 28 | 11 | 951 | 21 | na | na | na | na | na |
| 7 | 27 | 6 | 790 | 5 | na | na | na | na | na |
| 7 | 34 | 3 | 1205 | na | na | na | na | na | na |
| 7 | 29 | 4 | 1100 | na | na | na | na | na | na |
| 7 | 28 | 4 | 890 | 5 | na | na | na | na | na |
| | | | | | | | | | |
| 5 | 18 | 2 | 362 | 0 | 5.5 | * | * | 4 | 8 |
| 6 | 19 | 1 | 340 | 0 | 5 | * | * | 4 | 8 |
| 6 | 18 | 0 | 578 | 0 | na | * | * | 4 | 8 |
| 3 | 0 | 2 | 65 | 53 | 0 | na | na | na | na |
| | | | | | | | | | |
| 6 | 20 | 2 | 530 | na | na | * | 10 | 4 | 10 |
| 6 | 20 | 2 | 480 | na | na | * | 10 | 4 | 10 |
| 7 | 20 | 2 | 490 | na | na | na | na | na | na |
| 6 | 15 | 0 | 330 | na | na | na | na | na | na |
| 5 | 8 | 1 | 200 | 0 | 2.5 | * | * | 3 | 7 |

| FOOD NAME | Serving Size | Calories |
|---|---|---|
| Old El Paso with Green Chilies | ¼ cup | 50 |
| Old El Paso with Sausage | ¼ cup | 180 |
| RELISH | | |
| Claussen Pickle | 1 oz | 26 |
| Heinz Hamburger | 1 oz | 30 |
| Heinz Hot Dog | 1 oz | 35 |
| Heinz India | 1 oz | 35 |
| Heinz Piccallili | 1 oz | 30 |
| Heinz Sweet | 1 oz | 35 |
| Vlasic Dill | 1 oz | 2 |
| Vlasic Hamburger | 1 oz | 40 |
| Vlasic Hot Dog | 1 oz | 40 |
| Vlasic Hot Piccalilli | 1 oz | 35 |
| Vlasic India | 1 oz | 30 |
| Vlasic Sweet | 1 oz | 30 |
| RHUBARB  Cooked, sweetened | ½ cup | 140 |
| RICE  Cooked | | |
| Basmati (Texmati) | ½ cup | 110 |
| Brown, long grain (Carolina) | ½ cup | 110 |
| Brown, long grain (River) | ½ cup | 110 |
| Brown, long grain (Uncle Ben's) | ½ cup | 97 |
| Brown, medium grain | ½ cup | 110 |
| White, long grain (Carolina) | ½ cup | 100 |
| White, long grain (Minute) | ⅔ cup | 120 |
| White, long grain (Minute Boil-in-Bag) | ½ cup | 90 |

| Protein (g) | Carbohydrates (g) | Fat (g) | Sodium (mg) | Cholesterol (mg) | Fiber (g) | Vitamin A (%) | Vitamin C (%) | Calcium (%) | Iron (%) |
|---|---|---|---|---|---|---|---|---|---|
| 5 | 16 | 1 | 400 | na | 2.5 | * | * | * | 7 |
| 6 | 8 | 8 | 300 | na | na | * | * | * | 8 |
|  |  |  |  |  |  |  |  |  |  |
| Tr | 6 | Tr | 170 | 0 | na | na | na | na | na |
| 0 | 7 | 0 | 325 | 0 | na | na | na | * | * |
| 0 | 8 | 0 | 200 | 0 | na | na | na | * | * |
| 0 | 9 | 0 | 215 | 0 | na | na | na | * | * |
| 0 | 7 | 0 | 145 | 0 | na | na | na | na | na |
| 0 | 9 | 0 | 205 | 0 | na | na | na | * | * |
| 0 | 1 | 0 | 415 | na | na | * | * | * | * |
| 0 | 9 | 0 | 255 | na | na | 2 | * | * | * |
| 0 | 8 | 1 | 255 | na | na | * | 2 | * | 2 |
| 0 | 8 | 0 | 165 | na | na | 2 | * | * | * |
| 0 | 8 | 0 | 205 | na | na | * | * | * | * |
| 0 | 8 | 0 | 220 | na | na | * | * | * | * |
| <1 | 37 | Tr | 2 | 0 | 1 | 2 | 13 | 10 | 4 |
|  |  |  |  |  |  |  |  |  |  |
| 3 | 31 | 0 | 0 | 0 | na | na | na | na | na |
| 2 | 23 | 0 | 0 | 0 | 1.7 | * | * | 1 | 3 |
| 2 | 23 | 0 | na | 0 | 1.7 | * | * | 1 | 3 |
| 3 | 21 | 0 | 0 | 0 | 1.7 | * | * | 1 | 3 |
| 2 | 23 | <1 | 1 | 0 | 1.5 | na | na | na | na |
| 2 | 22 | 0 | <10 | 0 | 0.5 | * | * | * | 5 |
| 3 | 27 | 0 | 0 | 0 | 0.5 | * | * | 6 | * |
| 2 | 20 | 0 | 0 | 0 | 0.5 | * | * | 4 | * |

| FOOD NAME | Serving Size | Calories |
|---|---|---|
| White, long grain (Minute Premium) | ⅔ cup | 120 |
| White, long grain (River) | ½ cup | 100 |
| White, long grain (Uncle Ben's) | ⅔ cup | 130 |
| White, medium grain | ½ cup | 135 |
| Wild | 1 cup | 166 |
| **RICE DISH** | | |
| Birds Eye for One, with Broccoli Au Gratin | 5.75 oz | 180 |
| Birds Eye Country Style | 3.3 oz | 90 |
| Birds Eye French Style | 3.3 oz | 110 |
| Birds Eye Spanish Style | 3.3 oz | 110 |
| Birds Eye Vegetables with Wild Rice | 4.6 oz | 100 |
| Green Giant Asparagus Pilaf | 1 pkg | 190 |
| Green Giant Pilaf | ½ cup | 110 |
| Green Giant with Broccoli | ½ cup | 120 |
| Green Giant Florentine | ½ cup | 140 |
| Green Giant Medley | ½ cup | 100 |
| Green Giant White 'n Wild | ½ cup | 130 |
| La Choy Chicken Fried | ½ cup | 209 |
| Lipton Beef Flavor | ½ cup | 150 |
| Lipton Chicken Flavor | ½ cup | 150 |
| Lipton Herb and Butter | ½ cup | 140 |
| Lipton Spanish | ½ cup | 140 |

| Protein (g) | Carbohydrates (g) | Fat (g) | Sodium (mg) | Cholesterol (mg) | Fiber (g) | Vitamin A (%) | Vitamin C (%) | Calcium (%) | Iron (%) |
|---|---|---|---|---|---|---|---|---|---|
| 3 | 27 | 0 | 0 | 0 | 0.5 | * | * | 6 | * |
| 2 | 22 | 0 | <10 | 0 | 0.5 | * | * | * | 5 |
| 3 | 28 | 1 | 0 | 0 | 0.5 | na | na | na | na |
| <3 | 30 | Tr | <1 | 0 | 0.5 | na | na | na | na |
| 7 | 35 | <1 | 6 | 0 | 2.4 | na | na | na | na |
|  |  |  |  |  |  |  |  |  |  |
| 6 | 27 | 6 | 430 | 5 | 1 | 45 | 25 | 10 | 2 |
| 2 | 19 | 0 | 380 | 0 | 1 | 6 | 10 | * | 2 |
| 3 | 23 | 0 | 610 | 0 | na | * | 2 | * | 6 |
| 3 | 24 | 0 | 540 | 0 | na | 8 | 45 | * | 4 |
|  |  |  |  |  |  |  |  |  |  |
| 3 | 19 | 0 | 510 | 0 | 1 | 110 | 20 | 2 | 4 |
| 5 | 37 | 4 | 610 | 10 | 3 | 60 | 20 | 4 | 25 |
| 2 | 21 | 1 | 530 | 2 | na | * | * | * | 4 |
| 3 | 18 | 4 | 510 | 5 | na | 20 | 10 | 4 | 8 |
| 4 | 22 | 4 | 400 | 10 | na | 10 | * | 8 | 4 |
| 3 | 19 | 1 | 310 | 5 | na | * | * | * | 4 |
| 3 | 24 | 2 | 540 | 0 | na | * | * | * | 4 |
| 7 | 40 | 2 | 1153 | na | na | na | na | na | na |
| 3 | 26 | 3 | 600 | na | na | 2 | * | * | 4 |
| 3 | 25 | 4 | 470 | na | na | 2 | * | * | 4 |
| 3 | 22 | 4 | 800 | na | na | 2 | * | * | 4 |
| 3 | 26 | 3 | 570 | na | na | 6 | 2 | * | 4 |

| FOOD NAME | Serving Size | Calories |
|---|---|---|
| Minute Drumstick | ½ cup | 120 |
| Minute Fried Rice | ½ cup | 120 |
| Minute Long Grain & Wild | ½ cup | 120 |
| Minute Rib Roast | ½ cup | 120 |
| Minute Microwave Beef Flavored | ½ cup | 140 |
| Minute Microwave Cheese and Broccoli | ½ cup | 140 |
| Minute Microwave Chicken Flavored | ½ cup | 130 |
| Minute Microwave French Style Pilaf | ½ cup | 110 |
| Rice-a-Roni Beef Flavor | ½ cup | 170 |
| Rice-a-Roni Chicken Flavor | ½ cup | 170 |
| Rice-a-Roni Green Bean Almondine | ½ cup | 210 |
| Rice-a-Roni Spanish | ½ cup | 150 |
| Rice-a-Roni Stroganoff | ½ cup | 190 |
| Rice-a-Roni Vegetables and Cheese | ½ cup | 170 |
| Uncle Ben's Long Grain & Wild | ½ cup | 120 |
| RICE CAKE | | |
| Hain Plain | 1 | 40 |
| Hain Plain Mini | ½ oz | 50 |
| Hain Apple Cinnamon Mini | ½ oz | 50 |
| Hain Barbecue Mini | ½ oz | 70 |
| Hain Cheese Mini | ½ oz | 60 |
| Hain Sesame | 1 | 40 |

| Protein (g) | Carbohydrates (g) | Fat (g) | Sodium (mg) | Cholesterol (mg) | Fiber (g) | Vitamin A (%) | Vitamin C (%) | Calcium (%) | Iron (%) |
|---|---|---|---|---|---|---|---|---|---|
| 3 | 25 | 0 | 650 | 0 | na | * | * | 6 | * |
| 3 | 25 | 0 | 550 | 0 | na | * | * | 6 | * |
| 3 | 25 | 0 | 530 | 0 | na | * | * | 10 | 6 |
| 3 | 25 | 0 | 680 | 0 | na | * | * | 6 | * |
| 4 | 28 | 0 | 530 | 0 | na | 8 | * | 6 | * |
| 4 | 26 | 2 | 500 | 5 | na | 2 | 4 | 4 | 6 |
| 3 | 27 | 1 | 640 | 0 | na | 10 | * | 6 | * |
| 2 | 24 | 0 | 390 | 0 | na | * | * | * | 4 |
| 4 | 27 | 5 | 930 | na | na | * | * | * | 6 |
| 4 | 28 | 5 | 780 | na | na | * | * | * | 8 |
| 5 | 22 | 11 | 490 | na | na | na | na | na | na |
| 4 | 25 | 4 | 1090 | na | na | * | * | na | 4 |
| 4 | 27 | 8 | 830 | na | na | na | na | na | na |
| 4 | 23 | 7 | 420 | na | na | na | na | na | na |
| 3 | 22 | 2 | 520 | na | na | 1 | * | 3 | 6 |
| <1 | 8 | <1 | 10 | 0 | 0 | * | * | * | * |
| 1 | 12 | <1 | 75 | 0 | 0 | * | * | * | * |
| 1 | 12 | <1 | 5 | 0 | 0 | na | na | na | na |
| 1 | 10 | 3 | 70 | 0 | 0 | na | na | na | na |
| 1 | 10 | 2 | 80 | 0 | 0 | na | na | na | na |
| <1 | 8 | <1 | 10 | 0 | na | na | na | na | na |

| FOOD NAME | Serving Size | Calories | |
|---|---|---|---|
| Hain Teriyaki Mini | ½ oz | 50 | |
| Pritikin Multigrain | 1 | 35 | |
| Quaker | 1 | 35 | |
| Quaker Corn | 1 | 35 | |
| Quaker Multigrain | 1 | 34 | |
| Quaker Rye | 1 | 34 | |
| Quaker Sesame | 1 | 35 | |
| ROCKFISH Broiled | 4 oz | 140 | |
| ROLLS | | | |
| *Brown & Serve* | | | |
| Pepperidge Farm Club Enriched | 1 | 100 | |
| Pepperidge Farm French Enriched | ½ roll | 120 | |
| Pepperidge Farm Hearth Enriched | 1 | 50 | |
| Sweetheart | 1 | 90 | |
| Weber's | 1 | 90 | |
| Arnold Party | 2 | 110 | |
| *Dinner* | | | |
| Awrey | 1 | 60 | |
| Home Pride | 2 | 170 | |
| Pepperidge Farm Country | | | |
| Style Classic | 1 | 50 | |
| Pepperidge Farm Finger Poppy | | | |
| Seed Enriched | 1 | 50 | |
| Pepperidge Farm Hearty | | | |
| Potato Classic | 1 | 90 | |

| Protein (g) | Carbohydrates (g) | Fat (g) | Sodium (mg) | Cholesterol (mg) | Fiber (g) | Vitamin A (%) | Vitamin C (%) | Calcium (%) | Iron (%) |
|---|---|---|---|---|---|---|---|---|---|
| 1 | 11 | <1 | 80 | 0 | 0 | na | na | na | na |
| 1 | 7 | 0 | 0 | 0 | <1 | * | * | * | * |
| <1 | 7 | Tr | 36 | 0 | 0.3 | * | * | * | * |
| <1 | 7 | Tr | 31 | 0 | 0.3 | na | na | na | na |
| 1 | 7 | Tr | 29 | 0 | 0.4 | na | na | na | na |
| 1 | 7 | Tr | 12 | 0 | 0.4 | na | na | na | na |
| 1 | 7 | Tr | 36 | 0 | 0.3 | na | na | na | na |
| 27 | 0 | 2 | 87 | 50 | 0 | 13 | 3 | 3 | 5 |
| | | | | | | | | | |
| 3 | 19 | 1 | 190 | 0 | 0.5 | * | * | 4 | 6 |
| 4 | 24 | 1 | 250 | 0 | 0.5 | * | * | 4 | 8 |
| 2 | 10 | 1 | 100 | 0 | Tr | * | * | 2 | 4 |
| 1 | 11 | 3 | 185 | na | na | * | * | 4 | 4 |
| 1 | 11 | 3 | 185 | na | na | * | * | 4 | 4 |
| 3 | 20 | 3 | 280 | na | 1 | * | * | * | 6 |
| | | | | | | | | | |
| 2 | 11 | 1 | 115 | 0 | 0 | na | na | na | na |
| 3 | 28 | 4 | 340 | na | na | * | * | 8 | 8 |
| | | | | | | | | | |
| 2 | 9 | 1 | 90 | 0 | 0 | * | * | * | 4 |
| | | | | | | | | | |
| 2 | 8 | 2 | 80 | <5 | Tr | * | * | 2 | 2 |
| | | | | | | | | | |
| 2 | 14 | 3 | 125 | 0 | 1 | * | * | * | 2 |

| FOOD NAME | Serving Size | Calories |
|---|---|---|
| Pepperidge Farm Old Fashioned Enriched | 1 | 50 |
| Pepperidge Farm Parker | | |
| House Enriched | 1 | 60 |
| Pepperidge Farm Party Enriched | 1 | 30 |
| Pepperidge Farm Soft | | |
| Family Enriched | 1 | 100 |
| Pillsbury Butter Flavored Butterflake | 1 | 140 |
| Pillsbury Crescent | 1 | 100 |
| Pillsbury Cornbread Twists | 1 | 70 |
| Pillsbury Soft Bread Sticks | 1 | 100 |
| Wonder | 2 | 200 |
| *Fancy* | | |
| Pepperidge Farm Butter | | |
| Crescent Enriched | 1 | 110 |
| Pepperidge Farm Golden | | |
| Twist Enriched | 1 | 110 |
| Pepperidge Farm French Style | 1 | 100 |
| Pepperidge Farm Sourdough | | |
| French Style | 1 | 100 |
| *Kaiser* | | |
| Wonder | 1 | 460 |
| *Pan* | | |
| Wonder | 2 | 200 |
| *Sandwich* | | |
| Butternut Hamburger | 1 | 80 |

| Protein (g) | Carbohydrates (g) | Fat (g) | Sodium (mg) | Cholesterol (mg) | Fiber (g) | Vitamin A (%) | Vitamin C (%) | Calcium (%) | Iron (%) |
|---|---|---|---|---|---|---|---|---|---|
| 2 | 7 | 3 | 85 | 5 | Tr | * | * | 2 | 2 |
| | | | | | | | | | |
| 2 | 9 | 1 | 80 | 5 | Tr | * | * | 2 | 2 |
| 1 | 5 | 1 | 50 | 0 | Tr | * | * | * | 2 |
| | | | | | | | | | |
| 4 | 18 | 2 | 190 | 0 | 0.5 | * | * | 4 | 6 |
| 3 | 20 | 0 | 530 | 0 | na | * | * | * | 6 |
| 2 | 11 | 6 | 230 | 0 | na | * | * | * | 2 |
| 1 | 8 | 3 | 150 | 0 | na | * | * | * | 2 |
| 3 | 17 | 2 | 230 | 0 | na | * | * | * | 6 |
| 3 | 34 | 4 | 375 | na | na | * | * | 10 | 10 |
| | | | | | | | | | |
| | | | | | | | | | |
| 2 | 13 | 6 | 150 | 15 | Tr | 2 | * | 2 | 4 |
| | | | | | | | | | |
| 2 | 14 | 5 | 150 | 5 | Tr | * | * | 2 | 4 |
| 4 | 20 | 1 | 230 | 0 | 0.5 | * | * | 4 | 6 |
| | | | | | | | | | |
| 4 | 19 | 1 | 240 | 0 | 0.5 | * | * | 2 | 6 |
| | | | | | | | | | |
| na | 82 | 8 | 870 | na | na | * | * | 25 | 25 |
| | | | | | | | | | |
| 3 | 34 | 4 | 375 | na | na | * | * | 10 | 10 |
| | | | | | | | | | |
| 2 | 14 | 1 | 170 | na | na | * | * | 4 | 4 |

| FOOD NAME | Serving Size | Calories |
|---|---|---|
| Butternut Hot Dog | 1 | 80 |
| Eddy's Hamburger | 1 | 80 |
| Eddy's Hot Dog | 1 | 80 |
| Millbrook Hamburger | 1 | 80 |
| Millbrook Hot Dog | 1 | 80 |
| Pepperidge Farm Dijon Frankfurter | 1 | 160 |
| Pepperidge Farm Frankfurter | 1 | 140 |
| Pepperidge Farm Onion with Poppy Seeds | 1 | 150 |
| Pepperidge Farm Potato Buns | 1 | 160 |
| Pepperidge Farm Salad | 1 | 110 |
| Pepperidge Farm with Sesame Seeds | 1 | 140 |
| Pepperidge Farm Sliced Hamburger | 1 | 130 |
| Pepperidge Farm Soft Hoagie | 1 | 210 |
| Sweetheart Hamburger | 1 | 80 |
| Sweetheart Hot Dog | 1 | 80 |
| Weber's Hamburger | 1 | 80 |
| Weber's Hot Dog | 1 | 80 |
| Wonder Hamburger | 1 | 120 |
| Wonder Hot Dog | 1 | 120 |
| *Sweet* | | |
| Dolly Madison Cherry | 1 | 180 |
| Dolly Madison Cinnamon | 1 | 180 |
| Hostess Butterhorn | 1 | 330 |
| Hostess Honey Buns | 1 | 450 |
| Hostess Raspberry | 1 | 300 |

| Protein (g) | Carbohydrates (g) | Fat (g) | Sodium (mg) | Cholesterol (mg) | Fiber (g) | Vitamin A (%) | Vitamin C (%) | Calcium (%) | Iron (%) |
|---|---|---|---|---|---|---|---|---|---|
| 2 | 14 | 1 | 170 | na | na | * | * | 4 | 4 |
| 2 | 14 | 1 | 170 | na | na | * | * | 4 | 4 |
| 2 | 14 | 1 | 170 | na | na | * | * | 4 | 4 |
| 2 | 14 | 1 | 170 | na | na | * | * | 4 | 4 |
| 2 | 14 | 1 | 170 | na | na | * | * | 4 | 4 |
| 5 | 23 | 5 | 230 | 0 | 2 | * | * | 6 | 10 |
| 5 | 24 | 3 | 270 | 0 | 0.5 | * | * | 6 | 8 |
| 5 | 26 | 3 | 260 | 0 | 0.5 | * | * | 4 | 8 |
| 4 | 28 | 4 | 260 | 0 | 1 | * | * | * | 6 |
| 4 | 16 | 4 | 150 | 10 | na | * | * | 4 | 8 |
| 5 | 23 | 3 | 230 | 0 | 0.5 | * | * | 4 | 8 |
| 5 | 22 | 2 | 240 | 0 | 0.5 | * | * | 4 | 8 |
| 8 | 34 | 5 | 320 | 0 | 1 | * | 2 | 6 | 8 |
| 2 | 114 | 1 | 170 | na | na | * | * | 4 | 4 |
| 2 | 14 | 1 | 170 | na | na | * | * | 4 | 4 |
| 2 | 14 | 1 | 170 | na | na | * | * | 4 | 4 |
| 2 | 14 | 1 | 170 | na | na | * | * | 4 | 4 |
| 3 | 22 | 3 | 230 | na | na | * | * | 4 | 4 |
| 3 | 22 | 3 | 230 | na | na | * | * | 6 | 6 |
| 2 | 33 | 4 | 165 | na | na | * | * | 2 | 6 |
| 2 | 28 | 6 | 220 | na | na | * | * | 2 | 6 |
| 3 | 39 | 18 | 520 | na | na | * | * | 2 | 8 |
| 3 | 49 | 27 | 650 | na | na | * | * | 2 | 8 |
| 3 | 48 | 10 | 360 | na | na | * | * | 16 | 10 |

| FOOD NAME | Serving Size | Calories |
|---|---|---|
| Hungry Jack Cinnamon | 1 | 290 |
| Pepperidge Farm Cinnamon | 1 | 280 |
| Pillsbury Caramel with Nuts | 1 | 160 |
| Pillsbury Cinnamon Raisin | 1 | 150 |
| Pillsbury Cinnamon with Icing | 1 | 110 |
| Pillsbury Orange with Icing | 1 | 150 |
| RUTABAGA Fresh, cooked | 1 cup | 60 |
| SALAD DRESSING | | |
| Bacon & Tomato (Kraft) | 1 tbsp | 70 |
| Blue Cheese (Roka) | 1 tbsp | 60 |
| Blue Cheese (Wish-Bone) | 1 tbsp | 70 |
| Buttermilk (Seven Seas) | 1 tbsp | 80 |
| Buttermilk (Wish-Bone) | 1 tbsp | 50 |
| Buttermilk Creamy (Kraft) | 1 tbsp | 80 |
| Buttermilk & Onion (Hidden Valley Ranch) | 1 tbsp | 70 |
| Caesar (Wish-Bone) | 1 tbsp | 70 |
| Cheddar and Bacon (Wish-Bone) | 1 tbsp | 70 |
| Choice Creamy (Rancher's) | 1 tbsp | 90 |
| Chunky Blue Cheese (Kraft) | 1 tbsp | 60 |
| Coleslaw (Kraft) | 1 tbsp | 70 |
| Creamy Cucumber (Kraft) | 1 tbsp | 70 |
| Creamy Cucumber (Wish-Bone) | 1 tbsp | 80 |
| Creamy French (Seven Seas) | 1 tbsp | 60 |
| Creamy Garlic (Kraft) | 1 tbsp | 50 |
| Creamy Italian (Kraft) | 1 tbsp | 50 |

| Protein (g) | Carbohydrates (g) | Fat (g) | Sodium (mg) | Cholesterol (mg) | Fiber (g) | Vitamin A (%) | Vitamin C (%) | Calcium (%) | Iron (%) |
|---|---|---|---|---|---|---|---|---|---|
| 2 | 37 | 14 | 570 | na | na | * | * | * | 4 |
| 4 | 34 | 14 | 190 | na | na | * | * | 2 | 6 |
| 2 | 19 | 8 | 240 | 0 | na | * | * | * | 4 |
| 2 | 20 | 7 | 230 | 0 | na | * | * | * | 2 |
| 1 | 17 | 5 | 260 | 0 | na | * | * | * | 2 |
| 2 | 19 | 7 | 250 | 0 | na | * | * | * | 4 |
| <2 | 14 | Tr | 7 | 0 | 5.5 | 20 | 70 | 10 | 2 |
| | | | | | | | | | |
| 0 | 1 | 7 | 130 | 0 | 0 | * | * | * | * |
| 1 | 1 | 6 | 170 | 10 | 0 | * | * | 2 | * |
| 1 | <1 | 8 | 150 | na | 0 | * | * | * | * |
| 0 | 1 | 8 | 130 | 5 | 0 | * | * | * | * |
| 0 | 2 | 5 | 150 | na | 0 | * | * | * | * |
| 0 | 1 | 8 | 120 | <5 | 0 | * | * | * | * |
| 0 | 2 | 7 | 127 | na | 0 | * | * | * | * |
| 0 | <1 | 8 | 250 | na | 0 | * | * | * | * |
| 0 | 1 | 7 | 110 | na | 0 | * | * | * | * |
| 0 | 1 | 10 | 140 | 5 | 0 | * | * | * | * |
| 1 | 2 | 6 | 230 | <5 | 0 | * | * | * | * |
| 0 | 4 | 6 | 200 | 10 | 0 | * | * | * | * |
| 0 | 1 | 8 | 190 | 0 | 0 | * | * | * | * |
| 0 | 1 | 8 | 125 | na | 0 | * | * | * | * |
| 0 | 2 | 6 | 240 | 0 | 0 | * | * | * | * |
| 0 | 1 | 5 | 170 | 0 | 0 | * | * | * | * |
| 0 | 1 | 5 | 120 | 0 | 0 | * | * | * | * |

| FOOD NAME | Serving Size | Calories |
|---|---|---|
| Creamy Italian (Seven Seas) | 1 tbsp | 70 |
| Creamy Russian (Kraft) | 1 tbsp | 60 |
| French (Kraft) | 1 tbsp | 60 |
| French Deluxe (Wish-Bone) | 1 tbsp | 50 |
| French Garlic (Wish-Bone) | 1 tbsp | 60 |
| French Herbal (Wish-Bone) | 1 tbsp | 60 |
| French Sweet 'n Spicy (Wish-Bone) | 1 tbsp | 70 |
| Garden Herb (Hidden Valley Ranch) | 1 tbsp | 70 |
| Garlic (Wish-Bone) | 1 tbsp | 80 |
| Golden Caesar (Kraft) | 1 tbsp | 70 |
| House Italian (Kraft) | 1 tbsp | 60 |
| Italian (Wish-Bone) | 1 tbsp | 70 |
| Italian Robusto (Wish-Bone) | 1 tbsp | 80 |
| Italian, Creamy (Wish-Bone) | 1 tbsp | 60 |
| Italian, Herbal (Wish-Bone) | 1 tbsp | 70 |
| Miracle French (Kraft) | 1 tbsp | 70 |
| Oil & Vinegar (Kraft) | 1 tbsp | 70 |
| Original (Hidden Valley Ranch) | 1 tbsp | 70 |
| Presto Italian (Kraft) | 1 tbsp | 70 |
| Red Wine Vinegar & Oil (Kraft) | 1 tbsp | 60 |
| Russian (Kraft) | 1 tbsp | 60 |
| Russian (Wish-Bone) | 1 tbsp | 45 |
| Sour Cream and Bacon (Wish-Bone) | 1 tbsp | 70 |
| Thousand Island (Kraft) | 1 tbsp | 60 |
| Thousand Island (Seven Seas) | 1 tbsp | 50 |

| Protein (g) | Carbohydrates (g) | Fat (g) | Sodium (mg) | Cholesterol (mg) | Fiber (g) | Vitamin A (%) | Vitamin C (%) | Calcium (%) | Iron (%) |
|---|---|---|---|---|---|---|---|---|---|
| 0 | 1 | 7 | 240 | 0 | 0 | * | * | * | * |
| 0 | 2 | 5 | 150 | 5 | 0 | * | * | * | * |
| 0 | 2 | 6 | 125 | 0 | 0 | 6 | * | * | * |
| 0 | 2 | 5 | 80 | na | 0 | * | * | * | * |
| 0 | 2 | 6 | 150 | na | 0 | * | * | * | * |
| 0 | 2 | 6 | 130 | na | 0 | * | * | * | * |
| 0 | 3 | 6 | 150 | na | 0 | * | * | * | * |
| 0 | 2 | 7 | 125 | na | 0 | * | * | * | * |
| 0 | <1 | 8 | 170 | na | 0 | * | * | * | * |
| 0 | 1 | 7 | 180 | 0 | 0 | * | * | * | * |
| 0 | 1 | 6 | 115 | 0 | 0 | * | * | * | * |
| 0 | 1 | 7 | 240 | na | 0 | * | * | * | * |
| 0 | 1 | 8 | 340 | na | 0 | * | * | * | * |
| 0 | 1 | 6 | 145 | na | 0 | * | * | * | * |
| 0 | 1 | 7 | 240 | na | 0 | * | * | * | * |
| 0 | 3 | 6 | 240 | 0 | 0 | * | * | * | * |
| 0 | 1 | 8 | 210 | 0 | 0 | * | * | * | * |
| 0 | 2 | 7 | 125 | na | 0 | * | * | * | * |
| 0 | 1 | 7 | 150 | 0 | 0 | * | * | * | * |
| 0 | 4 | 4 | 200 | 0 | 0 | * | * | * | * |
| 0 | 4 | 5 | 130 | 0 | 0 | 2 | * | * | * |
| 0 | 6 | 2 | 140 | na | 0 | * | * | * | * |
| 0 | 1 | 7 | 95 | na | 0 | * | * | * | * |
| 0 | 2 | 5 | 150 | 5 | 0 | * | * | * | * |
| 0 | 2 | 5 | 150 | 5 | 0 | * | * | * | * |

| FOOD NAME | Serving Size | Calories |
|---|---|---|
| Thousand Island & Bacon (Kraft) | 1 tbsp | 60 |
| Thousand Island (Wish-Bone) | 1 tbsp | 60 |
| Thousand Island with Bacon (Wish-Bone) | 1 tbsp | 60 |
| Thousand Island Southern Recipe (Wish-Bone) | 1 tbsp | 70 |
| Viva Herb & Spice (Seven Seas) | 1 tbsp | 60 |
| Viva Italian (Seven Seas) | 1 tbsp | 50 |
| Viva Ranch (Seven Seas) | 1 tbsp | 80 |
| Viva Red Wine Vinegar & Oil (Seven Seas) | 1 tbsp | 70 |
| Zesty Italian (Kraft) | 1 tbsp | 50 |
| *Light* | | |
| Bacon & Tomato (Kraft) | 1 tbsp | 30 |
| Blue Cheese (Roka) | 1 tbsp | 16 |
| Blue Cheese (Wish-Bone) | 1 tbsp | 40 |
| Buttermilk (Kraft) | 1 tbsp | 30 |
| Buttermilk Recipe Ranch! (Seven Seas) | 1 tbsp | 50 |
| Catalina | 1 tbsp | 18 |
| Chunky Blue Cheese (Kraft) | 1 tbsp | 30 |
| Creamy Bacon (Kraft) | 1 tbsp | 30 |
| Creamy Cucumber (Kraft) | 1 tbsp | 25 |
| Creamy Cucumber (Wish-Bone) | 1 tbsp | 40 |
| Creamy Italian (Kraft) | 1 tbsp | 25 |
| French (Kraft) | 1 tbsp | 20 |
| French! (Seven Seas) | 1 tbsp | 35 |
| French Style (Wish-Bone) | 1 tbsp | 30 |
| French Style Sweet 'n Spicy (Wish-Bone) | 1 tbsp | 30 |

| Protein (g) | Carbohydrates (g) | Fat (g) | Sodium (mg) | Cholesterol (mg) | Fiber (g) | Vitamin A (%) | Vitamin C (%) | Calcium (%) | Iron (%) |
|---|---|---|---|---|---|---|---|---|---|
| 0 | 2 | 6 | 100 | 0 | 0 | * | * | * | * |
| 0 | 2 | 6 | 130 | na | 0 | * | * | * | * |
| 0 | 2 | 6 | 95 | na | 0 | * | * | * | * |
| 0 | 3 | 6 | 90 | na | 0 | * | * | * | * |
| 0 | 1 | 6 | 170 | 0 | 0 | * | * | * | * |
| 0 | 1 | 5 | 240 | 0 | 0 | * | * | * | * |
| 0 | 1 | 8 | 135 | 5 | 0 | * | * | * | * |
| 0 | 1 | 7 | 290 | 0 | 0 | * | * | * | * |
| 0 | 1 | 5 | 260 | 0 | 0 | * | * | * | * |
| | | | | | | | | | |
| 0 | 2 | 2 | 150 | 0 | 0 | * | * | * | * |
| 1 | 1 | 1 | 280 | 5 | 0 | * | * | 2 | * |
| 0 | 3 | 3 | 190 | na | 0 | * | * | * | * |
| 0 | 1 | 3 | 125 | <5 | 0 | * | * | * | * |
| 0 | 1 | 5 | 135 | 0 | 0 | * | * | * | * |
| 0 | 3 | 1 | 120 | 0 | 0 | 6 | * | * | * |
| 0 | 2 | 2 | 240 | <5 | 0 | * | * | * | * |
| 0 | 2 | 2 | 150 | 0 | 0 | * | * | * | * |
| 0 | 1 | 2 | 220 | 0 | 0 | * | * | * | * |
| 0 | 1 | 4 | 165 | na | 0 | * | * | * | * |
| 0 | 1 | 2 | 120 | 0 | 0 | * | * | * | * |
| 0 | 3 | 1 | 120 | 0 | 0 | 8 | * | * | * |
| 0 | 2 | 3 | 210 | 0 | 0 | * | * | * | * |
| 0 | 2 | 2 | 70 | na | 0 | * | * | * | * |
| 0 | 4 | 2 | 150 | na | 0 | * | * | * | * |

| FOOD NAME | Serving Size | Calories | |
|---|---|---|---|
| House Italian (Kraft) | 1 tbsp | 30 | |
| Italian (Wish-Bone) | 1 tbsp | 30 | |
| Italian, Creamy (Wish-Bone) | 1 tbsp | 30 | |
| Oil-Free Italian (Kraft) | 1 tbsp | 4 | |
| Onion & Chive (Wish-Bone) | 1 tbsp | 40 | |
| (Rancher's Choice) | 1 tbsp | 30 | |
| Russian (Kraft) | 1 tbsp | 30 | |
| Russian (Wish-Bone) | 1 tbsp | 25 | |
| Thousand Island (Kraft) | 1 tbsp | 20 | |
| Thousand Island! (Seven Seas) | 1 tbsp | 30 | |
| Thousand Island (Wish-Bone) | 1 tbsp | 25 | |
| Viva Creamy Italian! (Seven Seas) | 1 tbsp | 45 | |
| Viva Herbs & Spices! (Seven Seas) | 1 tbsp | 30 | |
| Viva Italian! (Seven Seas) | 1 tbsp | 30 | |
| Viva Ranch! (Seven Seas) | 1 tbsp | 50 | |
| Viva Red Wine Vinegar & Oil! (Seven Seas) | 1 tbsp | 45 | |
| Zesty Italian (Kraft) | 1 tbsp | 20 | |
| *Nonfat* | | | |
| Catalina (Kraft Free) | 1 tbsp | 16 | |
| French (Kraft Free) | 1 tbsp | 20 | |
| Italian (Kraft Free) | 1 tbsp | 6 | |
| Ranch (Kraft Free) | 1 tbsp | 16 | |
| Ranch (Seven Seas Free) | 1 tbsp | 16 | |
| Red Wine Vinegar (Seven Seas Free) | 1 tbsp | 6 | |

| Protein (g) | Carbohydrates (g) | Fat (g) | Sodium (mg) | Cholesterol (mg) | Fiber (g) | Vitamin A (%) | Vitamin C (%) | Calcium (%) | Iron (%) |
|---|---|---|---|---|---|---|---|---|---|
| 0 | 1 | 2 | 115 | 0 | 0 | * | * | * | * |
| 0 | 1 | 3 | 210 | na | 0 | * | * | * | * |
| 0 | 1 | 3 | 200 | na | 0 | * | * | * | * |
| 0 | 1 | 0 | 220 | 0 | 0 | * | * | * | * |
| 0 | 3 | 3 | 160 | na | 0 | * | * | * | * |
| 0 | 1 | 3 | 150 | 5 | 0 | * | * | * | * |
| 0 | 4 | 1 | 130 | 0 | 0 | * | * | * | * |
| 0 | 5 | <1 | 140 | na | 0 | * | * | * | * |
| 0 | 3 | 1 | 135 | 0 | 0 | * | * | * | * |
| 0 | 3 | 2 | 160 | 5 | 0 | * | * | * | * |
| 0 | 3 | 2 | 160 | na | 0 | * | * | * | * |
| 0 | 1 | 4 | 230 | 0 | 0 | * | * | * | * |
| 0 | 1 | 3 | 200 | 0 | 0 | * | * | * | * |
| 0 | 1 | 3 | 230 | 0 | 0 | * | * | * | * |
| 0 | 2 | 5 | 125 | 5 | 0 | * | * | * | * |
| 0 | 1 | 4 | 190 | 0 | 0 | * | * | * | * |
| 0 | 1 | 2 | 230 | 0 | 0 | * | * | * | * |
| 0 | 3 | 0 | 120 | 0 | 0 | 6 | * | * | * |
| 0 | 4 | 0 | 120 | 0 | 0 | 6 | * | * | *. |
| 0 | 1 | 0 | 210 | 0 | 0 | * | * | * | * |
| 0 | 3 | 0 | 150 | 0 | 0 | * | * | * | * |
| 0 | 4 | 0 | 120 | 0 | 0 | * | * | * | * |
| 0 | 1 | 0 | 190 | 0 | 0 | * | * | * | * |

| FOOD NAME | Serving Size | Calories |
|---|---|---|
| Thousand Island (Kraft Free) | 1 tbsp | 20 |
| Viva Italian (Seven Seas Free) | 1 tbsp | 4 |
| **SALAMI** | | |
| Beef (Boar's Head) | 1 oz | 60 |
| Beef (Hebrew National) | 1 oz | 80 |
| Beer (Eckrich) | 1 oz | 70 |
| Cooked (Eckrich) | 1 oz | 70 |
| Cotto (Eckrich) | 1 oz | 70 |
| Cotto (Oscar Mayer) | 1 sl | 50 |
| Cotto Beef (Eckrich) | 1 sl | 50 |
| Cotto Beef (Oscar Mayer) | 1 sl | 50 |
| Dry (Hormel) | 1 oz | 110 |
| For Beer (Oscar Mayer) | 1 sl | 55 |
| For Beer, Beef (Oscar Mayer) | 1 sl | 75 |
| Genoa (Hickory Farms) | 1 oz | 110 |
| Genoa (Oscar Mayer) | 1 sl | 34 |
| Hard (Eckrich) | 1 sl | 130 |
| Hard (Oscar Mayer) | 1 sl | 35 |
| **SALMON** | | |
| Fresh, broiled | 4 oz | 208 |
| Pink, canned (Del Monte) | ½ cup | 160 |
| Red, canned (Del Monte) | ½ cup | 180 |
| Smoked | 1 oz | 50 |
| **SALSA** | | |
| (Prima Meat) | ½ cup | 120 |

| Protein (g) | Carbohydrates (g) | Fat (g) | Sodium (mg) | Cholesterol (mg) | Fiber (g) | Vitamin A (%) | Vitamin C (%) | Calcium (%) | Iron (%) |
|---|---|---|---|---|---|---|---|---|---|
| 0 | 5 | 0 | 135 | 0 | 0 | * | * | * | * |
| 0 | 1 | 0 | 220 | 0 | 0 | * | * | * | * |
| | | | | | | | | | |
| 5 | <1 | 4 | 288 | 20 | 0 | * | * | * | 2 |
| 7 | <1 | 7 | 230 | 15 | 0 | * | * | * | 2 |
| 4 | 1 | 6 | 330 | na | 0 | * | * | * | 2 |
| 3 | 1 | 6 | 360 | na | 0 | * | * | * | 2 |
| 4 | 1 | 6 | 380 | na | 0 | * | * | * | 2 |
| 3 | 4 | 4 | 245 | na | 0 | * | 6 | * | 3 |
| 2 | 1 | 4 | 240 | na | 0 | * | 5 | * | 2 |
| 3 | <1 | 4 | 280 | na | 0 | * | 6 | * | 2 |
| 7 | 0 | 11 | 463 | na | 0 | na | na | na | na |
| 3 | Tr | 4 | 282 | na | 0 | * | 11 | * | * |
| 2 | Tr | 7 | 234 | na | 0 | * | 6 | * | * |
| 6 | 0 | 10 | 540 | 20 | 0 | na | na | na | na |
| 2 | Tr | 3 | 164 | 9 | 0 | na | na | na | na |
| 4 | 1 | 12 | 600 | na | 0 | * | * | * | 2 |
| 1 | Tr | 3 | 167 | na | 0 | * | 3 | * | * |
| | | | | | | | | | |
| 31 | 0 | 8 | 132 | 56 | 0 | 4 | * | 13 | 6 |
| 20 | 0 | 7 | 660 | na | 0 | * | * | 20 | 4 |
| 21 | 0 | 9 | 660 | na | 0 | 4 | * | 25 | 4 |
| 5 | 0 | 3 | na | na | 0 | * | * | * | 2 |
| | | | | | | | | | |
| 4 | 20 | 3 | na | na | 0 | 30 | 20 | * | 2 |

| FOOD NAME | Serving Size | Calories |
|---|---|---|
| (Prima Mushroom) | ½ cup | 110 |
| SALT | 1 tsp | 0 |
| *Seasoned* | | |
| Butter Flavor (French's) | 1 tsp | 8 |
| Celery (French's) | 1 tsp | 2 |
| Garlic (French's) | 1 tsp | 4 |
| Garlic Parsley (French's) | 1 tsp | 6 |
| Hickory Smoke (French's) | 1 tsp | 2 |
| Onion (French's) | 1 tsp | 6 |
| (Lawry's) | 1 tsp | 4 |
| (Lawry's Lite) | 1 tsp | 8 |
| (McCormick/Schilling) | 1 tsp | 4 |
| (Morton) | 1 tsp | 4 |
| (Morton Nature's Seasons) | 1 tsp | 3 |
| SALT SUBSTITUTE | | |
| (Lawry's) | 1 tsp | 10 |
| (Morton) | 1 tsp | <1 |
| SARDINES | | |
| *Canned* | | |
| In oil | 4 oz | 200 |
| In mustard sauce (Underwood) | 1 can | 230 |
| Norwegian brisling (S&W) | 1.5 oz | 130 |
| In soya bean oil (Underwood) | 1 can | 380 |
| In tomato sauce (Del Monte) | ½ cup | 360 |
| In tomato sauce (Underwood) | 1 can | 230 |

| Protein (g) | Carbohydrates (g) | Fat (g) | Sodium (mg) | Cholesterol (mg) | Fiber (g) | Vitamin A (%) | Vitamin C (%) | Calcium (%) | Iron (%) |
|---|---|---|---|---|---|---|---|---|---|
| 3 | 20 | 3 | na | na | 0 | 30 | 20 | * | 2 |
| 0 | 0 | 0 | 2132 | 0 | 0 | * | * | * | * |
| | | | | | | | | | |
| 0 | 0 | 1 | 1125 | 0 | 0 | * | * | * | * |
| 0 | 0 | 0 | 1505 | 0 | 0 | * | * | * | * |
| 0 | 1 | 0 | 2050 | 0 | 0 | * | * | * | * |
| 0 | 1 | 0 | 1125 | 0 | 0 | * | * | * | * |
| 0 | 0 | 0 | 1145 | 0 | 0 | * | * | * | * |
| 0 | 1 | 0 | 1590 | 0 | 0 | * | * | * | * |
| Tr | <1 | Tr | 1367 | 0 | 0.1 | * | * | * | * |
| Tr | <2 | Tr | 357 | 0 | 0.1 | * | * | * | * |
| Tr | <1 | na | 980 | 0 | na | * | * | * | * |
| <1 | <1 | Tr | 1300 | 0 | na | * | * | * | * |
| Tr | <1 | Tr | 1400 | 0 | na | * | * | * | * |
| | | | | | | | | | |
| Tr | <2 | Tr | 2 | 0 | 0.4 | * | * | * | * |
| 0 | Tr | 0 | <1 | 0 | na | * | * | * | * |
| | | | | | | | | | |
| | | | | | | | | | |
| 27 | 0 | 12 | 700 | 160 | 0 | 5 | 8 | 50 | 19 |
| 19 | na | 17 | 850 | na | 0 | 6 | * | 25 | 6 |
| 10 | 0 | 10 | 220 | na | 0 | na | na | na | na |
| 19 | na | 34 | 800 | na | 0 | 6 | * | 25 | 6 |
| 19 | 45 | 12 | 540 | na | na | * | 8 | 30 | 20 |
| 19 | 1 | 17 | 850 | na | 0 | 6 | 2 | 25 | 6 |

| FOOD NAME | Serving Size | Calories |
|---|---|---|
| **SAUCE** | | |
| Au Gratin mix for Potatoes (French's) | ⅙ pkg | 55 |
| Cheese mix (French's) | ¼ cup | 80 |
| Chili (Del Monte) | ¼ cup | 70 |
| Cocktail (Kraft Sauceworks) | 1 tbsp | 14 |
| Enchilada, Green Chili (Old El Paso) | ¼ cup | 17 |
| Enchilada, Hot (Del Monte) | ½ cup | 45 |
| Enchilada, Hot (Old El Paso) | ¼ cup | 27 |
| Enchilada, Mild (Del Monte) | ½ cup | 45 |
| Enchilada, Mild (Old El Paso) | ¼ cup | 25 |
| 57 (Heinz) | 1 tbsp | 15 |
| Hollandaise mix (French's) | 3 tbsp | 45 |
| Pizza (Contadina) | ½ cup | 80 |
| Pizza (Contadina with Cheese) | ½ cup | 90 |
| Pizza (Contadina with Pepperoni) | ½ cup | 80 |
| Pizza (Contadina with Tomato Chunks) | ½ cup | 50 |
| Scalloped mix for Potatoes (French's) | ⅙ pkg | 40 |
| Seafood Cocktail (Del Monte) | ¼ cup | 70 |
| Sloppy Joe (Hunt's) | 5 tbsp | 40 |
| Sloppy Joe (Hunt's Mexican) | 5 tbsp | 40 |
| Sour Cream & Chives mix for Potatoes (French's) | ⅙ pkg | 65 |
| Sour Cream mix (French's) | ¼ cup | 96 |
| Stroganoff mix (French's) | ¼ cup | 82 |
| Sweet 'n Sour (Contadina) | 4 fl oz | 150 |

| Protein (g) | Carbohydrates (g) | Fat (g) | Sodium (mg) | Cholesterol (mg) | Fiber (g) | Vitamin A (%) | Vitamin C (%) | Calcium (%) | Iron (%) |
|---|---|---|---|---|---|---|---|---|---|
| 0 | 5 | 3 | 670 | na | na | * | * | * | * |
| 3 | 7 | 4 | 425 | na | 0 | * | * | 10 | * |
| 1 | 17 | 0 | 835 | na | na | 6 | 10 | * | 4 |
| 0 | 3 | 0 | 170 | 0 | na | 2 | 2 | * | * |
| 0 | 4 | 0 | 400 | na | na | * | * | * | 6 |
| 1 | 11 | 0 | 1090 | na | na | 15 | 10 | 2 | 4 |
| 0 | 4 | 1 | 247 | na | na | * | * | * | 20 |
| 1 | 11 | 0 | 1150 | na | na | 15 | 6 | 2 | 6 |
| 0 | 4 | 1 | 250 | na | na | * | * | * | 6 |
| 0 | 3 | 0 | 265 | na | na | na | na | na | na |
| Tr | 2 | 4 | 290 | na | na | * | * | 2 | * |
| 2 | 10 | 4 | 700 | na | na | 20 | 15 | 2 | 6 |
| 2 | 11 | 4 | 750 | na | na | 25 | 20 | 4 | 4 |
| 2 | 9 | 4 | 715 | na | na | 25 | 20 | 2 | 4 |
| 2 | 10 | 0 | 600 | na | na | 16 | 20 | 4 | 4 |
| 0 | 8 | 0 | 650 | na | na | * | * | * | * |
| 0 | 17 | 0 | 765 | na | na | 10 | 8 | * | 2 |
| 1 | 10 | 0 | 405 | na | na | 20 | 25 | * | 6 |
| 1 | 9 | 0 | 470 | na | na | 25 | 20 | * | 6 |
| 0 | 17 | 0 | 765 | na | na | * | * | * | * |
| 3 | 8 | 8 | 208 | na | na | * | * | 10 | * |
| 4 | 8 | 4 | 367 | na | na | 2 | * | 8 | * |
| 0 | 30 | 3 | 500 | na | na | 4 | * | 2 | 2 |

| FOOD NAME | Serving Size | Calories |
|-----------|--------------|----------|
| Sweet 'n Sour mix (French's) | ½ cup | 55 |
| Sweet 'n Sour (Kraft Sauceworks) | 1 tbsp | 25 |
| Sweet 'n Sour (La Choy) | ¼ cup | 131 |
| Swiss Steak (Contadina) | ¼ cup | 20 |
| Taco, Hot (Del Monte) | ¼ cup | 15 |
| Taco, Hot (Old El Paso) | 2 tbsp | 11 |
| Taco, Mild (Del Monte) | ¼ cup | 15 |
| Taco, Mild (Old El Paso) | 2 tbsp | 11 |
| Taco Starter (Del Monte) | 8 fl oz | 140 |
| Tartar (Kraft Sauceworks) | 1 tbsp | 50 |
| Tartar (Kraft Sauceworks Natural | | |
| Lemon and Herb Flavor) | 1 tbsp | 70 |
| Teriyaki mix (French's) | ¼ cup | 70 |
| Welsh Rarebit Cheese (Snow's) | ½ cup | 170 |
| White | ¼ cup | 100 |
| Worcestershire (French's) | 1 tbsp | 10 |
| Worcestershire (French's Smoky) | 1 tbsp | 10 |
| SAUERKRAUT | | |
| (Del Monte) | 1 oz | 4 |
| Sauerkraut (Vlasic) | 1 oz | 4 |
| SAUSAGE | | |
| Beef | 1 slice | 35 |
| Beef (Oscar Mayer) | 1 slice | 35 |
| Brown 'n Serve (Swift Premium) | 1 link | 130 |
| Cheese Smoked (Eckrich) | 2 oz | 180 |

| Protein (g) | Carbohydrates (g) | Fat (g) | Sodium (mg) | Cholesterol (mg) | Fiber (g) | Vitamin A (%) | Vitamin C (%) | Calcium (%) | Iron (%) |
|---|---|---|---|---|---|---|---|---|---|
| 0 | 14 | 0 | 135 | na | na | * | * | * | * |
| 0 | 5 | 0 | 50 | 0 | na | * | * | * | * |
| 0 | 32 | 0 | 320 | na | na | na | na | na | na |
| 1 | 5 | 0 | 319 | na | na | * | 2 | 2 | 2 |
| 0 | 4 | 0 | 440 | na | na | 6 | 2 | * | 2 |
| 0 | 2 | 0 | 131 | na | na | * | * | * | * |
| 0 | 4 | 0 | 480 | na | na | 4 | * | * | 2 |
| 0 | 2 | 0 | 125 | na | na | * | 2 | * | * |
| 2 | 28 | 1 | 2180 | na | na | 100 | 15 | 6 | 15 |
| 0 | 2 | 5 | 85 | 5 | na | * | * | * | * |
|  |  |  |  |  |  |  |  |  |  |
| 0 | 0 | 8 | 85 | 5 | na | * | * | * | * |
| 2 | 14 | 0 | 2360 | na | na | * | * | 4 | 8 |
| 7 | 10 | 11 | 460 | na | na | * | * | 25 | 2 |
| 3 | 6 | 8 | 87 | na | na | 6 | 1 | 7 | 1 |
| 0 | 2 | 0 | 165 | na | na | * | * | * | * |
| 0 | 2 | 0 | 165 | na | na | * | * | * | * |
|  |  |  |  |  |  |  |  |  |  |
| 0 | 1 | 0 | 280 | 0 | na | * | 4 | * | 2 |
| 0 | 1 | 0 | 280 | 0 | na | * | 4 | * | 2 |
|  |  |  |  |  |  |  |  |  |  |
| 3 | <1 | 2 | 295 | 18 | 0 | * | 8 | * | * |
| 3 | <1 | 2 | 295 | na | 0 | * | 8 | * | * |
| 4 | 1 | 12 | 240 | na | 0 | * | na | * | na |
| 7 | 2 | 15 | 500 | na | 0 | * | 20 | 4 | 4 |

| FOOD NAME | Serving Size | Calories |
|---|---|---|
| Ham Roll (Oscar Mayer) | 1 slice | 35 |
| Honey Roll Beef (Oscar Mayer) | 1 slice | 40 |
| Luncheon Roll (Oscar Mayer) | 1 slice | 35 |
| Minced Roll (Eckrich) | 1 slice | 80 |
| Pork (Eckrich) | 2 oz | 260 |
| Pork (Hormel) | 2 links | 143 |
| Pork (Jones) | 1 link | 140 |
| Pork Patties (Oscar Mayer) | 1 | 125 |
| Pork Roll (Eckrich) | 2 oz | 240 |
| Smoked (Eckrich Skinless) | 1 link | 180 |
| Smoked (Hillshire Farm) | 2 oz | 180 |
| Smokies (Oscar Mayer Beef) | 1 link | 123 |
| Smokies (Oscar Mayer Cheese) | 1 link | 127 |
| SAUSAGE SUBSTITUTE | | |
| Morningstar Breakfast Link | 3 | 186 |
| Morningstar Breakfast Patties | 2 | 221 |
| SCALLIONS | 6 | 15 |
| SCALLOPS | | |
| Steamed | 4 oz | 130 |
| Fried (Mrs. Paul's) | 3 oz | 160 |
| SEASONING | | |
| Barbecue (French's) | 1 tsp | 6 |
| Beef Stew (French's) | ⅙ pkg | 25 |
| Beef Stock Base (French's) | 1 tsp | 8 |
| Chicken Stock Base (French's) | 1 tsp | 8 |

| Protein (g) | Carbohydrates (g) | Fat (g) | Sodium (mg) | Cholesterol (mg) | Fiber (g) | Vitamin A (%) | Vitamin C (%) | Calcium (%) | Iron (%) |
|---|---|---|---|---|---|---|---|---|---|
| 4 | <1 | 2 | 270 | na | 0 | * | 8 | * | * |
| 4 | <1 | 2 | 304 | na | 0 | * | 6 | * | 2 |
| 3 | Tr | 2 | 244 | na | 0 | * | 8 | * | * |
| 4 | 1 | 7 | 300 | na | 0 | * | 10 | * | 2 |
| 5 | 1 | 26 | na | na | 0 | * | * | * | 2 |
| 7 | 0 | 13 | 327 | na | 0 | * | * | * | na |
| 3 | Tr | 14 | 176 | 24 | 0 | * | * | * | na |
| 6 | 0 | 11 | 282 | na | 0 | * | * | * | 3 |
| 7 | 1 | 26 | na | na | 0 | * | * | * | 4 |
| 7 | 2 | 16 | 420 | na | 0 | * | 15 | * | 4 |
| 8 | 2 | 16 | 570 | na | 0 | * | na | * | na |
| 5 | <1 | 11 | 430 | 27 | 0 | * | 13 | * | 2 |
| 6 | <1 | 11 | 453 | 29 | 0 | * | 12 | 2 | 2 |
|  |  |  |  |  |  |  |  |  |  |
| 16 | 1 | 14 | 598 | 0 | na | * | * | 3 | 19 |
| 16 | 6 | 14 | 818 | 0 | na | * | * | 5 | 24 |
| 0 | 3 | 0 | 2 | 0 | 1.2 | * | 13 | 1 | 1 |
|  |  |  |  |  |  |  |  |  |  |
| 26 | 0 | 2 | 300 | na | 0 | * | * | 13 | 19 |
| 8 | 18 | 7 | 320 | 10 | 0 | * | * | 2 | * |
|  |  |  |  |  |  |  |  |  |  |
| 0 | 1 | 0 | 70 | na | na | * | * | * | * |
| 0 | 5 | 0 | 765 | 0 | na | * | * | 2 | 2 |
| 0 | 2 | 0 | 500 | na | na | * | * | * | * |
| 0 | 1 | 0 | 475 | na | na | * | * | * | * |

| FOOD NAME | Serving Size | Calories |
|---|---|---|
| Chili-O (French's) | ⅙ pkg | 25 |
| Ground Beef with Onions (French's) | ¼ pkg | 25 |
| Hamburger (French's) | ¼ pkg | 25 |
| Meat Marinade (French's) | ⅛ pkg | 10 |
| Meat Tenderizer (French's) | 1 tsp | 2 |
| Meat Tenderizer, Seasoned (French's) | 1 tsp | 2 |
| Meatball (French's) | ¼ pkg | 35 |
| Meat Loaf (Contadina) | 1 tbsp | 35 |
| Meat Loaf (French's) | ⅛ pkg | 20 |
| Pepper (French's) | 1 tsp | 8 |
| Pepper & Lemon (French's) | 1 tsp | 6 |
| Pizza (French's) | 1 tsp | 4 |
| Salad Onions (French's) | 1 tbsp | 15 |
| Seafood (French's) | 1 tsp | 2 |
| Sloppy Joe (French's) | ⅛ pkg | 16 |
| Taco (French's) | ⅙ pkg | 20 |
| Vegetable Flakes (French's) | 1 tbsp | 12 |
| **SEASONING MIXTURE** | | |
| Extra Crispy for Chicken (Shake 'n Bake) | ¼ pkg | 110 |
| Homestyle for Chicken (Shake 'n Bake) | ¼ pkg | 80 |
| Italian Herb (Shake 'n Bake) | ¼ pkg | 80 |
| Original Recipe for Chicken (Shake 'n Bake) | ¼ pkg | 80 |
| Original Recipe for Fish (Shake 'n Bake) | ¼ pkg | 70 |
| Original Recipe for Pork (Shake 'n Bake) | ⅛ pkg | 40 |

| Protein (g) | Carbohydrates (g) | Fat (g) | Sodium (mg) | Cholesterol (mg) | Fiber (g) | Vitamin A (%) | Vitamin C (%) | Calcium (%) | Iron (%) |
|---|---|---|---|---|---|---|---|---|---|
| 0 | 5 | 0 | 630 | na | na | * | * | * | * |
| 0 | 6 | 0 | 440 | na | na | * | * | * | * |
| 1 | 5 | 0 | 450 | na | na | * | 2 | * | * |
| 0 | 2 | 0 | 540 | na | na | * | * | * | * |
| 0 | 0 | 0 | 1760 | na | na | * | * | * | * |
| 0 | 0 | 0 | 1550 | na | na | * | * | * | * |
| 1 | 7 | 0 | 825 | na | na | * | * | * | 2 |
| 1 | 7 | <1 | 430 | na | na | * | * | * | na |
| 0 | 5 | 0 | 615 | na | na | * | * | * | * |
| 0 | 1 | 0 | 5 | na | na | * | * | * | * |
| 0 | 1 | 0 | 805 | na | na | * | * | * | * |
| 0 | 1 | 0 | 400 | na | na | * | * | * | * |
| 0 | 3 | 0 | 2 | na | na | * | * | * | * |
| 0 | 0 | 0 | 1410 | na | na | * | * | * | * |
| 0 | 4 | 0 | 390 | na | na | * | * | * | * |
| 1 | 4 | 0 | 365 | na | na | * | * | * | * |
| 0 | 3 | 0 | 20 | na | na | * | * | * | * |
| | | | | | | | | | |
| 3 | 20 | 2 | 810 | 0 | na | 4 | 2 | 6 | 2 |
| 1 | 15 | 2 | 970 | 0 | na | 4 | * | 2 | 2 |
| 2 | 14 | 1 | 620 | 0 | na | 2 | 2 | 2 | * |
| | | | | | | | | | |
| 2 | 14 | 2 | 450 | 0 | na | 6 | * | * | 2 |
| 1 | 14 | 1 | 410 | 0 | na | 2 | * | 2 | * |
| 1 | 8 | 1 | 300 | 0 | na | * | * | * | * |

| FOOD NAME | Serving Size | Calories | |
|---|---|---|---|
| Original Barbecue Recipe for Chicken (Shake 'n Bake) | ¼ pkg | 90 | |
| Original Barbecue Recipe for Pork (Shake 'n Bake) | ⅛ pkg | 40 | |
| SESAME CHIPS (Flavor Tree) | 1 oz | 150 | |
| SESAME NUTS (Flavor Tree) | 1 oz | 180 | |
| SESAME STICKS | | | |
| Flavor Tree | 1 oz | 150 | |
| No Salt (Flavor Tree) | 1 oz | 160 | |
| With Bran (Flavor Tree) | 1 oz | 160 | |
| SHAD Baked with butter | 4 oz | 230 | |
| SHRIMP | | | |
| Canned | 4 oz | 130 | |
| Fried (Mrs. Paul's) | 3 oz | 170 | |
| SNACK MIX | | | |
| Classic (Pepperidge Farm) | 1 oz | 140 | |
| Lightly Smoked (Pepperidge Farm) | 1 oz | 150 | |
| Spicy (Pepperidge Farm) | 1 oz | 140 | |
| Sunflower Sesame (Flavor Tree) | 1 oz | 170 | |
| Pretzel (Pepperidge Farm) | 8 | 120 | |
| Pumpernickel (Pepperidge Farm) | 8 | 140 | |
| Sesame (Pepperidge Farm) | 8 | 140 | |
| Three Cheese (Pepperidge Farm) | 8 | 130 | |
| SOFT DRINK | | | |
| Bitter Lemon (Schweppes) | 6 fl oz | 84 | |

| Protein (g) | Carbohydrates (g) | Fat (g) | Sodium (mg) | Cholesterol (mg) | Fiber (g) | Vitamin A (%) | Vitamin C (%) | Calcium (%) | Iron (%) |
|---|---|---|---|---|---|---|---|---|---|
| 1 | 18 | 2 | 840 | 0 | na | 8 | * | 2 | * |
| | | | | | | | | | |
| 0 | 7 | 1 | 350 | 0 | na | 2 | * | * | * |
| 2 | 13 | 10 | 410 | na | na | * | * | 6 | 2 |
| 4 | 8 | 14 | 185 | na | na | * | * | 6 | 6 |
| | | | | | | | | | |
| 2 | 13 | 10 | 405 | na | na | * | * | 6 | 2 |
| 2 | 12 | 11 | 10 | na | na | * | * | 6 | 2 |
| 3 | 11 | 11 | 370 | na | na | * | * | 6 | 4 |
| 26 | 0 | 13 | 90 | na | 0 | 1 | na | 3 | 4 |
| | | | | | | | | | |
| 28 | 1 | 1 | 2607 | na | 0 | 1 | na | 13 | 19 |
| 9 | 17 | 11 | 480 | na | na | * | * | 2 | 2 |
| | | | | | | | | | |
| 4 | 14 | 8 | 360 | 0 | na | * | * | 4 | 4 |
| 4 | 13 | 9 | 350 | 0 | na | * | * | 4 | 2 |
| 4 | 14 | 8 | 340 | <5 | na | * | * | 2 | * |
| 5 | 8 | 13 | na | na | na | * | * | 4 | 10 |
| 3 | 23 | 3 | 430 | 0 | na | * | * | * | * |
| 3 | 20 | 6 | 330 | 0 | na | * | * | * | 4 |
| 4 | 19 | 5 | 280 | 0 | na | * | * | 6 | 4 |
| 4 | 19 | 5 | 400 | 0 | na | * | * | 4 | * |
| | | | | | | | | | |
| 0 | 20 | 0 | 2 | 0 | 0 | * | * | * | * |

| FOOD NAME | Serving Size | Calories |
|---|---|---|
| Club Soda (Canada Dry No Sodium) | 6 fl oz | 0 |
| Club Soda (Schweppes) | 6 fl oz | 0 |
| Cola (Coke Classic) | 6 fl oz | 72 |
| Cola (Caffeine-Free Coca-Cola) | 6 fl oz | 76 |
| Cola (Diet Coke) | 6 fl oz | <1 |
| Cola (Caffeine-Free Diet Coke) | 6 fl oz | <1 |
| Cola (Pepsi) | 6 fl oz | 80 |
| Cola (Diet Pepsi) | 6 fl oz | <1 |
| Cola (RC 100 Caffeine Free) | 6 fl oz | 78 |
| Cola (Diet RC 100 Caffeine Free) | 6 fl oz | <1 |
| Cola (Royal Crown) | 6 fl oz | 78 |
| Cola (Shasta) | 6 fl oz | 73 |
| Cola (Shasta Free) | 6 fl oz | 75 |
| Cola (Spree) | 6 fl oz | 74 |
| Fresca | 6 fl oz | 2 |
| Ginger Ale (Canada Dry) | 8 fl oz | 90 |
| Ginger Ale (Canada Dry Golden) | 8 fl oz | 100 |
| Ginger Ale (Fanta) | 6 fl oz | 63 |
| Ginger Ale (Shasta) | 6 fl oz | 60 |
| Ginger Ale (Spree) | 6 fl oz | 60 |
| Ginger Ale (Schweppes) | 6 fl oz | 65 |
| Ginger Ale (Schweppes Sugar Free) | 6 fl oz | 2 |
| Ginger Ale, Raspberry (Schweppes) | 6 fl oz | 65 |
| Ginger Beer (Schweppes) | 6 fl oz | 72 |
| Grape (Canada Dry) | 8 fl oz | 130 |

| Protein (g) | Carbohydrates (g) | Fat (g) | Sodium (mg) | Cholesterol (mg) | Fiber (g) | Vitamin A (%) | Vitamin C (%) | Calcium (%) | Iron (%) |
|---|---|---|---|---|---|---|---|---|---|
| 0 | 0 | 0 | 0 | 0 | 0 | * | * | * | * |
| 0 | 0 | 0 | 26 | 0 | 0 | * | * | * | * |
| 0 | 19 | 0 | 7 | 0 | 0 | * | * | * | * |
| 0 | 20 | 0 | 3 | 0 | 0 | * | * | * | * |
| 0 | Tr | 0 | 13 | 0 | 0 | * | * | * | * |
| 0 | Tr | 0 | 13 | 0 | 0 | * | * | * | * |
| 0 | 20 | 0 | 1 | 0 | 0 | * | * | * | * |
| 0 | 0 | 0 | 35 | 0 | 0 | * | * | * | * |
| 0 | 19 | 0 | Tr | 0 | 0 | * | * | * | * |
| 0 | Tr | 0 | 11 | 0 | 0 | * | * | * | * |
| 0 | 19 | 0 | Tr | 0 | 0 | * | * | * | * |
| 0 | 20 | 0 | <2 | 0 | 0 | * | * | * | * |
| 0 | 20 | 0 | 1 | 0 | 0 | * | * | * | * |
| 0 | 20 | 0 | <1 | 0 | 0 | * | * | * | * |
| 0 | 0 | 0 | 18 | 0 | 0 | * | * | * | * |
| 0 | 21 | 0 | 7 | 0 | 0 | * | * | * | * |
| 0 | 24 | 0 | 24 | 0 | 0 | * | * | * | * |
| 0 | 0 | 0 | 14 | 0 | 0 | * | * | * | * |
| 0 | 17 | 0 | 12 | 0 | 0 | * | * | * | * |
| 0 | 17 | 0 | <1 | 0 | 0 | * | * | * | * |
| 0 | 16 | 0 | 10 | 0 | 0 | * | * | * | * |
| 0 | 0 | 0 | 20 | 0 | 0 | * | * | * | * |
| 0 | 16 | 0 | 10 | 0 | 0 | * | * | * | * |
| 0 | 17 | 0 | 14 | 0 | 0 | * | * | * | * |
| 0 | 32 | 0 | 21 | 0 | 0 | * | * | * | * |

| FOOD NAME | Serving Size | Calories |
|---|---|---|
| Grape (Fanta) | 6 fl oz | 86 |
| Grape (Hi-C) | 6 fl oz | 78 |
| Grape (Nehi) | 6 fl oz | 87 |
| Grape (Schweppes) | 6 fl oz | 95 |
| Grape (Shasta) | 6 fl oz | 88 |
| Grapefruit (Schweppes) | 6 fl oz | 80 |
| Grapefruit (Spree) | 6 fl oz | 77 |
| Grapefruit (Wink) | 8 fl oz | 120 |
| Half & Half (Canada Dry) | 8 fl oz | 110 |
| Kiwi-Passion Fruit (Schweppes) | 6 fl oz | 35 |
| Lemon (Hi-C) | 6 fl oz | 78 |
| Lemon, Bitter (Schweppes) | 6 fl oz | 82 |
| Lemon, Dry (Schweppes) | 10 fl oz | 161 |
| Lemon, Sour (Schweppes) | 6 fl oz | 79 |
| Lemon-Lime (Schweppes) | 6 fl oz | 72 |
| Lemon-Lime (Shasta) | 6 fl oz | 73 |
| Lemon-Lime (Spree) | 6 fl oz | 77 |
| Lime, Mandarin (Spree) | 6 fl oz | 77 |
| Mello Yellow | 6 fl oz | 86 |
| Mineral Water (Schweppes) | 6 fl oz | 0 |
| Mountain Dew | 6 fl oz | 80 |
| Mr. Pibb | 6 fl oz | 71 |
| Orange (Fanta) | 6 fl oz | 88 |
| Orange (Hi-C) | 6 fl oz | 77 |
| Orange (Nehi) | 6 fl oz | 93 |

| Protein (g) | Carbohydrates (g) | Fat (g) | Sodium (mg) | Cholesterol (mg) | Fiber (g) | Vitamin A (%) | Vitamin C (%) | Calcium (%) | Iron (%) |
|---|---|---|---|---|---|---|---|---|---|
| 0 | 22 | 0 | 7 | 0 | 0 | * | * | * | * |
| 0 | 20 | 0 | 6 | 0 | 0 | * | 60 | * | * |
| 0 | 22 | 0 | 8 | 0 | 0 | * | * | * | * |
| 0 | 23 | 0 | 15 | 0 | 0 | * | * | * | * |
| 0 | 24 | 0 | 17 | 0 | 0 | * | * | * | * |
| 0 | 20 | 0 | 28 | 0 | 0 | * | * | * | * |
| 0 | 21 | 0 | <1 | 0 | 0 | * | * | * | * |
| 0 | 30 | 0 | 19 | 0 | 0 | * | * | * | * |
| 0 | 26 | 0 | 17 | 0 | 0 | * | * | * | * |
| 0 | 8 | 0 | <5 | 0 | 0 | * | * | * | * |
| 0 | 20 | 0 | 6 | 0 | 0 | * | * | * | * |
| 0 | 20 | 0 | 13 | 0 | 0 | * | * | * | * |
| 0 | 40 | 0 | 25 | 0 | 0 | * | * | * | * |
| 0 | 19 | 0 | 12 | 0 | 0 | * | * | * | * |
| 0 | 18 | 0 | 30 | 0 | 0 | * | * | * | * |
| 0 | 20 | 0 | 10 | 0 | 0 | * | * | * | * |
| 0 | 211 | 0 | <1 | 0 | 0 | * | * | * | * |
| 0 | 21 | 0 | <1 | 0 | 0 | * | * | * | * |
| 0 | 22 | 0 | 14 | 0 | 0 | * | * | * | * |
| 0 | 0 | 0 | 3 | 0 | 0 | * | * | * | * |
| 0 | 22 | 0 | 15 | 0 | 0 | * | * | * | * |
| 0 | 19 | 0 | 10 | 0 | 0 | * | * | * | * |
| 0 | 23 | 0 | 7 | 0 | 0 | * | * | * | * |
| 0 | 20 | 0 | 7 | 0 | 0 | * | 60 | * | * |
| 0 | 23 | 0 | 12 | 0 | 0 | * | * | * | * |

| FOOD NAME | Serving Size | Calories |
|---|---|---|
| Orange (Minute Maid) | 6 fl oz | 87 |
| Orange (Schweppes) | 6 fl oz | 88 |
| Red Pop (Shasta) | 6 fl oz | 78 |
| Red Creme (Schweppes) | 10 fl oz | 127 |
| Rondo (Schweppes) | 10 fl oz | 127 |
| Rondo Sugar Free (Schweppes) | 10 fl oz | 0 |
| Root Beer (Fanta) | 6 fl oz | 78 |
| Root Beer (Nehi) | 6 fl oz | 87 |
| Root Beer (Ramblin') | 6 fl oz | 88 |
| Root Beer (Schweppes) | 6 fl oz | 76 |
| Root Beer (Shasta) | 6 fl oz | 77 |
| Root Beer (Spree) | 6 fl oz | 77 |
| Seltzer (Canada Dry Original) | 6 fl oz | 0 |
| Seltzer (Schweppes Low Sodium) | 6 fl oz | 0 |
| Seltzer, Flavored (Schweppes, all flavors) | 6 fl oz | 0 |
| 7UP | 6 fl oz | 72 |
| 7UP Cherry | 6 fl oz | 74 |
| Diet 7UP | 6 fl oz | 2 |
| Sprite | 6 fl oz | 71 |
| Diet Sprite | 6 fl oz | 1 |
| Strawberry (Nehi) | 6 fl oz | 87 |
| Strawberry (Shasta) | 6 fl oz | 73 |
| TAB | 6 fl oz | <1 |
| TAB Caffeine Free | 6 fl oz | <1 |
| Teem | 8 fl oz | 99 |

| Protein (g) | Carbohydrates (g) | Fat (g) | Sodium (mg) | Cholesterol (mg) | Fiber (g) | Vitamin A (%) | Vitamin C (%) | Calcium (%) | Iron (%) |
|---|---|---|---|---|---|---|---|---|---|
| 0 | 22 | 0 | Tr | 0 | 0 | * | * | * | * |
| 0 | 22 | 0 | 17 | 0 | 0 | * | * | * | * |
| 0 | 22 | 0 | 10 | 0 | 0 | * | * | * | * |
| 0 | 33 | 0 | 22 | 0 | 0 | * | * | * | * |
| 0 | 33 | 0 | 22 | 0 | 0 | * | * | * | * |
| 0 | 0 | 0 | 36 | 0 | 0 | * | * | * | * |
| 0 | 20 | 0 | 10 | 0 | 0 | * | * | * | * |
| 0 | 22 | 0 | 9 | 0 | 0 | * | * | * | * |
| 0 | 23 | 0 | 17 | 0 | 0 | * | * | * | * |
| 0 | 19 | 0 | 17 | 0 | 0 | * | * | * | * |
| 0 | 21 | 0 | 15 | 0 | 0 | * | * | * | * |
| 0 | 21 | 0 | 1 | 0 | 0 | * | * | * | * |
| 0 | 0 | 0 | 0 | 0 | 0 | * | * | * | * |
| 0 | 0 | 0 | 7 | 0 | 0 | * | * | * | * |
| 0 | 0 | 0 | <5 | 0 | 0 | * | * | * | * |
| 0 | 18 | 0 | 16 | 0 | 0 | * | * | * | * |
| 0 | 18 | 0 | 16 | 0 | 0 | * | * | * | * |
| 0 | 0 | 0 | 18 | 0 | 0 | * | * | * | * |
| 0 | 18 | 0 | 23 | 0 | 0 | * | * | * | * |
| 0 | 0 | 0 | 21 | 0 | 0 | * | * | * | * |
| 0 | 22 | 0 | 0 | 0 | 0 | * | * | * | * |
| 0 | 20 | 0 | 18 | 0 | 0 | * | * | * | * |
| 0 | Tr | 0 | 15 | 0 | 0 | * | * | * | * |
| 0 | Tr | 0 | 15 | 0 | 0 | * | * | * | * |
| 0 | 25 | 0 | 21 | 0 | 0 | * | * | * | * |

| FOOD NAME | Serving Size | Calories |
|---|---|---|
| Tonic (Canada Dry) | 8 fl oz | 90 |
| Tonic (Schweppes) | 6 fl oz | 66 |
| Tonic, Sugar Free (Schweppes) | 6 fl oz | 1 |
| Tropical Blend (Spree) | 6 fl oz | 73 |
| Vichy Water (Schweppes) | 6 fl oz | 0 |
| **SOFT DRINK MIX** | | |
| Cherry (Kool-Aid) | 8 fl oz | 80 |
| Grape (Kool-Aid) | 8 fl oz | 80 |
| Lemonade (Kool-Aid) | 8 fl oz | 80 |
| Mountain Berry Punch (Kool-Aid) | 8 fl oz | 80 |
| Orange (Kool-Aid) | 8 fl oz | 80 |
| Purplesaurus Rex (Kool-Aid) | 8 fl oz | 80 |
| Rainbow Punch (Kool-Aid) | 8 fl oz | 80 |
| Raspberry (Kool-Aid) | 8 fl oz | 80 |
| Strawberry (Kool-Aid) | 8 fl oz | 80 |
| SharkleBerry Fin (Kool-Aid) | 8 fl oz | 80 |
| Tropical Punch (Kool-Aid) | 8 fl oz | 80 |
| *Sugar Free* | | |
| Berry Blue (Kool-Aid) | 8 fl oz | 4 |
| Cherry (Kool-Aid) | 8 fl oz | 4 |
| Grape (Kool-Aid) | 8 fl oz | 4 |
| Lemonade (Kool-Aid) | 8 fl oz | 4 |
| Mountain Berry Punch (Kool-Aid) | 8 fl oz | 4 |
| Purplesaurus Rex (Kool-Aid) | 8 fl oz | 4 |
| SharkleBerry Fin (Kool-Aid) | 8 fl oz | 4 |

| Protein (g) | Carbohydrates (g) | Fat (g) | Sodium (mg) | Cholesterol (mg) | Fiber (g) | Vitamin A (%) | Vitamin C (%) | Calcium (%) | Iron (%) |
|---|---|---|---|---|---|---|---|---|---|
| 0 | 22 | 0 | 7 | 0 | 0 | * | * | * | * |
| 0 | 16 | 0 | 4 | 0 | 0 | * | * | * | * |
| 0 | 0 | 0 | 37 | 0 | 0 | * | * | * | * |
| 0 | 20 | 0 | 1 | 0 | 0 | * | * | * | * |
| 0 | 0 | 0 | 80 | 0 | 0 | * | * | * | * |
| | | | | | | | | | |
| 0 | 20 | 0 | 0 | 0 | 0 | * | 10 | * | * |
| 0 | 20 | 0 | 25 | 0 | 0 | * | 10 | * | * |
| 0 | 20 | 0 | 0 | 0 | 0 | * | 10 | * | * |
| 0 | 20 | 0 | 15 | 0 | 0 | * | 10 | * | * |
| 0 | 20 | 0 | 0 | 0 | 0 | * | 10 | * | * |
| 0 | 21 | 0 | 5 | 0 | 0 | * | 10 | * | * |
| 0 | 21 | 0 | 20 | 0 | 0 | * | 10 | * | * |
| 0 | 20 | 0 | 25 | 0 | 0 | * | 10 | * | * |
| 0 | 20 | 0 | 0 | 0 | 0 | * | 10 | * | * |
| 0 | 21 | 0 | 0 | 0 | 0 | * | 10 | * | * |
| 0 | 21 | 0 | 0 | 0 | 0 | * | 10 | * | * |
| | | | | | | | | | |
| 0 | 0 | 0 | 5 | 0 | 0 | * | 10 | * | * |
| 0 | 0 | 0 | 0 | 0 | 0 | * | 10 | * | * |
| 0 | 0 | 0 | 0 | 0 | 0 | * | 10 | * | * |
| 0 | 0 | 0 | 0 | 0 | 0 | * | 10 | * | * |
| 0 | 0 | 0 | 35 | 0 | 0 | * | 10 | * | * |
| 0 | 0 | 0 | 5 | 0 | 0 | * | 10 | * | * |
| 0 | 0 | 0 | 0 | 0 | 0 | * | 10 | * | * |

| FOOD NAME | Serving Size | Calories | |
|---|---|---|---|
| Surfin' Berry Punch (Kool-Aid) | 8 fl oz | 4 | |
| Tropical Punch (Kool-Aid) | 8 fl oz | 4 | |
| *Unsweetened* | | | |
| Berry Blue (Kool-Aid) | 8 fl oz | 2 | |
| Black Cherry (Kool-Aid) | 8 fl oz | 2 | |
| Cherry (Kool-Aid) | 8 fl oz | 2 | |
| Grape (Kool-Aid) | 8 fl oz | 2 | |
| Lemon-Lime (Kool-Aid) | 8 fl oz | 2 | |
| Lemonade, Pink (Kool-Aid) | 8 fl oz | 2 | |
| Mountain Berry Punch (Kool-Aid) | 8 fl oz | 2 | |
| Orange (Kool-Aid) | 8 fl oz | 2 | |
| Purplesaurus Rex (Kool-Aid) | 8 fl oz | 2 | |
| Rainbow Punch (Kool-Aid) | 8 fl oz | 2 | |
| Raspberry (Kool-Aid) | 8 fl oz | 2 | |
| SharkleBerry Fin (Kool-Aid) | 8 fl oz | 2 | |
| Strawberry (Kool-Aid) | 8 fl oz | 2 | |
| Surfin' Berry Punch (Kool-Aid) | 8 fl oz | 2 | |
| Tropical Punch (Kool-Aid) | 8 fl oz | 2 | |
| SOLE | | | |
| Fresh, baked, broiled or microwaved | 4 oz | 133 | |
| Frozen (Mrs. Paul's) | 1 fillet | 240 | |
| SORBET (Sherbet) | 1 cup | 270 | |
| SOUP   *Note: All soups are prepared with water, unless otherwise noted.* | | | |
| *Canned, condensed* | | | |
| Asparagus, Cream of (Campbell's) | 8 oz | 80 | |

| Protein (g) | Carbohydrates (g) | Fat (g) | Sodium (mg) | Cholesterol (mg) | Fiber (g) | Vitamin A (%) | Vitamin C (%) | Calcium (%) | Iron (%) |
|---|---|---|---|---|---|---|---|---|---|
| 0 | 0 | 0 | 25 | 0 | 0 | * | 10 | * | * |
| 0 | 0 | 0 | 10 | 0 | 0 | * | 10 | * | * |
| 0 | 0 | 0 | 0 | 0 | 0 | * | 10 | * | * |
| 0 | 0 | 0 | 0 | 0 | 0 | * | 10 | * | * |
| 0 | 0 | 0 | 0 | 0 | 0 | * | 10 | * | * |
| 0 | 0 | 0 | 0 | 0 | 0 | * | 10 | * | * |
| 0 | 0 | 0 | 0 | 0 | 0 | * | 10 | * | * |
| 0 | 0 | 0 | 0 | 0 | 0 | * | 10 | * | * |
| 0 | 0 | 0 | 15 | 0 | 0 | * | 10 | * | * |
| 0 | 0 | 0 | 0 | 0 | 0 | * | 10 | * | * |
| 0 | 0 | 0 | 5 | 0 | 0 | * | 10 | * | * |
| 0 | 0 | 0 | 0 | 0 | 0 | * | 10 | * | * |
| 0 | 0 | 0 | 25 | 0 | 0 | * | 10 | * | * |
| 0 | 0 | 0 | 0 | 0 | 0 | * | 10 | * | * |
| 0 | 0 | 0 | 25 | 0 | 0 | * | 10 | * | * |
| 0 | 0 | 0 | 25 | 0 | 0 | * | 10 | * | * |
| 0 | 0 | 0 | 0 | 0 | 0 | * | 10 | * | * |
| 27 | 0 | 2 | 120 | 77 | 0 | 1 | * | 2 | 6 |
| 16 | 20 | 10 | 450 | 50 | <1 | 2 | * | 4 | 4 |
| 2 | 60 | 4 | 90 | 0 | 0 | 4 | 7 | 10 | 2 |
| 2 | 10 | 4 | 820 | na | na | 4 | 2 | 2 | 2 |

| FOOD NAME | Serving Size | Calories |
|---|---|---|
| Bean with Bacon (Campbell's) | 8 oz | 140 |
| Bean, Homestyle (Campbell's) | 8 oz | 130 |
| Beef (Campbell's) | 8 oz | 80 |
| Beef Bouillon (Campbell's) | 8 oz | 16 |
| Beef Noodle (Campbell's) | 8 oz | 70 |
| Beef Noodle, Homestyle (Campbell's) | 8 oz | 80 |
| Beefy Mushroom (Campbell's) | 8 oz | 60 |
| Broccoli, Cream of (Campbell's) | 8 oz | 80 |
| Broccoli, Cream of *prepared with 2% low-fat milk* (Campbell's) | 8 oz | 140 |
| Celery, Cream of (Campbell's) | 8 oz | 100 |
| Cheddar Cheese (Campbell's) | 8 oz | 110 |
| Chicken Alphabet (Campbell's) | 8 oz | 80 |
| Chicken Barley (Campbell's) | 8 oz | 70 |
| Chicken Broth (Campbell's) | 8 oz | 30 |
| Chicken Broth & Noodles (Campbell's) | 8 oz | 45 |
| Chicken, Cream of (Campbell's) | 8 oz | 110 |
| Chicken 'n Dumplings (Campbell's) | 8 oz | 80 |
| Chicken Gumbo (Campbell's) | 8 oz | 60 |
| Chicken Mushroom, Creamy (Campbell's) | 8 oz | 120 |
| Chicken Noodle (Campbell's) | 8 oz | 60 |
| Chicken Noodle Homestyle (Campbell's) | 8 oz | 70 |
| Chicken Noodle-O's (Campbell's) | 8 oz | 70 |
| Chicken with Rice (Campbell's) | 8 oz | 60 |

| Protein (g) | Carbohydrates (g) | Fat (g) | Sodium (mg) | Cholesterol (mg) | Fiber (g) | Vitamin A (%) | Vitamin C (%) | Calcium (%) | Iron (%) |
|---|---|---|---|---|---|---|---|---|---|
| 6 | 21 | 4 | 840 | na | na | 15 | * | 6 | 10 |
| 6 | 25 | 1 | 700 | na | na | 15 | 4 | 6 | 8 |
| 5 | 10 | 2 | 830 | na | na | 20 | 2 | * | 4 |
| 3 | 1 | 0 | 820 | na | na | * | * | * | * |
| 4 | 7 | 3 | 830 | na | na | 4 | * | * | 4 |
| 5 | 7 | 4 | 810 | na | na | * | 2 | * | 4 |
| 4 | 5 | 3 | 960 | na | na | * | * | * | 2 |
| 1 | 8 | 5 | 790 | na | na | 2 | 10 | 2 | 2 |
| | | | | | | | | | |
| 5 | 14 | 7 | 850 | na | na | 6 | 10 | 15 | 2 |
| 2 | 8 | 7 | 820 | na | na | 6 | * | 2 | * |
| 4 | 10 | 6 | 810 | na | na | 15 | * | 10 | 2 |
| 3 | 10 | 3 | 800 | na | na | 15 | * | * | 4 |
| 3 | 10 | 2 | 850 | na | na | 20 | * | * | 2 |
| 1 | 2 | 2 | 710 | na | na | * | * | * | * |
| 1 | 8 | 1 | 860 | na | na | 8 | * | * | * |
| 2 | 9 | 7 | 810 | na | na | 10 | * | 2 | * |
| 4 | 9 | 3 | 960 | na | na | 8 | * | * | 2 |
| 2 | 8 | 2 | 900 | na | na | 2 | * | 2 | * |
| | | | | | | | | | |
| 3 | 8 | 8 | 920 | na | na | 15 | * | 2 | 2 |
| 3 | 8 | 2 | 900 | na | na | 6 | * | * | 2 |
| 3 | 8 | 3 | 880 | na | na | 15 | 2 | * | 4 |
| 3 | 9 | 2 | 820 | na | na | 8 | * | * | 2 |
| 2 | 7 | 3 | 790 | na | na | 8 | * | * | * |

| FOOD NAME | Serving Size | Calories |
|---|---|---|
| Chicken & Stars (Campbell's) | 8 oz | 60 |
| Chicken Vegetable (Campbell's) | 8 oz | 70 |
| Chili Beef (Campbell's) | 8 oz | 140 |
| Clam Chowder, Manhattan Style (Campbell's) | 8 oz | 70 |
| Clam Chowder, New England (Campbell's) | 8 oz | 80 |
| Clam Chowder, New England *prepared with 2% low-fat milk* (Campbell's) | 8 oz | 150 |
| Consomme (Campbell's) | 8 oz | 25 |
| Curly Noodle with Chicken (Campbell's) | 8 oz | 80 |
| French Onion (Campbell's) | 8 oz | 60 |
| Green Pea (Campbell's) | 8 oz | 160 |
| Minestrone (Campbell's) | 8 oz | 80 |
| Mushroom, Cream of (Campbell's) | 8 oz | 100 |
| Mushroom, Golden (Campbell's) | 8 oz | 70 |
| Nacho Cheese (Campbell's) | 8 oz | 110 |
| Noodles & Ground Beef (Campbell's) | 8 oz | 90 |
| Onion, Cream of (Campbell's) | 8 oz | 100 |
| Oyster Stew (Campbell's) | 8 oz | 70 |
| Pepper Pot (Campbell's) | 8 oz | 90 |
| Potato, Cream of (Campbell's) | 8 oz | 80 |
| Scotch Broth (Campbell's) | 8 oz | 80 |
| Shrimp, Cream of (Campbell's) | 8 oz | 90 |
| Split Pea with Ham & Bacon (Campbell's) | 8 oz | 160 |

| Protein (g) | Carbohydrates (g) | Fat (g) | Sodium (mg) | Cholesterol (mg) | Fiber (g) | Vitamin A (%) | Vitamin C (%) | Calcium (%) | Iron (%) |
|---|---|---|---|---|---|---|---|---|---|
| 3 | 7 | 2 | 870 | na | na | 8 | * | * | 2 |
| 3 | 8 | 3 | 850 | na | na | 50 | * | * | 4 |
| 5 | 20 | 5 | 840 | na | na | 10 | 4 | 2 | 8 |
| 2 | 10 | 2 | 820 | na | na | 30 | 8 | 2 | 2 |
| 3 | 12 | 3 | 870 | na | na | * | 2 | 2 | 4 |
| 7 | 17 | 7 | 930 | na | na | 2 | 4 | 10 | 4 |
| 4 | 2 | 0 | 750 | na | na | * | * | * | 2 |
| 3 | 11 | 3 | 800 | na | na | 15 | * | * | 4 |
| 2 | 9 | 2 | 900 | na | na | * | 4 | 2 | 2 |
| 8 | 25 | 3 | 820 | na | na | * | * | * | 8 |
| 3 | 13 | 2 | 900 | na | na | 45 | 6 | 2 | 4 |
| 2 | 8 | 7 | 820 | na | na | * | * | 2 | * |
| 2 | 9 | 3 | 870 | na | na | 15 | * | * | 2 |
| 4 | 8 | 8 | 740 | na | na | 25 | 10 | 4 | * |
| 4 | 10 | 4 | 820 | na | na | 15 | * | * | 4 |
| 2 | 12 | 5 | 830 | na | na | 6 | * | 2 | * |
| 2 | 5 | 5 | 840 | na | na | * | 8 | * | 8 |
| 5 | 9 | 4 | 970 | na | na | 20 | * | 2 | 4 |
| 1 | 12 | 3 | 870 | na | na | 4 | * | * | * |
| 4 | 9 | 3 | 870 | na | na | 45 | * | * | 2 |
| 2 | 8 | 6 | 810 | na | na | * | * | * | * |
| 9 | 24 | 4 | 780 | na | na | 8 | * | * | 10 |

| FOOD NAME | Serving Size | Calories |
|---|---|---|
| Teddy Bear (Campbell's) | 8 oz | 70 |
| Tomato (Campbell's) | 8 oz | 90 |
| Tomato *prepared with* | | |
| 2% *low-fat milk* (Campbell's) | 8 oz | 150 |
| Tomato Bisque (Campbell's) | 8 oz | 120 |
| Tomato, Homestyle Cream of (Campbell's) | 8 oz | 110 |
| Tomato, Zesty (Campbell's) | 8 oz | 100 |
| Tomato Rice (Campbell's) | 8 oz | 110 |
| Turkey Noodle (Campbell's) | 8 oz | 70 |
| Turkey Vegetable (Campbell's) | 8 oz | 70 |
| Vegetable (Campbell's) | 8 oz | 90 |
| Vegetable Beef (Campbell's) | 8 oz | 70 |
| Vegetable Homestyle (Campbell's) | 8 oz | 60 |
| Vegetable Old Fashioned (Campbell's) | 8 oz | 60 |
| Vegetarian Vegetable (Campbell's) | 8 oz | 80 |
| Won Ton (Campbell's) | 8 oz | 40 |
| *Canned, condensed* | | |
| Bean with Bacon | | |
| (Campbell's Special Request) | 8 oz | 140 |
| Chicken, Cream of | | |
| (Campbell's Special Request) | 8 oz | 110 |
| Chicken Noodle | | |
| (Campbell's Special Request) | 8 oz | 60 |
| Chicken with Rice | | |
| (Campbell's Special Request) | 8 oz | 60 |

| Protein (g) | Carbohydrates (g) | Fat (g) | Sodium (mg) | Cholesterol (mg) | Fiber (g) | Vitamin A (%) | Vitamin C (%) | Calcium (%) | Iron (%) |
|---|---|---|---|---|---|---|---|---|---|
| 3 | 11 | 2 | 790 | na | na | 15 | * | * | 4 |
| 3 | 11 | 2 | 790 | na | na | 10 | 45 | * | 2 |
| | | | | | | | | | |
| 5 | 22 | 4 | 740 | na | na | 15 | 45 | 15 | 4 |
| 2 | 22 | 3 | 820 | na | na | 10 | 30 | 4 | 2 |
| 1 | 20 | 3 | 810 | na | na | 10 | 40 | * | 2 |
| 1 | 20 | 2 | 760 | na | na | 25 | 30 | 2 | 4 |
| 1 | 22 | 2 | 730 | na | na | 8 | 20 | * | 2 |
| 3 | 9 | 2 | 880 | na | na | 10 | * | * | 2 |
| 2 | 8 | 3 | 710 | na | na | 50 | * | * | 2 |
| 3 | 14 | 2 | 830 | na | na | 40 | 6 | 2 | 2 |
| 4 | 10 | 2 | 780 | na | na | 40 | 4 | * | 4 |
| 2 | 9 | 2 | 880 | na | na | 45 | 6 | 2 | 2 |
| 2 | 9 | 2 | 880 | na | na | 50 | 2 | * | 2 |
| 2 | 13 | 2 | 790 | na | na | 40 | 6 | * | 4 |
| 2 | 5 | 1 | 850 | na | na | * | * | * | 2 |
| | | | | | | | | | |
| 6 | 21 | 4 | 470 | 5 | na | 15 | * | 6 | 10 |
| | | | | | | | | | |
| 3 | 9 | 7 | 490 | 10 | na | 15 | * | 2 | * |
| | | | | | | | | | |
| 3 | 8 | 2 | 440 | 15 | na | 6 | * | * | 2 |
| | | | | | | | | | |
| 2 | 7 | 3 | 480 | 10 | na | 8 | * | * | * |

| FOOD NAME | Serving Size | Calories | |
|---|---|---|---|
| Mushroom, Cream of | | | |
| (Campbell's Special Request) | 8 oz | 100 | |
| Tomato (Campbell's Special Request) | 8 oz | 90 | |
| Vegetable (Campbell's Special Request) | 8 oz | 90 | |
| Vegetable Beef | | | |
| (Campbell's Special Request) | 8 oz | 70 | |
| *Canned, ready-to-serve* | | | |
| Beef (Campbell's) | 9.5 oz | 170 | |
| Chicken Noodle (Campbell's) | 9.5 oz | 180 | |
| Chicken Corn Chowder (Campbell's) | 9.5 oz | 300 | |
| Chicken Nuggets (Campbell's) | 9.5 oz | 170 | |
| Chicken with Rice (Campbell's) | 9.5 oz | 140 | |
| Chicken Vegetable (Campbell's) | 9.5 oz | 170 | |
| Chili Beef (Campbell's) | 9.75 oz | 260 | |
| Clam Chowder, Manhattan (Campbell's) | 9.5 oz | 150 | |
| Clam Chowder, New England (Campbell's) | 9.5 oz | 260 | |
| Creamy Chicken Mushroom (Campbell's) | 9.38 oz | 240 | |
| Creole Style (Campbell's) | 9.5 oz | 220 | |
| Mediterranean Vegetable (Campbell's) | 9.5 oz | 170 | |
| Minestrone (Campbell's) | 9.5 oz | 160 | |
| Old Fashioned Bean with Ham (Campbell's) | 9.63 oz | 250 | |
| Old Fashioned Chicken (Campbell's) | 9.5 oz | 150 | |
| Old Fashioned Vegetable Beef (Campbell's) | 9.5 oz | 160 | |
| Pepper Steak (Campbell's) | 9.5 oz | 160 | |
| Sirloin Burger (Campbell's) | 9.5 oz | 200 | |

| Protein (g) | Carbohydrates (g) | Fat (g) | Sodium (mg) | Cholesterol (mg) | Fiber (g) | Vitamin A (%) | Vitamin C (%) | Calcium (%) | Iron (%) |
|---|---|---|---|---|---|---|---|---|---|
| 2 | 8 | 7 | 480 | <5 | na | * | * | 2 | * |
| 1 | 17 | 2 | 430 | 0 | na | 10 | 45 | * | 2 |
| 3 | 14 | 2 | 500 | <5 | na | 40 | 6 | 2 | 2 |
| 4 | 10 | 2 | 470 | 10 | na | 40 | 4 | * | 4 |
| 13 | 21 | 4 | 970 | na | na | 90 | 10 | 2 | 10 |
| 12 | 18 | 7 | 1000 | na | na | 20 | * | 2 | 10 |
| 12 | 21 | 19 | 1060 | na | na | 40 | * | 2 | 6 |
| 9 | 21 | 6 | 940 | na | na | 50 | 10 | 4 | 8 |
| 10 | 16 | 4 | 1060 | na | na | 120 | 6 | 4 | 4 |
| 10 | 19 | 6 | 1080 | na | na | 130 | 8 | 2 | 6 |
| 18 | 33 | 6 | 990 | na | na | 25 | 8 | 6 | 20 |
| 8 | 23 | 15 | 1060 | na | na | * | * | 6 | 10 |
| 8 | 23 | 15 | 1060 | na | na | * | * | 6 | 10 |
| 10 | 12 | 17 | 1140 | na | na | 15 | * | 2 | 4 |
| 10 | 28 | 7 | 800 | na | na | 6 | * | 6 | 10 |
| 4 | 24 | 6 | 1010 | na | na | 110 | 10 | 6 | 6 |
| 6 | 24 | 4 | 870 | na | na | 90 | 10 | 8 | 10 |
| 12 | 33 | 8 | 960 | na | na | 80 | 8 | 8 | 15 |
| 10 | 18 | 4 | 1070 | na | na | 110 | 10 | 4 | 8 |
| 12 | 17 | 5 | 970 | na | na | 100 | 10 | 4 | 10 |
| 12 | 21 | 3 | 920 | na | na | 45 | 15 | 2 | 10 |
| 11 | 20 | 8 | 1090 | na | na | 80 | 10 | 2 | 10 |

| FOOD NAME | Serving Size | Calories |
|---|---|---|
| Split Pea with Ham (Campbell's) | 9.5 oz | 210 |
| Steak and Potato (Campbell's) | 9.5 oz | 170 |
| Turkey Vegetable (Campbell's) | 9.38 oz | 150 |
| Vegetable (Campbell's) | 9.5 oz | 150 |
| *Canned, ready-to-serve low sodium* | | |
| Chicken Broth (Campbell's) | 10.5 oz | 30 |
| Chicken with Noodles (Campbell's) | 10.75 oz | 170 |
| Chunky Vegetable Beef (Campbell's) | 10.75 oz | 180 |
| Mushroom, Cream of (Campbell's) | 10.5 oz | 210 |
| Split Pea (Campbell's) | 10.75 oz | 230 |
| Tomato (Campbell's) | 10.5 oz | 190 |
| *Canned, ready-to-serve* | | |
| Bean and Ham (Home Cookin') | 9.5 oz | 180 |
| Beef with Vegetables and Pasta (Home Cookin') | 9.5 oz | 120 |
| Chicken Gumbo (Home Cookin') | 9.5 oz | 120 |
| Chicken Minestrone (Home Cookin') | 9.5 oz | 160 |
| Chicken with Noodles (Home Cookin') | 9.5 oz | 110 |
| Chicken Rice (Home Cookin') | 9.5 oz | 130 |
| Country Vegetable (Home Cookin') | 9.5 oz | 100 |
| Hearty Lentil (Home Cookin') | 9.5 oz | 140 |
| Minestrone (Home Cookin') | 9.5 oz | 120 |
| Split Pea with Ham (Home Cookin') | 9.5 oz | 200 |
| Tomato Garden (Home Cookin') | 9.5 oz | 130 |
| Vegetable Beef (Home Cookin') | 9.5 oz | 120 |

| Protein (g) | Carbohydrates (g) | Fat (g) | Sodium (mg) | Cholesterol (mg) | Fiber (g) | Vitamin A (%) | Vitamin C (%) | Calcium (%) | Iron (%) |
|---|---|---|---|---|---|---|---|---|---|
| 11 | 30 | 5 | 950 | na | na | 60 | 10 | 2 | 10 |
| 12 | 21 | 4 | 1000 | na | na | * | 8 | * | 10 |
| 9 | 16 | 6 | 1060 | na | na | 130 | 10 | 4 | 6 |
| 4 | 25 | 4 | 970 | na | na | 110 | 6 | 6 | 10 |
| | | | | | | | | | |
| 3 | 2 | 1 | 85 | na | na | * | * | 2 | 4 |
| 13 | 17 | 5 | 90 | na | na | 35 | 4 | 2 | 10 |
| 14 | 19 | 5 | 90 | na | na | 100 | 15 | 4 | 10 |
| 3 | 18 | 14 | 55 | na | na | * | * | 6 | 6 |
| 12 | 37 | 4 | 30 | na | na | 30 | 8 | 4 | 10 |
| 4 | 30 | 6 | 45 | na | na | 30 | 60 | 4 | 8 |
| | | | | | | | | | |
| 12 | 25 | 4 | 890 | na | na | 30 | * | 4 | 15 |
| | | | | | | | | | |
| 10 | 16 | 2 | 940 | na | na | 4 | 6 | 2 | 8 |
| 9 | 13 | 3 | 960 | na | na | 50 | * | 4 | 8 |
| 13 | 15 | 5 | 840 | na | na | 35 | 4 | 6 | 10 |
| 11 | 10 | 3 | 1020 | na | na | 60 | * | 2 | 8 |
| 12 | 9 | 5 | 960 | na | na | 25 | * | 2 | 6 |
| 3 | 18 | 2 | 940 | na | na | 80 | 15 | 4 | 6 |
| 9 | 24 | 1 | 820 | na | na | 70 | 6 | 4 | 20 |
| 4 | 20 | 3 | 1080 | na | na | 80 | 6 | 6 | 6 |
| 14 | 34 | 1 | 1150 | na | na | 45 | 10 | 4 | 15 |
| 2 | 25 | 2 | 820 | na | na | 40 | 20 | 8 | 8 |
| 11 | 15 | 2 | 1020 | na | na | 90 | 6 | 4 | 8 |

| FOOD NAME | Serving Size | Calories |
|---|---|---|
| *Microwave* | | |
| Bean with Bacon 'n Ham (Campbell's) | 7.5 oz | 230 |
| Chicken Noodle (Campbell's) | 7.5 oz | 100 |
| Chicken with Rice (Campbell's) | 7.5 oz | 100 |
| Chili Beef (Campbell's) | 7.5 oz | 190 |
| Vegetable Beef (Campbell's) | 7.5 oz | 100 |
| *Microwave Cup* | | |
| Beef Flavor Noodle (Campbell's) | 1.35 oz | 130 |
| Chicken Flavor Noodle (Campbell's) | 1.35 oz | 140 |
| Hearty Noodle with Vegetables (Campbell's) | 1.7 oz | 180 |
| Noodle Soup with Chicken Broth (Campbell's) | 1.35 oz | 130 |
| *Mix* | | |
| Chicken Noodle (Campbell's) | 8 oz | 100 |
| Chicken Noodle with White Meat (Campbell's) | 6 oz | 90 |
| Creamy Chicken with White Meat (Campbell's) | 6 oz | 90 |
| Hearty Noodle (Campbell's) | 8 oz | 90 |
| Noodle (Campbell's) | 8 oz | 110 |
| Noodle with Chicken Broth (Campbell's) | 6 oz | 90 |
| Onion (Campbell's) | 8 oz | 30 |
| Vegetable (Campbell's) | 8 oz | 40 |

| Protein (g) | Carbohydrates (g) | Fat (g) | Sodium (mg) | Cholesterol (mg) | Fiber (g) | Vitamin A (%) | Vitamin C (%) | Calcium (%) | Iron (%) |
|---|---|---|---|---|---|---|---|---|---|
| 8 | 38 | 5 | 830 | na | na | 15 | 2 | 6 | 10 |
| 5 | 11 | 4 | 870 | na | na | 25 | * | * | 4 |
| 3 | 14 | 4 | 820 | na | na | 30 | * | * | 20 |
| 7 | 32 | 4 | 870 | na | na | 20 | 2 | 4 | 10 |
| 5 | 16 | 2 | 830 | na | na | 25 | 4 | 2 | 6 |
| 6 | 23 | 2 | 1270 | na | na | 25 | 2 | 2 | 8 |
| 7 | 22 | 3 | 1340 | na | na | * | * | * | 8 |
| 7 | 32 | 2 | 1320 | na | na | 15 | 2 | 2 | 10 |
| 6 | 23 | 2 | 1360 | na | na | 25 | 2 | * | 8 |
| 5 | 16 | 2 | 710 | na | na | * | * | 2 | 6 |
| 6 | 12 | 2 | 770 | na | na | * | * | * | 4 |
| 3 | 12 | 4 | 1020 | na | na | * | * | 2 | * |
| 4 | 15 | 1 | 840 | na | na | 20 | * | 2 | 4 |
| 5 | 19 | 2 | 700 | na | na | * | * | 2 | 8 |
| 4 | 15 | 2 | 910 | na | na | 10 | * | 2 | 6 |
| 1 | 7 | 0 | 700 | na | na | * | * | * | * |
| 1 | 8 | 0 | 710 | na | na | 10 | 4 | 2 | * |

| FOOD NAME | Serving Size | Calories | |
|---|---|---|---|
| *Mix* | | | |
| Beef Flavor with Vegetables (Cup-A-Ramen) | 8 oz | 270 | |
| Chicken Flavor with Vegetables (Cup-A-Ramen) | 8 oz | 270 | |
| Oriental Flavor with Vegetables (Cup-A-Ramen) | 8 oz | 270 | |
| Shrimp Flavor with Vegetables (Cup-A-Ramen) | 8 oz | 280 | |
| Beef Flavor with Vegetables (Low-Fat Cup-A-Ramen) | 8 oz | 220 | |
| Chicken Flavor with Vegetables (Low-Fat Cup-A-Ramen) | 8 oz | 220 | |
| Oriental Flavor with Vegetables (Low-Fat Cup-A-Ramen) | 8 oz | 220 | |
| Shrimp Flavor with Vegetables (Low-Fat Cup-A-Ramen) | 8 oz | 230 | |
| *Mix* | | | |
| Beef Flavor (Low-Fat Block Ramen Noodle) | 8 oz | 160 | |
| Chicken Flavor (Low-Fat Block Ramen Noodle) | 8 oz | 160 | |
| Oriental Flavor (Low-Fat Block Ramen Noodle) | 8 oz | 150 | |
| Pork Flavor (Low-Fat Block Ramen Noodle) | 8 oz | 150 | |
| Beef Flavor (Ramen Noodle) | 8 oz | 190 | |

| Protein (g) | Carbohydrates (g) | Fat (g) | Sodium (mg) | Cholesterol (mg) | Fiber (g) | Vitamin A (%) | Vitamin C (%) | Calcium (%) | Iron (%) |
|---|---|---|---|---|---|---|---|---|---|
| 6 | 38 | 10 | 1530 | na | na | 20 | * | 2 | 10 |
| 6 | 38 | 10 | 1470 | na | na | 20 | 2 | 2 | 10 |
| 6 | 38 | 10 | 1210 | na | na | 15 | 2 | 2 | 15 |
| 6 | 40 | 10 | 1190 | na | na | 30 | 4 | 2 | 10 |
| 7 | 44 | 2 | 1600 | na | na | 40 | 2 | 2 | 10 |
| 7 | 44 | 2 | 1500 | na | na | 40 | 2 | 2 | 10 |
| 7 | 44 | 2 | 1400 | na | na | 40 | 2 | 2 | 10 |
| 7 | 45 | 2 | 1290 | na | na | 25 | 2 | 2 | 15 |
| 5 | 32 | 1 | 890 | na | na | * | * | * | 10 |
| 5 | 32 | 1 | 940 | na | na | * | * | * | 10 |
| 5 | 31 | 1 | 940 | na | na | * | * | * | 10 |
| 4 | 31 | 1 | 1140 | na | na | * | * | * | 15 |
| 5 | 26 | 8 | 1010 | na | na | * | * | 2 | 8 |

| FOOD NAME | Serving Size | Calories |
|---|---|---|
| Chicken Flavor (Ramen Noodle) | 8 oz | 190 |
| Oriental Flavor (Ramen Noodle) | 8 oz | 190 |
| Pork Flavor (Ramen Noodle) | 8 oz | 200 |
| SOUR CREAM | ¼ cup | 124 |
| Imitation | ¼ cup | 104 |
| Light (Land O' Lakes) | 2 tbsp | 40 |
| Light with Chives (Land O' Lakes) | 2 tbsp | 40 |
| SOY SAUCE | 1 tbsp | 12 |
| Kikkoman | 1 tbsp | 10 |
| La Choy | 1 tbsp | 8 |
| SOYBEANS Cooked | 1 cup | 234 |
| SOYBEAN CAKE (Tofu) | 4 oz | 82 |
| SPAGHETTI | | |
| *Dry* | 2 oz | 210 |
| Canned | | |
| In Tomato Sauce with Cheese | | |
| (Franco-American) | 7⅜ oz | 180 |
| With Meatballs in | | |
| Tomato Sauce (Franco-American) | 7⅜ oz | 220 |
| SpaghettiO's in Tomato & Cheese Sauce | 7½ oz | 170 |
| SpaghettiO's with Meatballs | 7⅜ oz | 220 |
| SpaghettiO's with Sliced Franks | 7⅜ oz | 220 |
| *Mix* | | |
| Mild American Spaghetti Dinner (Kraft) | 1 cup | 300 |
| With Meat Sauce Dinner (Kraft) | 1 cup | 360 |

| Protein (g) | Carbohydrates (g) | Fat (g) | Sodium (mg) | Cholesterol (mg) | Fiber (g) | Vitamin A (%) | Vitamin C (%) | Calcium (%) | Iron (%) |
|---|---|---|---|---|---|---|---|---|---|
| 5 | 26 | 8 | 970 | na | na | * | * | 2 | 10 |
| 5 | 26 | 8 | 930 | na | na | * | * | 2 | 10 |
| 5 | 26 | 8 | 860 | na | na | * | * | * | 8 |
| 2 | 3 | 12 | 29 | 25 | 0 | 9 | 1 | 7 | * |
| 2 | 3 | 10 | 61 | na | 0 | * | 1 | 7 | * |
| 2 | 4 | 2 | 35 | 5 | 0 | 4 | * | 4 | * |
| 2 | 4 | 2 | 150 | 5 | 0 | 8 | 2 | 4 | * |
| 1 | 2 | <1 | 1320 | 0 | 0 | * | * | 2 | 4 |
| 1 | 1 | Tr | 892 | 0 | 0 | * | * | 2 | 4 |
| 1 | 1 | 0 | 975 | 0 | 0 | * | * | 2 | 4 |
| 20 | 19 | 10 | 4 | 0 | 10 | 1 | * | 13 | 27 |
| 9 | 3 | 5 | 8 | 0 | 1.2 | * | * | 15 | 12 |
| 7 | 42 | 1 | 0 | 0 | na | * | * | * | 10 |
| 5 | 36 | 2 | 840 | na | na | 8 | * | 2 | 8 |
| 10 | 28 | 8 | 870 | na | na | 8 | * | 2 | 10 |
| 5 | 33 | 2 | 860 | na | na | 10 | * | 2 | 6 |
| 9 | 25 | 9 | 950 | na | na | 8 | * | 2 | 10 |
| 8 | 26 | 9 | 1000 | na | na | 8 | * | 2 | 8 |
| 10 | 50 | 7 | 630 | 0 | na | 20 | 6 | 15 | 15 |
| 12 | 47 | 14 | 880 | 15 | na | 10 | 10 | 15 | 15 |

| FOOD NAME | Serving Size | Calories | |
|---|---|---|---|
| Tangy Italian Style Spaghetti Dinner (Kraft) | 1 cup | 310 | |
| **SPAGHETTI SAUCE** | | | |
| Extra Chunky Garden Combination (Prego) | 4 oz | 80 | |
| Extra Chunky Mushroom and Green Pepper (Prego) | 4 oz | 100 | |
| Extra Chunky Mushroom and Onion (Prego) | 4 oz | 100 | |
| Extra Chunky Mushroom and Tomato (Prego)) | 4 oz | 110 | |
| Extra Chunky Mushroom with Extra Spice (Prego) | 4 oz | 100 | |
| Extra Chunky Sausage & Green Pepper (Prego) | 4 oz | 160 | |
| Extra Chunky Tomato and Onion (Prego) | 4 oz | 110 | |
| Italian, from mix (French's) | ½ cup | 80 | |
| Marinara (Prego) | 4 oz | 100 | |
| Meat Flavored (Prego) | 4 oz | 140 | |
| Mushroom (Prego) | 4 oz | 130 | |
| Mushroom, from mix (French's) | ½ cup | 100 | |
| No Salt Added (Hunt's) | 4 oz | 80 | |
| No Salt Added (Prego) | 4 oz | 110 | |
| Onion and Garlic (Prego) | 4 oz | 110 | |
| Ragu | 4 oz | 80 | |
| Regular (Prego) | 4 oz | 130 | |

| Protein (g) | Carbohydrates (g) | Fat (g) | Sodium (mg) | Cholesterol (mg) | Fiber (g) | Vitamin A (%) | Vitamin C (%) | Calcium (%) | Iron (%) |
|---|---|---|---|---|---|---|---|---|---|
| 111 | 49 | 8 | 670 | 5 | na | 20 | 8 | 15 | 15 |
| 2 | 14 | 2 | 420 | na | na | 20 | 40 | 4 | 6 |
| 2 | 14 | 4 | 410 | na | na | 15 | 20 | 2 | 6 |
| 2 | 13 | 4 | 490 | na | na | 10 | 20 | 2 | 6 |
| 1 | 14 | 5 | 500 | na | na | 10 | 20 | 2 | 6 |
| 2 | 17 | 3 | 450 | na | na | 15 | 35 | 4 | 6 |
| 3 | 19 | 8 | 500 | na | na | 20 | 30 | 4 | 6 |
| 2 | 14 | 5 | 490 | na | na | 10 | 20 | 2 | 6 |
| 2 | 12 | 3 | 720 | na | 0 | 28 | 24 | 2 | 6 |
| 2 | 10 | 6 | 620 | na | na | 15 | 30 | 2 | 4 |
| 2 | 20 | 6 | 660 | na | na | 20 | 25 | 4 | 6 |
| 2 | 20 | 5 | 630 | na | na | 20 | 25 | 4 | 4 |
| 2 | 13 | 4 | 1045 | na | 0 | 35 | 30 | 4 | 8 |
| 2 | 13 | 2 | 30 | na | na | 30 | 35 | 2 | 10 |
| 2 | 11 | 6 | 25 | na | na | 30 | 30 | 4 | 6 |
| 1 | 16 | 4 | 510 | na | na | 20 | 8 | 2 | 6 |
| 2 | 9 | 4 | 740 | 0 | na | 15 | 10 | 2 | 4 |
| 2 | 20 | 5 | 630 | na | na | 20 | 30 | 4 | 6 |

| FOOD NAME | Serving Size | Calories |
|---|---|---|
| Thick, from mix (French's) | ½ cup | 97 |
| Three Cheese (Prego) | 4 oz | 100 |
| Tomato & Basil (Prego) | 4 oz | 100 |
| Traditional (Hunt's) | 4 oz | 70 |
| SPINACH | | |
| *Raw*, chopped | 1 cup | 12 |
| *Cooked*, drained | 1 cup | 42 |
| *Canned* | | |
| Del Monte | ½ cup | 25 |
| Del Monte No Salt | ½ cup | 25 |
| *Frozen* | | |
| Birds Eye Chopped | 3.3 oz | 20 |
| Birds Eye Whole Leaf | 3.3 oz | 20 |
| Birds Eye, Creamed | 3 oz | 60 |
| Green Giant | ½ cup | 25 |
| Green Giant, in Butter Sauce | ½ cup | 40 |
| Green Giant, Creamed | ½ cup | 70 |
| Stouffer's, Creamed | 9 oz | 170 |
| Stouffer's, Souffle | 12 oz | 140 |
| SQUASH | | |
| Summer, cooked | 1 cup | 30 |
| Winter, cooked | 1 cup | 130 |
| Winter, frozen (Birds Eye) | 4 oz | 45 |
| STRAWBERRIES | | |
| *Fresh* | 1 cup | 46 |

| Protein (g) | Carbohydrates (g) | Fat (g) | Sodium (mg) | Cholesterol (mg) | Fiber (g) | Vitamin A (%) | Vitamin C (%) | Calcium (%) | Iron (%) |
|---|---|---|---|---|---|---|---|---|---|
| 2 | 14 | 4 | 831 | na | 0 | 29 | 29 | 1 | 6 |
| 3 | 17 | 2 | 410 | na | na | 15 | 35 | 4 | 8 |
| 2 | 18 | 2 | 370 | na | na | 20 | 35 | 4 | 6 |
| 2 | 12 | 2 | 530 | 0 | na | na | na | na | na |
| | | | | | | | | | |
| 2 | 2 | Tr | 44 | 0 | 1.4 | 90 | 45 | 6 | 10 |
| 5 | 7 | Tr | 126 | 0 | 4 | 292 | 80 | 15 | 20 |
| | | | | | | | | | |
| 2 | 4 | 0 | 355 | 0 | na | 164 | 20 | 10 | 8 |
| 2 | 4 | 0 | 35 | 0 | na | 164 | 20 | 10 | 8 |
| | | | | | | | | | |
| 3 | 3 | 0 | 90 | 0 | 3 | 150 | 35 | 10 | 10 |
| 3 | 4 | 0 | 90 | 0 | 3 | 150 | 45 | 10 | 10 |
| 2 | 5 | 4 | 310 | 0 | 1 | 80 | 20 | 8 | 6 |
| 4 | 5 | 0 | 170 | 0 | 3 | 50 | 10 | 10 | 8 |
| 3 | 6 | 2 | 380 | 5 | 3.5 | 140 | 40 | 10 | 10 |
| 3 | 10 | 3 | 480 | 2 | 2 | 35 | 4 | 10 | 4 |
| 4 | 7 | 14 | 380 | na | na | 60 | 4 | 10 | 6 |
| 6 | 8 | 9 | 500 | na | na | 30 | 4 | 8 | 6 |
| | | | | | | | | | |
| 2 | 7 | Tr | 2 | 0 | 2 | 15 | 35 | 6 | 4 |
| 3 | 32 | 1 | 2 | 0 | 6 | 170 | 45 | 6 | 8 |
| 1 | 11 | 0 | 0 | 0 | 2 | 90 | 20 | 2 | 4 |
| | | | | | | | | | |
| 1 | 10 | <1 | 2 | 0 | 3.8 | 2 | 150 | 4 | 8 |

| FOOD NAME | Serving Size | Calories | |
|---|---|---|---|
| *Frozen* | | | |
| Birds Eye, Halved in Syrup | 5 oz | 120 | |
| Birds Eye, Halved in Lite Syrup | 5 oz | 90 | |
| Birds Eye, Whole in Lite Syrup | 4 oz | 80 | |
| **STRAWBERRY JUICE DRINK** | | | |
| Kool-Aid | 8 fl oz | 80 | |
| Kool-Aid Unsweetened | 8 fl oz | 2 | |
| Tang Fruit Box | 8.5 oz | 120 | |
| **STUFFING** | | | |
| Americana San Francisco (Stove Top) | ½ cup | 100 | |
| Americana San Francisco, with butter and salt (Stove Top) | ½ cup | 170 | |
| Apple & Raisin (Pepperidge Farm) | 1 oz | 110 | |
| Beef (Stove Top) | ½ cup | 110 | |
| Beef, with butter and salt (Stove Top) | ½ cup | 180 | |
| Broccoli and Cheese (Stove Top Microwave) | ½ cup | 140 | |
| Broccoli and Cheese, with butter and salt (Stove Top Microwave) | ½ cup | 170 | |
| Chicken (Stove Top) | ½ cup | 110 | |
| Chicken, with butter and salt (Stove Top) | ½ cup | 180 | |
| Chicken (Stove Top Flexible Serving) | ½ cup | 120 | |
| Chicken, with butter and salt (Stove Top Flexible Serving) | ½ cup | 170 | |
| Chicken (Stove Top Microwave) | ½ cup | 130 | |

| Protein (g) | Carbohydrates (g) | Fat (g) | Sodium (mg) | Cholesterol (mg) | Fiber (g) | Vitamin A (%) | Vitamin C (%) | Calcium (%) | Iron (%) |
|---|---|---|---|---|---|---|---|---|---|
| 1 | 20 | 0 | 0 | 0 | 2 | * | 110 | * | 4 |
| 1 | 22 | 0 | 5 | 0 | 2 | * | 110 | * | 2 |
| 1 | 20 | 0 | 0 | 0 | 2 | * | 80 | * | * |
| 0 | 20 | 0 | 25 | 0 | 0 | * | 10 | * | * |
| 0 | 0 | 0 | 25 | 0 | 0 | * | 10 | * | * |
| 0 | 32 | 0 | 10 | 0 | 0 | * | 100 | * | * |
| 4 | 20 | 1 | 570 | 0 | na | 2 | 2 | 4 | 4 |
| 4 | 20 | 9 | 650 | 20 | na | 8 | 2 | 4 | 4 |
| 3 | 21 | 1 | 410 | na | na | * | 2 | 2 | 10 |
| 4 | 21 | 1 | 520 | 0 | na | 4 | 4 | 4 | 4 |
| 4 | 21 | 9 | 590 | 20 | na | 10 | 4 | 4 | 4 |
| 4 | 20 | 5 | 540 | 5 | na | * | 6 | 4 | 8 |
| 4 | 20 | 8 | 580 | 15 | na | 4 | 6 | 4 | 8 |
| 4 | 20 | 1 | 490 | 0 | na | * | 4 | 4 | 4 |
| 4 | 20 | 9 | 570 | 20 | na | 6 | 4 | 4 | 4 |
| 4 | 20 | 3 | 520 | 0 | na | * | 2 | 4 | 4 |
| 4 | 20 | 9 | 580 | 15 | na | 6 | 2 | 4 | 4 |
| 4 | 20 | 4 | 440 | 0 | na | * | 2 | 4 | 4 |

| FOOD NAME | Serving Size | Calories | |
|---|---|---|---|
| Chicken, with butter and salt | | | |
| (Stove Top Microwave) | ½ cup | 160 | |
| Classic Chicken (Pepperidge Farm) | 1 oz | 110 | |
| Cornbread (Stove Top) | ½ cup | 110 | |
| Cornbread, with butter and salt | | | |
| (Stove Top) | ½ cup | 170 | |
| Cornbread (Stove Top | | | |
| Flexible Serving) | ½ cup | 130 | |
| Cornbread, with butter and salt | | | |
| (Stove Top Flexible Serving) | ½ cup | 180 | |
| Cornbread, with butter and salt | | | |
| (Stove Top Microwave) | ½ cup | 1160 | |
| Cornbread, Homestyle | | | |
| (Stove Top Microwave) | ½ cup | 120 | |
| Country Garden Herb | | | |
| (Pepperidge Farm) | 1 oz | 120 | |
| Harvest Vegetable & Almond | | | |
| (Pepperidge Farm) | 1 oz | 110 | |
| Homestyle Herb (Stove Top | | | |
| Flexible Serving) | ½ cup | 120 | |
| Homestyle Herb, with butter and salt | | | |
| (Stove Top Flexible Serving) | ½ cup | 170 | |
| Long Grain and Wild Rice (Stove Top) | ½ cup | 110 | |
| Long Grain and Wild Rice, | | | |
| with butter and salt (Stove Top) | ½ cup | 180 | |

| Protein (g) | Carbohydrates (g) | Fat (g) | Sodium (mg) | Cholesterol (mg) | Fiber (g) | Vitamin A (%) | Vitamin C (%) | Calcium (%) | Iron (%) |
|---|---|---|---|---|---|---|---|---|---|
| 4 | 20 | 7 | 480 | 10 | na | 4 | 2 | 4 | 4 |
| 4 | 20 | 1 | 410 | na | na | 6 | 8 | 4 | 8 |
| 3 | 21 | 1 | 490 | 0 | na | * | 2 | 4 | 4 |
| 3 | 21 | 9 | 570 | 20 | na | 6 | 2 | 4 | 4 |
| 4 | 22 | 3 | 540 | 0 | na | * | 2 | 4 | 4 |
| 4 | 22 | 9 | 600 | 15 | na | 6 | 2 | 4 | 4 |
| 3 | 20 | 7 | 450 | 10 | na | 4 | * | 4 | 2 |
| 3 | 20 | 3 | 410 | 0 | na | * | * | 4 | 2 |
| 4 | 18 | 4 | 300 | na | na | * | 4 | 4 | 10 |
| 4 | 19 | 3 | 250 | na | na | * | 10 | 4 | 15 |
| 4 | 20 | 3 | 460 | 0 | na | * | 4 | 6 | 4 |
| 4 | 20 | 9 | 520 | 15 | na | 6 | 4 | 6 | 4 |
| 4 | 22 | 1 | 480 | 0 | na | * | 2 | 4 | 4 |
| 4 | 22 | 9 | 560 | 20 | na | 6 | 2 | 4 | 4 |

| FOOD NAME | Serving Size | Calories |
|---|---|---|
| Mushroom and Onion (Stove Top) | ½ cup | 110 |
| Mushroom and Onion, with butter and salt (Stove Top) | ½ cup | 180 |
| Mushroom and Onion Flavor (Stove Top Microwave) | ½ cup | 130 |
| Mushroom and Onion Flavor, with butter and salt (Stove Top Microwave) | ½ cup | 170 |
| Pork (Stove Top) | ½ cup | 110 |
| Pork, with butter and salt (Stove Top) | ½ cup | 170 |
| Pork (Stove Top Flexible Serving) | ½ cup | 120 |
| Pork, with butter and salt (Stove Top Flexible Serving) | ½ cup | 170 |
| Savory Herbs (Stove Top) | ½ cup | 110 |
| Savory Herbs, with butter and salt (Stove Top) | ½ cup | 170 |
| Turkey (Stove Top) | ½ cup | 110 |
| Turkey, with butter and salt (Stove Top) | ½ cup | 170 |
| Wild Rice (Stove Top) | ½ cup | 110 |
| Wild Rice, with butter and salt (Stove Top) | ½ cup | 180 |
| SUGAR | | |
| Brown | 1 cup | 820 |
| White | 1 cup | 770 |
| White | 1 tsp | 13 |
| SUNFLOWER SEEDS  Kernels | 1 oz | 160 |

| Protein (g) | Carbohydrates (g) | Fat (g) | Sodium (mg) | Cholesterol (mg) | Fiber (g) | Vitamin A (%) | Vitamin C (%) | Calcium (%) | Iron (%) |
|---|---|---|---|---|---|---|---|---|---|
| 4 | 20 | 1 | 410 | 0 | na | * | 2 | 4 | 4 |
| 4 | 20 | 9 | 490 | 20 | na | 6 | 2 | 4 | 4 |
| 4 | 21 | 3 | 470 | 0 | na | * | 2 | 4 | 4 |
| 4 | 21 | 7 | 510 | 10 | na | 4 | 2 | 4 | 4 |
| 4 | 20 | 1 | 490 | 0 | na | 4 | 4 | 6 | 4 |
| 4 | 20 | 9 | 570 | 20 | na | 8 | 4 | 6 | 4 |
| 4 | 20 | 3 | 580 | 0 | na | * | 4 | 6 | 4 |
| 4 | 20 | 9 | 630 | 15 | na | 6 | 4 | 6 | 4 |
| 4 | 20 | 1 | 510 | 0 | na | * | 4 | 6 | 4 |
| 4 | 20 | 9 | 590 | 20 | na | 6 | 4 | 6 | 4 |
| 4 | 20 | 1 | 560 | 0 | na | * | 4 | 4 | 4 |
| 4 | 20 | 9 | 640 | 20 | na | 6 | 4 | 4 | 4 |
| 4 | 22 | 1 | 490 | 0 | na | * | 2 | 4 | 4 |
| 4 | 22 | 9 | 570 | 20 | na | 6 | 2 | 4 | 4 |
| 0 | 210 | 0 | 66 | 0 | 0 | * | * | 20 | 40 |
| 0 | 200 | 0 | 2 | 0 | 0 | * | * | * | 2 |
| 0 | 4 | 0 | Tr | 0 | 0 | * | * | * | * |
| 7 | 6 | 13 | 3 | 0 | 4.4 | * | * | 3 | 11 |

| FOOD NAME | Serving Size | Calories | |
|---|---|---|---|
| **SWEET POTATO** | | | |
| Baked in skin | 1 | 120 | |
| Mashed | ½ cup | 170 | |
| **SWORDFISH** Broiled in butter | 3 oz | 140 | |
| **SYRUP** | | | |
| Corn, Dark (Karo) | 1 tbsp | 60 | |
| Corn, Light (Karo) | 1 tbsp | 60 | |
| Fruit (Smucker's) | 2 tbsp | 100 | |
| Maple (Log Cabin) | 1 oz | 100 | |
| Maple (Log Cabin Country Kitchen) | 1 oz | 100 | |
| Maple (Log Cabin Lite) | 1 oz | 50 | |
| Pancake (Golden Griddle) | 1 tbsp | 50 | |
| Pancake (Karo) | 1 tbsp | 60 | |
| Sorghum | 1 tbsp | 60 | |
| **TACO SAUCE** | | | |
| Hot (Del Monte) | ¼ cup | 15 | |
| Hot (Old El Paso) | 2 tbsp | 11 | |
| Mild (Del Monte) | ¼ cup | 15 | |
| Mild (Old El Paso) | 2 tbsp | 11 | |
| **TACO SHELL** (Old El Paso) | 1 | 51 | |
| **TACO STARTER** (Del Monte) | 8 fl oz | 140 | |
| **TAMALES** (Old El Paso) | 2 | 232 | |
| **TANGERINE** | 1 | 40 | |
| **TANGERINE JUICE** | | | |
| Frozen (Minute Maid) | 6 fl oz | 85 | |

| Protein (g) | Carbohydrates (g) | Fat (g) | Sodium (mg) | Cholesterol (mg) | Fiber (g) | Vitamin A (%) | Vitamin C (%) | Calcium (%) | Iron (%) |
|---|---|---|---|---|---|---|---|---|---|
| 2 | 28 | Tr | 12 | 0 | 3.9 | 185 | 42 | 5 | 6 |
| 3 | 40 | <1 | 21 | 0 | 3 | 239 | 43 | 5 | 6 |
| 24 | 0 | 6 | na | 45 | 0 | 35 | * | 2 | 6 |
| | | | | | | | | | |
| 0 | 15 | 0 | 40 | 0 | 0 | * | * | * | * |
| 0 | 15 | 0 | 30 | 0 | 0 | * | * | * | * |
| 0 | 26 | 0 | <10 | na | na | * | * | * | * |
| 0 | 26 | 0 | 35 | 0 | 0 | * | * | * | * |
| 0 | 26 | 0 | 20 | 0 | 0 | * | * | * | * |
| 0 | 13 | 0 | 90 | 0 | 0 | * | * | * | * |
| 0 | 13 | 0 | 20 | 0 | 0 | * | * | * | * |
| 0 | 15 | 0 | 35 | 0 | 0 | * | * | * | * |
| 0 | 14 | 0 | na | 0 | na | * | * | 4 | 15 |
| | | | | | | | | | |
| 0 | 4 | 0 | 440 | na | na | 6 | 2 | * | 2 |
| 0 | 2 | 0 | 131 | na | na | * | * | * | * |
| 0 | 4 | 0 | 480 | na | na | 4 | * | * | 2 |
| 0 | 2 | 0 | 125 | na | na | * | 2 | * | * |
| 1 | 7 | 2 | 50 | na | na | * | * | * | 2 |
| 2 | 28 | 1 | 2180 | na | na | 100 | 15 | 6 | 15 |
| 6 | 23 | 13 | na | na | na | 2 | * | 3 | 25 |
| 1 | 10 | 0 | 1 | 0 | 0.3 | 7 | 45 | 3 | 2 |
| | | | | | | | | | |
| 1 | 22 | Tr | 19 | 0 | na | 10 | 60 | 2 | 2 |

| FOOD NAME | Serving Size | Calories | |
|---|---|---|---|
| **TARTAR SAUCE** | | | |
| (Kraft Sauceworks) | 1 tbsp | 50 | |
| Natural Lemon and Herb Flavor | | | |
| (Kraft Sauceworks) | 1 tbsp | 70 | |
| **TEA** | | | |
| Brewed Bag (Lipton) | 1 cup | 2 | |
| Brewed Instant (Lipton) | 8 fl oz | 2 | |
| Flavored (Bigelow, all varieties) | 5¼ fl oz | 1 | |
| Flavored (Celestial Seasonings, | | | |
| most varieties) | 8 fl oz | <4 | |
| Herbal (Bigelow, most varieties) | 5 fl oz | <2 | |
| Herbal (Celestial Seasonings, | | | |
| most varieties) | 8 fl oz | <6 | |
| Herbal (Lipton, most varieties) | 8 fl oz | <5 | |
| Iced Mix (Crystal Light) | 8 fl oz | 4 | |
| Iced Mix (Crystal Light Decaffeinated) | 8 fl oz | 4 | |
| Iced Mix (Nestea, all flavors) | 6 fl oz | 6 | |
| Iced Mix, Lemon (Lipton) | 6 fl oz | 55 | |
| **TERIYAKI SAUCE** (French's mix) | ¼ cup | 70 | |
| **TOFU** | 4 oz | 82 | |
| **TOMATO** | | | |
| Raw | 1 | 26 | |
| Cooked | 1 cup | 60 | |
| *Canned* | | | |
| Whole (Hunt's) | 4 oz | 20 | |

| Protein (g) | Carbohydrates (g) | Fat (g) | Sodium (mg) | Cholesterol (mg) | Fiber (g) | Vitamin A (%) | Vitamin C (%) | Calcium (%) | Iron (%) |
|---|---|---|---|---|---|---|---|---|---|
| 0 | 2 | 5 | 85 | 5 | na | * | * | * | * |
| 0 | 0 | 8 | 85 | 5 | na | * | * | * | * |
| 0 | 0 | 0 | 0 | 0 | 0 | * | * | * | * |
| 0 | 0 | 0 | 0 | 0 | 0 | * | 8 | * | * |
| 0 | 0 | 0 | 0 | 0 | 0 | * | * | * | * |
| Tr | <1 | Tr | <3 | 0 | 0 | * | * | * | * |
| Tr | Tr | Tr | <4 | 0 | 0 | * | * | * | * |
| Tr | <2 | Tr | <9 | 0 | 0 | * | * | * | * |
| 0 | <2 | 0 | 0 | 0 | 0 | * | * | * | * |
| 0 | 0 | 0 | 0 | 0 | 0 | * | 10 | * | * |
| 0 | 0 | 0 | 0 | 0 | 0 | * | * | * | * |
| 0 | 1 | 0 | 0 | 0 | 0 | * | * | * | * |
| 0 | 14 | 0 | 1 | 0 | 0 | * | * | * | * |
| 2 | 14 | 0 | 2360 | na | na | * | * | 4 | 8 |
| 9 | 3 | 5 | 8 | 0 | 1.2 | * | * | 15 | 12 |
| 1 | 6 | Tr | 11 | 0 | 1.6 | 35 | 70 | 2 | 4 |
| 3 | 14 | 1 | 26 | 0 | 2 | 50 | 100 | 4 | 8 |
| 0 | 5 | 0 | 415 | 0 | na | 15 | 20 | 4 | 4 |

| FOOD NAME | Serving Size | Calories | |
|---|---|---|---|
| Whole (Hunt's No Salt) | 4 oz | 20 | |
| Whole, peeled (Contadina) | ½ cup | 25 | |
| Whole, peeled (Del Monte) | ½ cup | 25 | |
| Wedges (Del Monte) | ½ cup | 30 | |
| Stewed (Contadina) | ½ cup | 35 | |
| Stewed (Del Monte) | ½ cup | 35 | |
| Stewed (Del Monte No Salt) | ½ cup | 35 | |
| Stewed (Hunt's) | 4 oz | 35 | |
| Stewed (Hunt's No Salt) | 4 oz | 35 | |
| **TOMATO PASTE** | | | |
| *Canned* | | | |
| Contadina | 6 oz | 150 | |
| Del Monte | ¾ cup | 150 | |
| Del Monte No Salt | 6 oz | 150 | |
| Hunt's | 2 oz | 45 | |
| Hunt's No Salt | 2 oz | 45 | |
| Italian Style (Contadina) | 2 oz | 70 | |
| Italian Style (Hunt's) | 2 oz | 50 | |
| **TOMATO PUREE** | | | |
| Contadina | ½ cup | 50 | |
| Hunt's | 4 oz | 45 | |
| **TOMATO SAUCE** | | | |
| Contadina | ½ cup | 45 | |
| Hunt's | ½ cup | 35 | |
| Hunt's Herb | ½ cup | 80 | |

| Protein (g) | Carbohydrates (g) | Fat (g) | Sodium (mg) | Cholesterol (mg) | Fiber (g) | Vitamin A (%) | Vitamin C (%) | Calcium (%) | Iron (%) |
|---|---|---|---|---|---|---|---|---|---|
| 0 | 5 | 0 | 15 | 0 | na | 15 | 20 | 4 | 4 |
| 0 | 6 | 0 | 390 | 0 | na | 15 | 30 | 4 | 2 |
| 0 | 5 | 0 | 220 | 0 | na | 10 | 30 | 2 | 2 |
| 0 | 8 | 0 | 355 | 0 | na | 10 | 25 | 2 | 2 |
| 0 | 9 | 0 | 405 | 0 | na | 10 | 25 | 4 | 2 |
| 0 | 8 | 0 | 355 | 0 | na | 10 | 30 | 2 | 2 |
| 0 | 8 | 0 | 45 | 0 | na | 10 | 30 | 2 | 2 |
| 2 | 8 | 0 | 460 | 0 | na | 15 | 30 | 4 | 6 |
| 2 | 8 | 0 | 20 | 0 | na | 15 | 30 | 4 | 6 |
| | | | | | | | | | |
| 6 | 35 | 0 | 135 | 0 | na | 90 | 80 | 4 | 10 |
| 4 | 34 | 1 | 110 | 0 | na | 90 | 60 | 6 | 15 |
| 4 | 34 | 1 | 110 | 0 | na | 90 | 60 | 6 | 15 |
| 2 | 11 | 0 | 150 | 0 | na | 40 | 45 | 2 | 10 |
| 2 | 11 | 0 | 25 | 0 | na | 40 | 45 | 2 | 10 |
| 2 | 12 | 1 | 710 | 0 | na | 20 | 10 | 2 | 4 |
| 2 | 11 | 0 | 525 | 0 | na | 40 | 45 | 2 | 10 |
| | | | | | | | | | |
| 2 | 11 | 0 | 90 | 0 | na | 25 | 25 | * | 4 |
| 2 | 10 | 0 | 185 | 0 | na | 35 | 45 | 2 | 10 |
| | | | | | | | | | |
| 2 | 9 | 0 | 680 | 0 | na | 25 | 15 | * | 4 |
| 1 | 8 | 0 | 665 | 0 | na | 20 | 10 | * | 2 |
| 2 | 12 | 4 | 495 | 0 | na | 20 | 15 | 2 | 4 |

| FOOD NAME | Serving Size | Calories |
|---|---|---|
| Hunt's Special | ½ cup | 40 |
| Hunt's with Bits | ½ cup | 35 |
| Hunt's with Cheese | ½ cup | 70 |
| Hunt's with Mushrooms | ½ cup | 40 |
| TOPPING | | |
| Butterscotch (Kraft) | 1 tbsp | 60 |
| Caramel (Kraft) | 1 tbsp | 60 |
| Chocolate (Kraft) | 1 tbsp | 50 |
| Cool Whip (Birds Eye Extra Creamy) | 1 tbsp | 14 |
| Cool Whip Lite (Birds Eye) | 1 tbsp | 8 |
| Cool Whip Non-Dairy (Birds Eye) | 1 tbsp | 12 |
| Dream Whip mix, prepared with whole milk | 1 tbsp | 10 |
| D-Zerta Reduced Calorie Whipped | 1 tbsp | 8 |
| Hot Fudge (Kraft) | 1 tbsp | 70 |
| Pineapple (Kraft) | 1 tbsp | 50 |
| Real Cream (Kraft) | ¼ cup | 30 |
| Strawberry (Kraft) | 1 tbsp | 50 |
| Whipped (Kraft) | ¼ cup | 35 |
| TUNA | | |
| Canned in water | 4 oz | 144 |
| Canned in oil | 4 oz | 227 |
| TURKEY | | |
| Breast, Barbecued (Louis Rich) | 1 oz | 40 |
| Breast (Louis Rich) | 1 oz | 45 |

| Protein (g) | Carbohydrates (g) | Fat (g) | Sodium (mg) | Cholesterol (mg) | Fiber (g) | Vitamin A (%) | Vitamin C (%) | Calcium (%) | Iron (%) |
|---|---|---|---|---|---|---|---|---|---|
| 1 | 10 | 0 | na | 0 | na | 15 | 15 | * | 2 |
| 1 | 8 | 0 | 695 | 0 | na | 20 | 20 | * | 2 |
| 3 | 10 | 2 | 795 | 0 | na | 20 | 10 | 4 | 4 |
| 1 | 9 | 0 | 710 | 0 | na | 20 | 25 | * | 4 |
| | | | | | | | | | |
| 0 | 13 | 1 | 70 | 0 | 0 | * | * | * | * |
| 1 | 13 | 0 | 45 | 0 | 0 | * | * | 4 | * |
| 11 | 11 | 0 | 15 | 0 | 0 | * | * | * | * |
| 0 | 1 | 1 | 0 | 0 | 0 | * | * | * | * |
| 0 | 1 | <1 | 0 | 0 | 0 | * | * | * | * |
| 0 | 1 | 1 | 0 | 0 | 0 | * | * | * | * |
| | | | | | | | | | |
| 0 | 1 | 0 | 0 | 0 | 0 | * | * | * | * |
| 0 | 0 | 1 | 5 | 0 | 0 | * | * | * | * |
| 1 | 11 | 2 | 50 | 0 | 0 | * | * | * | * |
| 0 | 13 | 0 | 0 | 0 | 0 | * | * | * | * |
| 0 | 2 | 2 | 5 | 10 | 0 | 2 | * | * | * |
| 0 | 14 | 0 | 5 | 0 | 0 | * | 2 | * | * |
| 0 | 2 | 3 | 10 | 0 | 0 | * | * | * | * |
| | | | | | | | | | |
| 32 | 0 | 1 | 450 | na | 0 | * | * | * | 10 |
| 32 | 0 | 9 | 400 | na | 0 | 2 | * | 1 | 12 |
| | | | | | | | | | |
| 5 | 0 | 1 | 156 | 10 | 0 | na | na | * | * |
| 8 | 0 | 2 | 25 | 15 | 0 | na | na | * | * |

| FOOD NAME | Serving Size | Calories |
|---|---|---|
| Breast, Hickory Smoked (Louis Rich) | 1 oz | 35 |
| Breast, Oven Roasted (Louis Rich) | 1 slice | 30 |
| Chopped or diced | 1 cup | 238 |
| Dark meat only | 4 oz | 233 |
| Dark and light meat | 4 oz | 193 |
| Drumsticks (Louis Rich) | 1 oz | 60 |
| Light meat only | 4 oz | 200 |
| Wings (Louis Rich) | 1 oz | 55 |
| TURKEY, PROCESSED | | |
| Bologna (Louis Rich) | 2 slices | 120 |
| Breast (Louis Rich) | 2 slices | 60 |
| Franks (Louis Rich) | 1 | 100 |
| Ham (Louis Rich) | 2 slices | 70 |
| Pastrami (Louis Rich) | 2 slices | 70 |
| TURNIP Cooked | 1 cup | 35 |
| TURNOVER | | |
| Apple (Pepperidge Farm) | 1 | 300 |
| Apple (Pillsbury) | 1 | 170 |
| Blueberry (Pepperidge Farm) | 1 | 310 |
| Cherry (Pepperidge Farm) | 1 | 310 |
| Cherry (Pillsbury) | 1 | 170 |
| Peach (Pepperidge Farm) | 1 | 310 |
| Raspberry (Pepperidge Farm) | 1 | 310 |
| V-8 JUICE | | |
| Original | 6 fl oz | 35 |

| Protein (g) | Carbohydrates (g) | Fat (g) | Sodium (mg) | Cholesterol (mg) | Fiber (g) | Vitamin A (%) | Vitamin C (%) | Calcium (%) | Iron (%) |
|---|---|---|---|---|---|---|---|---|---|
| 5 | <1 | 1 | 208 | 10 | 0 | na | na | * | * |
| 5 | Tr | 1 | 214 | na | 0 | na | na | * | * |
| 41 | 0 | 7 | 99 | 107 | 0 | 2 | * | 2 | 10 |
| 35 | 0 | 9 | 112 | 96 | 0 | 5 | * | 3 | 15 |
| 33 | 0 | 6 | 79 | 86 | 0 | * | * | 3 | 11 |
| 8 | 0 | 3 | 24 | 20 | 0 | na | na | * | 3 |
| 37 | 0 | 4 | 59 | 78 | 0 | 3 | * | * | 7 |
| 7 | 0 | 3 | 21 | 15 | 0 | na | na | * | * |
| | | | | | | | | | |
| 7 | 1 | 9 | 444 | na | 0 | na | na | 4 | 4 |
| 12 | 0 | 2 | 380 | na | 0 | na | na | * | * |
| 6 | 1 | 8 | 472 | na | 0 | na | na | 5 | 4 |
| 11 | 0 | 2 | 576 | na | 0 | na | na | * | 4 |
| 11 | 0 | 3 | 556 | na | 0 | na | na | * | 4 |
| 1 | 8 | 0 | 17 | 0 | 4.6 | * | 57 | 5 | 3 |
| | | | | | | | | | |
| 3 | 34 | 17 | 210 | na | na | * | 4 | * | 4 |
| 2 | 23 | 8 | 330 | 0 | na | * | * | * | 4 |
| 3 | 32 | 19 | 230 | na | na | * | 10 | * | 4 |
| 3 | 32 | 19 | 280 | na | na | * | 8 | * | 4 |
| 2 | 24 | 8 | 330 | 0 | na | * | 6 | * | 4 |
| 3 | 34 | 18 | 260 | na | na | 6 | 60 | * | 2 |
| 4 | 36 | 17 | 260 | na | na | * | 20 | * | 4 |
| | | | | | | | | | |
| 1 | 8 | 0 | 640 | na | na | 35 | 45 | 2 | 4 |

| FOOD NAME | Serving Size | Calories | |
|---|---|---|---|
| Low Sodium | 6 fl oz | 40 | |
| Spicy Hot | 6 fl oz | 40 | |
| **VEAL** | | | |
| *Cutlet* Broiled | 4 oz | 250 | |
| *Chop* | | | |
| Loin, lean only | 4 oz | 235 | |
| Loin, lean and fat | 4 oz | 480 | |
| Rib, lean only | 4 oz | 245 | |
| Rib, lean and fat | 4 oz | 360 | |
| **VEGETABLES, MIXED** | | | |
| *Canned* | | | |
| Del Monte | ½ cup | 40 | |
| *Frozen* | | | |
| Birds Eye Bavarian Style | 3.3 oz | 100 | |
| Birds Eye Chinese Style | 3.3 oz | 35 | |
| Birds Eye Oriental Style | 3.3 oz | 70 | |
| Birds Eye Italian Style | 3.3 oz | 100 | |
| Birds Eye Japanese Style | 3.3 oz | 90 | |
| Birds Eye New England Style | 3.3 oz | 130 | |
| Birds Eye Pasta Primavera Style | 3.3 oz | 120 | |
| Birds Eye San Francisco Style | 3.3 oz | 100 | |
| Birds Eye With Authentic Oriental | | | |
| Sauce for Beef | 4.6 oz | 90 | |
| Birds Eye With Creamy Mushroom | | | |
| Sauce for Beef | 4.6 oz | 60 | |

| Protein (g) | Carbohydrates (g) | Fat (g) | Sodium (mg) | Cholesterol (mg) | Fiber (g) | Vitamin A (%) | Vitamin C (%) | Calcium (%) | Iron (%) |
|---|---|---|---|---|---|---|---|---|---|
| 1 | 9 | 0 | 60 | na | na | 35 | 45 | 2 | 4 |
| 1 | 8 | 0 | 660 | na | na | 35 | 45 | 2 | 4 |
| 31 | 0 | 12 | 75 | 120 | 0 | * | * | 1 | 20 |
| 39 | 0 | 8 | 74 | 120 | 0 | * | * | 2 | 27 |
| 26 | 0 | 41 | 50 | 119 | 0 | * | * | 1 | 18 |
| 39 | 0 | 10 | 68 | 130 | 0 | * | * | 2 | 27 |
| 31 | 0 | 25 | 56 | 125 | 0 | * | * | 2 | 22 |
| 2 | 7 | 0 | 355 | 0 | na | 100 | 6 | 2 | 4 |
| 2 | 11 | 5 | 350 | 10 | 2 | 10 | 6 | 4 | 4 |
| 2 | 8 | 0 | 540 | 0 | 2 | 45 | 25 | 4 | 6 |
| 2 | 8 | 4 | 300 | 0 | 1 | 30 | 25 | 4 | 4 |
| 2 | 11 | 5 | 490 | 0 | 2 | 10 | 45 | 4 | 4 |
| 2 | 10 | 5 | 420 | 0 | 2 | 15 | 30 | 2 | 2 |
| 3 | 14 | 7 | 430 | 0 | 2 | 15 | 15 | 2 | 2 |
| 5 | 14 | 5 | 340 | 5 | 2 | 80 | 30 | 10 | 4 |
| 2 | 11 | 5 | 400 | 0 | 1 | 10 | 15 | 2 | 2 |
| 6 | 11 | 4 | 350 | 0 | 2 | 35 | 70 | 4 | 6 |
| 3 | 9 | 2 | 450 | 5 | 2 | 20 | 25 | 4 | 4 |

| FOOD NAME | Serving Size | Calories | |
|---|---|---|---|
| Birds Eye With Delicate Herb Sauce | | | |
|   for Chicken or Shrimp | 4.6 oz | 90 | |
| Birds Eye With Dijon Mustard Sauce | | | |
|   for Chicken or Fish | 4.6 oz | 70 | |
| Birds Eye With Savory Tomato Basil | | | |
|   Sauce for Chicken | 4.6 oz | 110 | |
| Birds Eye With Wild Rice in White | | | |
|   Wine Sauce for Chicken | 4.6 oz | 100 | |
| Green Giant California Style | ½ cup | 25 | |
| Green Giant Heartland Style | ½ cup | 25 | |
| Green Giant Manhattan Style | ½ cup | 25 | |
| Green Giant New England Style | ½ cup | 70 | |
| Green Giant San Francisco Style | ½ cup | 25 | |
| Green Giant Santa Fe Style | ½ cup | 70 | |
| Green Giant Seattle Style | ½ cup | 25 | |
| Green Giant Western Style | ½ cup | 60 | |
| Green Giant With Butter Sauce | ½ cup | 60 | |
| VINEGAR | 2 tbsp | 0 | |
| WAFFLES | | | |
|   Blueberry (Aunt Jemima) | 1 | 80 | |
|   Hot 'n Buttery (Downyflake) | 1 | 65 | |
|   Jumbo (Aunt Jemima) | 1 | 80 | |
|   Jumbo Original (Aunt Jemima) | 1 | 80 | |
| WALNUTS Chopped | ⅓ cup | 260 | |
| WATERCRESS | 10 sprigs | 3 | |

| Protein (g) | Carbohydrates (g) | Fat (g) | Sodium (mg) | Cholesterol (mg) | Fiber (g) | Vitamin A (%) | Vitamin C (%) | Calcium (%) | Iron (%) |
|---|---|---|---|---|---|---|---|---|---|
| 3 | 8 | 5 | 460 | 0 | 2 | 80 | 40 | 2 | 4 |
| 4 | 9 | 3 | 310 | 5 | 1 | 250 | 30 | 4 | 6 |
| 5 | 17 | 3 | 360 | 0 | 1 | 10 | 20 | 4 | 6 |
| 3 | 19 | 0 | 510 | 0 | 1 | 110 | 20 | 2 | 4 |
| 2 | 6 | 0 | 40 | 0 | 2 | 140 | 40 | 2 | * |
| 1 | 6 | 0 | 35 | 0 | 2.5 | 45 | 55 | 2 | 2 |
| 2 | 5 | 0 | 15 | 0 | 2 | 8 | 60 | 2 | 2 |
| 3 | 14 | 1 | 75 | 0 | 4 | 80 | 15 | * | 4 |
| 1 | 7 | 0 | 35 | 0 | 2.5 | 40 | 45 | 2 | 2 |
| 2 | 16 | 1 | 0 | 0 | 2 | 10 | 25 | * | 2 |
| 2 | 7 | 0 | 35 | 0 | 2 | 100 | 35 | 2 | * |
| 2 | 12 | 2 | 25 | 0 | 2 | 8 | 20 | 2 | 2 |
| 2 | 11 | 2 | 300 | 5 | 2 | 80 | 6 | 2 | 4 |
| 0 | 1 | 0 | 0 | 0 | 0 | na | na | * | 1 |
| 2 | 14 | 2 | 315 | 5 | 1.3 | * | * | 4 | 10 |
| 2 | 11 | 3 | na | na | na | * | * | * | 5 |
| 2 | 14 | 2 | 350 | 7 | 1.3 | * | * | 4 | 10 |
| 2 | 14 | 2 | 340 | na | na | * | * | 4 | 10 |
| 9 | 6 | 25 | 1 | 0 | 2.1 | 3 | * | na | 14 |
| <1 | Tr | Tr | 10 | 0 | 0.6 | 35 | 45 | 6 | 4 |

| FOOD NAME | Serving Size | Calories |
|---|---|---|
| Chopped | ½ cup | 2 |
| WATERMELON | 1 slice | 150 |
| WHITEFISH Smoked | 4 oz | 175 |
| WINE | | |
| Dessert | 1 fl oz | 41 |
| Table | 1 fl oz | 25 |
| YAM Cooked | ½ cup | 80 |
| YOGURT | | |
| Cherry (Dannon) | 1 cup | 260 |
| Cherry (Yoplait Custard Style) | 6 oz | 180 |
| Cherry Vanilla (Borden) | 8 oz | 270 |
| Coffee (Dannon) | 1 cup | 200 |
| Fruit Flavors (Y.E.S.) | 6 oz | 190 |
| Fruit Flavors (Yoplait Custard Style) | 6 oz | 190 |
| Fruit Flavors (Yoplait Custard Style) | 4 oz | 130 |
| Fruit Flavors (Yoplait Fat Free) | 6 oz | 150 |
| Fruit Flavors (Yoplait Light) | 6 oz | 80 |
| Fruit Flavors (Yoplait Light) | 4 oz | 60 |
| Fruit Flavors (Yoplait Original) | 6 oz | 190 |
| Fruit Flavors (Yoplait Original) | 4 oz | 120 |
| Lemon (Borden) | 8 oz | 320 |
| Lemon (Dannon) | 1 cup | 200 |
| Mixed Berry (Yoplait Custard Style) | 6 oz | 180 |
| Peach (Dannon) | 1 cup | 260 |
| Pineapple (Borden) | 8 oz | 260 |

| Protein (g) | Carbohydrates (g) | Fat (g) | Sodium (mg) | Cholesterol (mg) | Fiber (g) | Vitamin A (%) | Vitamin C (%) | Calcium (%) | Iron (%) |
|---|---|---|---|---|---|---|---|---|---|
| Tr | Tr | Tr | 7 | 0 | 0.4 | 60 | 85 | 10 | 5 |
| 3 | 35 | 2 | 10 | 0 | 1.9 | 50 | 50 | 3 | 12 |
| 24 | 0 | 8 | 1156 | 37 | 0 | na | na | 3 | na |
| | | | | | | | | | |
| Tr | 2 | 0 | 1 | 0 | 0 | * | * | * | * |
| Tr | 1 | 0 | 1 | 0 | 0 | * | * | * | * |
| 1 | 19 | Tr | 6 | 0 | na | na | na | na | na |
| | | | | | | | | | |
| 9 | 49 | 3 | na | na | 0 | * | * | 35 | * |
| 7 | 30 | 4 | 95 | 20 | 0 | * | * | 20 | * |
| 9 | 54 | 2 | 160 | na | 0 | * | * | 30 | * |
| 11 | 32 | 4 | na | na | 0 | 2 | * | 35 | * |
| 7 | 33 | 4 | 40-90 | na | 0 | 2 | * | 30 | * |
| 7 | 32 | 4 | 95 | 20 | 0 | 2 | * | 20 | * |
| 5 | 21 | 3 | 60 | 15 | 0 | * | * | 15 | * |
| 7 | 31 | 0 | 95 | 5 | 0 | * | * | 25 | * |
| 7 | 13 | 0 | 80 | <5 | 0 | * | * | 15 | * |
| 5 | 9 | 0 | 50 | <5 | 0 | * | * | 10 | * |
| 8 | 32 | 3 | 110 | 10 | 0 | * | * | 25 | * |
| 5 | 21 | 2 | 75 | 5 | 0 | * | * | 15 | * |
| 9 | 69 | 2 | 115 | na | 0 | * | * | 30 | * |
| 11 | 32 | 4 | na | na | 0 | 2 | * | 25 | * |
| 7 | 30 | 4 | 95 | 20 | 0 | * | * | 20 | * |
| 9 | 49 | 3 | na | na | 0 | * | * | 35 | * |
| 9 | 51 | 2 | 115 | na | 0 | * | * | 30 | * |

| FOOD NAME | Serving Size | Calories |
|---|---|---|
| Plain (Dannon) | 1 cup | 150 |
| Plain (Lite-Line) | 8 oz | 180 |
| Plain (Yoplait Nonfat) | 8 oz | 120 |
| Plain (Yoplait Original) | 6 oz | 130 |
| Strawberry (Borden) | 8 oz | 230 |
| Strawberry (Dannon) | 1 cup | 260 |
| Vanilla (Dannon) | 1 cup | 200 |
| Vanilla (Yoplait Custard Style) | 6 oz | 180 |
| Vanilla (Yoplait Custard Style) | 4 oz | 130 |
| Vanilla (Yoplait Nonfat) | 8 oz | 180 |
| Vanilla (Yoplait Original) | 6 oz | 180 |
| YOGURT, FROZEN | | |
| Blueberry (Danny) | 1 cup | 210 |
| Chocolate (Danny) | 1 cup | 190 |
| Raspberry (Danny) | 1 cup | 210 |
| Strawberry (Danny) | 1 cup | 210 |
| Vanilla (Danny) | 1 cup | 180 |
| YOGURT, FROZEN BAR | | |
| Chocolate, Chocolate Coated (Danny) | 1 | 130 |
| Vanilla, Chocolate Coated (Danny) | 1 | 130 |
| ZUCCHINI Cooked | 1 cup | 22 |

| Protein (g) | Carbohydrates (g) | Fat (g) | Sodium (mg) | Cholesterol (mg) | Fiber (g) | Vitamin A (%) | Vitamin C (%) | Calcium (%) | Iron (%) |
|---|---|---|---|---|---|---|---|---|---|
| 13 | 17 | 4 | 115 | na | 0 | 2 | * | 40 | * |
| 11 | 24 | 4 | 145 | na | 0 | 2 | * | 35 | * |
| 13 | 18 | 0 | 160 | 5 | 0 | * | * | 45 | * |
| 10 | 15 | 3 | 140 | 15 | 0 | 2 | * | 30 | * |
| 9 | 46 | 2 | 145 | na | 0 | * | * | 30 | * |
| 9 | 49 | 3 | na | na | 0 | * | * | 35 | * |
| 11 | 32 | 4 | na | na | 0 | 2 | * | 35 | * |
| 7 | 30 | 4 | 110 | 20 | 0 | 2 | * | 25 | * |
| 5 | 20 | 3 | 70 | 15 | 0 | * | * | 15 | * |
| 11 | 35 | 0 | 140 | 5 | 0 | * | * | 40 | * |
| 9 | 29 | 3 | 120 | 10 | 0 | * | * | 25 | * |
| | | | | | | | | | |
| 7 | 42 | 2 | na | na | 0 | * | * | 20 | * |
| 9 | 32 | 3 | na | na | 0 | * | * | 30 | * |
| 7 | 42 | 2 | na | na | 0 | * | * | 20 | * |
| 7 | 42 | 2 | na | na | 0 | * | * | 20 | * |
| 7 | 33 | 2 | na | na | 0 | * | * | 25 | * |
| | | | | | | | | | |
| | | | | | | | | | |
| 4 | 12 | 8 | na | na | na | * | na | 15 | * |
| 3 | 11 | 8 | na | na | na | * | na | 13 | * |
| 2 | 5 | 0 | 2 | 0 | 1 | 11 | 27 | 5 | 4 |
| | | | | | | | | | |
| | | | | | | | | | |
| | | | | | | | | | |